Essential Quick Review

ORTHODONTICS

Essential Quick Review
ORTHODONTICS

Editior-in-Chief

Priya Verma Gupta MDS FPFA
Professor
Department of Pedodontics and Preventive Dentistry
Divya Jyoti College of Dental Sciences and Research
Ghaziabad, Uttar Pradesh, India

Co-Author

MS Kannan BDS MDS
Professor
Department of Orthodontics
Sree Balaji Dental College and Hospital
Chennai, Tamil Nadu, India

JAYPEE
The Health Sciences Publisher
New Delhi | London | Philadelphia | Panama

Jaypee Brothers Medical Publishers (P) Ltd

Headquarters

Jaypee Brothers Medical Publishers (P) Ltd
4838/24, Ansari Road, Daryaganj
New Delhi 110 002, India
Phone: +91-11-43574357
Fax: +91-11-43574314
Email: jaypee@jaypeebrothers.com

Overseas Offices

J.P. Medical Ltd
83 Victoria Street, London
SW1H 0HW (UK)
Phone: +44 20 3170 8910
Fax: +44 (0)20 3008 6180
Email: info@jpmedpub.com

Jaypee-Highlights Medical Publishers Inc.
City of Knowledge, Bld. 235, 2nd Floor, Clayton
Panama City, Panama
Phone: +1 507-301-0496
Fax: +1 507-301-0499
Email: cservice@jphmedical.com

Jaypee Medical Inc.
325 Chestnut Street
Suite 412, Philadelphia, PA 19106, USA
Phone: +1 267-519-9789
Email: support@jpmedus.com

Jaypee Brothers Medical Publishers (P) Ltd
17/1-B Babar Road, Block-B, Shaymali
Mohammadpur, Dhaka-1207
Bangladesh
Mobile: +08801912003485
Email: jaypeedhaka@gmail.com

Jaypee Brothers Medical Publishers (P) Ltd
Bhotahity, Kathmandu, Nepal
Phone: +977-9741283608
Email: kathmandu@jaypeebrothers.com

Website: www.jaypeebrothers.com
Website: www.jaypeedigital.com

Inquiries for bulk sales may be solicited at: jaypee@jaypeebrothers.com

Essential Quick Review: Orthodontics

First Edition: **2016**

ISBN: 978-93-86056-17-7

Printed at Rajkamal Electric Press, Plot No. 2, Phase-IV, Kundli, Haryana.

Editorial Board

Preface

I am very pleased to introduce you to the first edition of Essential Quick Review; A series for final year undergraduate students.

The series will be available in eight subjects, i.e., Periodontics, Operative Dentistry and Endodontics, Pedodontics, Prosthodontics, Oral Surgery, Oral Medicine and Radiology, Orthodontics and Public Health Dentistry covering essential parts of each subject. This book will not only help the student to attain the knowledge, but will also give an idea how to attempt a question during the examination, covering entire syllabus in a limited period of time.

The book gives a complete outline for writing an essay type, a short answer type or a viva-voce type of question. The language used is very simple enabling a better understanding with well-illustrated diagrams wherever possible. Each book also carries a section that contains recently asked questions covering majority of the universities in India.

What makes it different from other books is, that it is supported with a supplementary booklet for each subject that contains three sections, i.e., definitions, classifications and viva-voce covering the entire syllabus enabling the student to undergo a quick revision.

The study material provided in this book is an attempt to provide an additional help to students for easy retention and reproduction of subject in the examination. This book is in no way a replacement to standard text books.

I thank all my subject matter experts for their valued suggestions and contributions. A very special word of thanks to my family for being the source of constant encouragement. I profusely thank Shri Jitendar P Vij (CEO), Mr Ankit Vij (Group President), and production team of M/S Jaypee Brothers Medical Publishers (P) Ltd, New Delhi for their enthusiasm and constant efforts in bringing out this book.

Dr Priya Verma Gupta

Contents

Section 1 Orthodontics

Section 2 Recently Asked Questions

SECTION 1

ORTHODONTICS

CHAPTER 1 Introduction to Orthodontics

SHORT NOTES

Question 1

Define Orthodontics, preventive orthodontics and interceptive orthodontics?

Answer

The word Orthodontics has been derived from Greek words "orthos" meaning "correct" and "odontos" meaning teeth.

Orthodontics

It is that branch of dentistry concerned with prevention, interception and correction of malocclusion and other abnormalities of the dento-facial region.

Preventive Orthodontics

According to Graber, "Preventive orthodontics is the action taken to preserve the integrity of what appears to be normal at a specific time. Any procedures that ward off untoward environmental attacks or anything that would change the normal course of events".

Interceptive Orthodontics

- According to Popovich and Hiles: It is defined as any procedure that eliminates or reduces the severity of or malocclusion in the developing dentition
- According to Ackerman and Proffit: It is defined as all simple procedures that eliminate the developing malocclusion.

Question 2

What are the aims of orthodontic treatment/Jackson's Triad?

Answer

The aims of orthodontic treatment summarised by Jackson are as follows:

- Functional efficiency
- Aesthetic harmony
- Structural balance.

Functional Efficiency

The goal of the orthodontic treatment should be to achieve proper functioning of the orofacial apparatus.

Aesthetic Harmony

Orthodontic therapy should result in the enhancement of the aesthetics.

Structural Balance

Orthodontic therapy should aim at achieving a balance between the skeletal, dental and soft tissues.

CHAPTER 2

Growth and Development: General Principles

LONG ESSAYS

Question 1

Define growth and development. Describe in detail various theories of growth?

Answer

Growth is defined as:

- According to Todd: Growth refers to increase in size
- According to Moyers: Growth may be defined as the normal changes in the amount of living substance
- According to Profitt: Growth usually refers to an increase in size and the number.

Development can be defined as:

- According to Todd: Development is progress towards maturity
- According to Enlow: Development connotes a maturation process involving progressive differentiation at the cellular and tissue levels.

Growth Theories

- Genetic theory
- Sutural theory
- Cartilagnous theory
- Functional matrix theory
- Composite theory.

Genetic Theory

According to this theory the basic control of growth, both in magnitude and timing is located in the genes. The potential for growth is genetic.

The common ground shared by all the genetic studies has led the orthodontic specialty in general to conclude that genes are fundamental in causing malocclusion.

However the genetic theory is not complete in explaining the role of environmental and epigenetic factors influence on the characteristics of an individual including the dentofacial forms.

Sutural Theory

Proposed by Sicher in 1955.

According to Sicher, "The primary event in sutural growth is the proliferation of the connective tissue between the two bones. If sutural tissue proliferates, it creates the space for appositional growth at the border of the bones".

In Sicher's view all bone-forming elements, cartilage, sutures and periosteum are growth centres, which are responsible for facial growth and assumed all were under tight intrinsic genetic control.

He felt that the connective tissue in suture of both the nasomaxillary complex and vault produced forces that separated the bones, just as the synchondroses expanded the cranial base and the epiphyseal plates lengthened long bones.

Evidences Against Sicher's Theory

- Auto transplants of sutures fail to grow in cultural medium though provided with same environment and conditions
- Extirpation of sutures has no appreciable effect on growth of skeleton
- The shape and growth within sutures is dependent on external stimuli
- It is possible to bring the sutural growth to halt by mechanical stresses applied across the sutures.

Cartilaginous Theory (James Scott–1956)

Scott hypothesis emphasises that the intrinsic growth controlling factors are present in the cartilage and in the periosteum, with the sutures being only secondary and dependent on extrasutural influences. According to this theory, the determinant of craniofacial growth is growth of cartilages.

According the Scott

- Spheno-occipital synchondrosis cartilage is responsible for the growth of cranial base
- Nasal septal cartilage is responsible for the growth of maxilla
- Condylar cartilage is responsible for the growth of mandible.

Sutural growth, Scott felt, came in response to the growth of the other structures including cartilaginous elements, brain, the eyes and so forth. Sutural growth is responsive to synchondrosis proliferation and local environmental factors that is, sutures are passive and secondary.

His theory expounds cartilage and periosteum as growth centres and classifies sutures as passive and secondary. The cartilaginous parts of the skull must be recognised as primary centres of growth, with the nasal septum being a major contributor in maxillary growth, per se.

Spheno-occipital Synchodrosis

Important growth centre of craniofacial skeleton, especially cranial base.

Cartilage of Nasal Septum

- Growth of maxilla is difficult to explain on the cartilage theory. Proponents of the cartilage theory hypothesise that the cartilaginous nasal septum serves as a pacemaker for other aspects of maxillary growth
- Two kinds of experiments have been carried out to test the idea that cartilage can serve as a true growth centre.
  - Transplanting nasal cartilage to cultural medium or any other place did not give equivocal results— that is sometime it grew, sometimes it did not. Indicating doubtful growth potential of the nasal septal cartilage whereas, if a piece of the epiphyseal plate of a long bone is transplanted, it will continue to grow in a new location or in culture, indicating that these cartilages do have innate potential
  - It was demonstrated that after the fracture of the mandibular condyle in a child, there was an excellent chance that the condylar process would regenerate to approximately its original size and a small chance that it would overgrow after the injury despite the damage to the condylar cartilage.

Cartilaginous theory was successful in explaining the growth of the cranial base and to a great extent maxilla too, it could not explain the growth of mandible and relate the growth of mandible to the condylar cartilage satisfactorily.

Functional Matrix Theory

Proposed by Melvin C Moss in 1965.

According to Moss, "the origin, growth and maintenance of all skeletal tissues and organs are always secondary, compensatory and obligatory to temporally and operational prior events or processes that occur in specifically related non-skeletal tissues, organs or functional spaces".

Each of these functions is completely carried out by *functional cranial component* **(Flowchart 2.1)**.

- *Functional matrix*: Consisting of the soft tissue and space, which completely performs a particular function.
- *Skeletal unit*: A related skeletal unit that acts biomechanically to protect and/or support its functional matrix.

Functional Matrix

Functional matrices provide the extrinsic (environmental) influences which are morphogenetically primary for the form, growth, position and maintenance in being of all skeletal units.

This consist of soft tissue-muscle, gland, nerve, vessels, fat and non-skeletal cartilages.

There are two distinct types of functional matrix.

1. The periosteal matrix
2. The capsular matrix.

Periosteal Functional Matrix

This term relates the matrix to those tissues that influence the bone directly through the periosteum.

Muscles are attached to the periosteum and consequently are excellent examples of this kind of matrix. Blood vessels and nerves lying in grooves or entering or exiting through foramen can also exert a periosteal influence on the skeletal unit.

Periosteal functional matrices are virtually self-defining.

All periosteal matrices act homologously, usually by means of the processes of osseous deposition and resorption. They

Flowchart 2.1: Different components of functional matrix theory

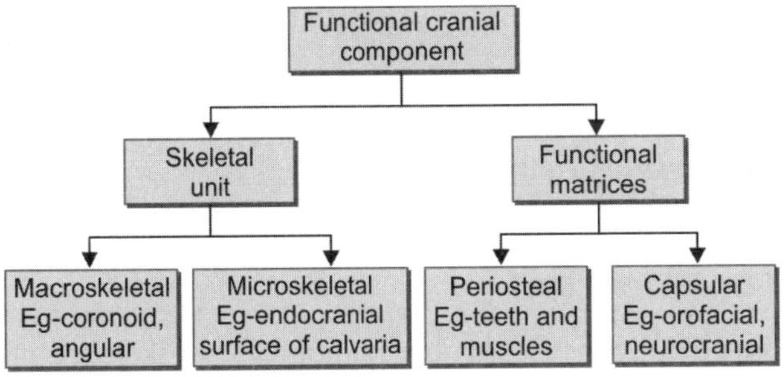

act to alter either or both the size and shape of skeletal units per se.

The periosteal matrix affects a microskeletal unit meaning that the sphere of influences is usually limited to a part of one bone.

Capsular Functional Matrix

This is the second type of functional matrix. Included in this class of matrix are those masses and spaces that are surrounded by capsules.

All functional cranial components (skeletal units plus functional matrices) arise, grow, operate and are maintained within a series of cranial capsules.

Four capsules are present:

1. Neuro cranial
2. Orofacial
3. Otic
4. Orbital.

Each of these capsules is an envelope, which contains a series of functional cranial components (skeletal units plus their related functional matrices), which as a whole, are sandwiched in between two covering layers.

All spaces intervening between functional components themselves, and between them and the limits of the capsule, are filled with indifferent loose connective tissue.

These capsules tend to influence macroskeletal units, which mean that portions of several bones are simultaneously affected.

Capsular functional matrices act indirectly and passively on their related skeletal units, producing a secondary, compensatory translation in space.

Example: The inner surface of calvarium.

The neural mass within its capsules elicit a reaction on the surface of the calvarium that transcends a localised area. As a result, apposition on the occipital, parietal, temporal and frontal occurs as if all of them were but one bone. This sharing of reaction by several adjacent bones constitutes a macroskeletal unit.

Skeletal Units

Skeletal units may be composed of bone, cartilage, or tendinous tissues.

Moss divided the skeletal units into:

1. Microskeletal units
2. Macroskeletal units.

Microskeletal Unit

Formed by bones consisting of number of small skeletal units.

Maxilla

- Orbital
- Pneumatic
- Palatal
- Basal

Mandible

- Coronoid
- Angular
- Alveolar
- Basal

Macroskeletal Unit

When adjoining portions of a number of neighbouring bones united to function as a single cranial component, we term this as macroskeletal unit.

Van Limborgh's Composite Theory

It is a theory that unifies all the factors contributing to growth, namely the genetic, the epigenetic and the environmental factors.

Van Limborgh's summarisation:

- Intrinsic control of growth is at synchondroses
- Synchondroses act as Growth centre
- Sutural growth is controlled in part by growth of cranial base
- Periosteal bone growth (vault) is controlled epigenetically by adjacent structures
- Growth of cranial vault is also controlled by local environmental factors (muscle forces inclusive) **(Fig. 2.1).**

Enlow's Principles

Two important principles regarding growth were put forward by Enlow. They are:

1. Counterpart principle
2. 'V' principle.

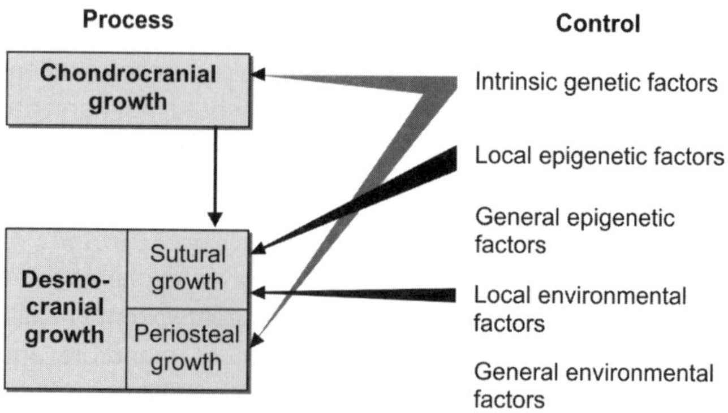

Fig. 2.1: Composite theory of Van Limborgh

Counterpart Principle of Craniofacial Growth

This principle states that the growth of any given facial or cranial part relates specifically to other structural and geometric "counterparts" in the face and cranium.

- Maxilla: Mandible
- Anterior cranial fossa: Palate
- Palate: Maxillary apical bases
- Middle cranial fossa: Ramus: Zygomatic arch.

These are regional relationships throughout the whole face and cranium.

If each regional part and its particular counterpart enlarge to the same extent, balanced growth between them is the result.

This is the key to what determines the presence or lack of balance in any region.

Imbalances are produced by differences in respective amounts or direction of growth between parts and counterparts.

"V" principle: "V" principle is the most useful and basic concept in facial growth. Many facial and cranial bones, or part of bones, have a V-shaped configuration.

Bone deposition occurs on the inner side of the "V", resorption takes place on the outside surface **(Fig. 2.2)**.

The "V" thereby moves from position A to B and, at same time, increases in overall dimensions.

The direction of movement is towards the wide end of the "V" thus, a simultaneous growth movement and enlargement occurs by additions of bone on the inside with removal from the outside.

The outcome of these growth processes is **(Fig. 2.3)**:

- Enlargement in overall size of the "V"-shaped area
- Movement of the entire "V" structure towards its own wide end
- Continuous relocation.

Maxillary Arch

The anterior part of the bony maxillary arch has a periosteal surface that is resorptive because this area grows straight downwards.

The labial (external) side of the premaxillary region faces away from the downward direction of growth, and it is thus resorptive. The lingual side faces towards the downwards growth directions and is depository **(Fig 2.4)**.

This growth pattern also provides for the remodelling of the alveolar bone as it adapts to the variable positions of the incisors.

If the midsagittal section of the maxilla is displayed as a shallow "V" the inside or palatal side is found to be depository,

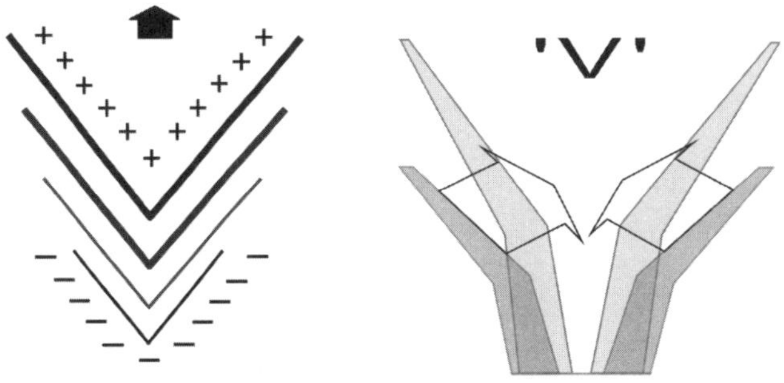

Fig. 2.2: Bone growth as described by Enlow's V- principle with deposition of bone occurring on the inner aspect of V and resorption of bone on outer aspect of V

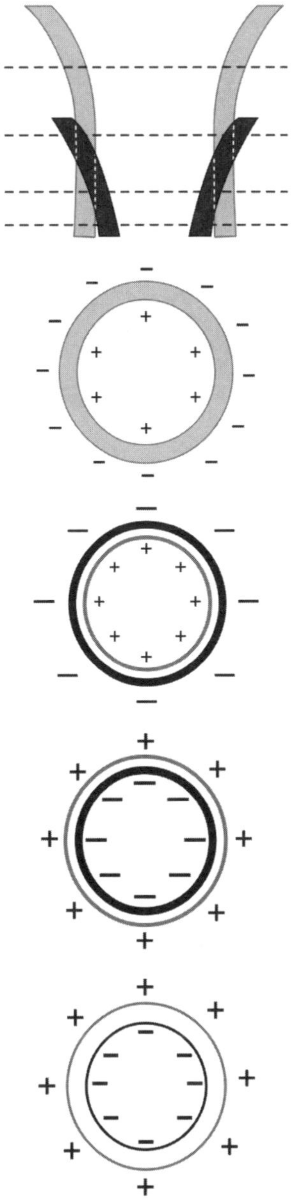

Fig. 2.3: Enlargement of Bone according to V-principle

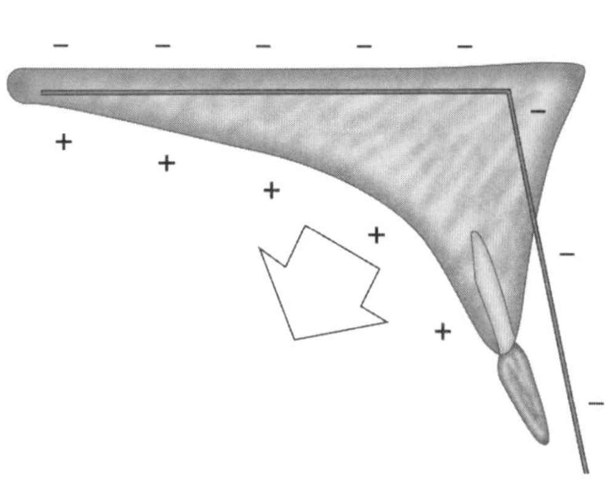

Fig. 2.4: Growth of maxilla in downward direction according to V principle

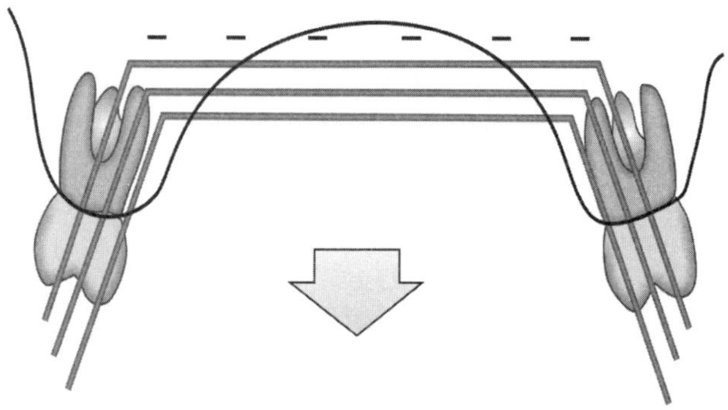

Fig. 2.5: Growth of palate in downward direction with deposition on the inferior aspect and resorption on the superior aspect

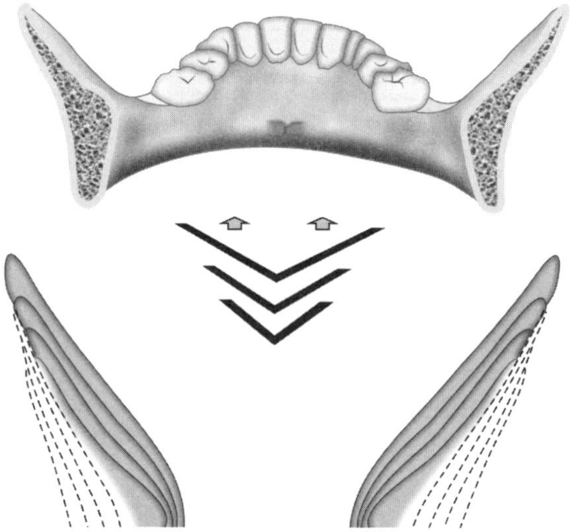

Fig. 2.6: Growth of mandible according to V principle in coronoid region

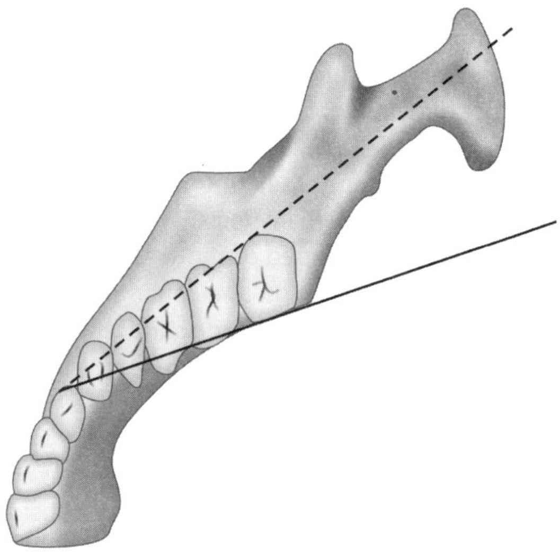

Fig. 2.7: Growth of lateral aspect of ramus from above view

while the floor of the nasal cavity and the surface just above the maxillary incisors (both of which are on the side opposite to the direction of growth) are resorptive **(Fig. 2.5)**.

Mandibular Growth

If we take a cross section of the mandible through the coronoid processes, we can see that the coronoid processes is an example of an ever-expanding "V" with the inside surface undergoing apposition and the outer surface resorption. Here the "V" is oriented vertically.

These same deposits of bone on the lingual side also bring about a posterior direction of growth movement, because this surface also faces posteriorly.

This produces a backward movement of the two coronoid processes, even though deposits are added on the inside (lingual) surface **(Fig. 2.6)**.

This is also an example of the expanding "V" principle, with the "V" oriented horizontally.

These same deposits of bone on the lingual side also bring about a posterior direction of growth movement, because this surface also faces posteriorly. This produces a backwards movement of the two coronoid processes, even though deposits are added on the inside (lingual) surface. This is also an example of the expanding "V" principle, with the "V" oriented horizontally.

Further applications of the "V" explain the apposition on the buccal surface of the ramus and the resorption of the lingual surface beneath the mylohyoid ridge.

These combined activities profoundly influence the shape of the mandible in two ways. First, the lateral ramus deposition is part of the drift that leads to the square jaw of the adult. Second, when one looks at the mandible from above **(Fig. 2.7)** it is apparent that the process is designed to

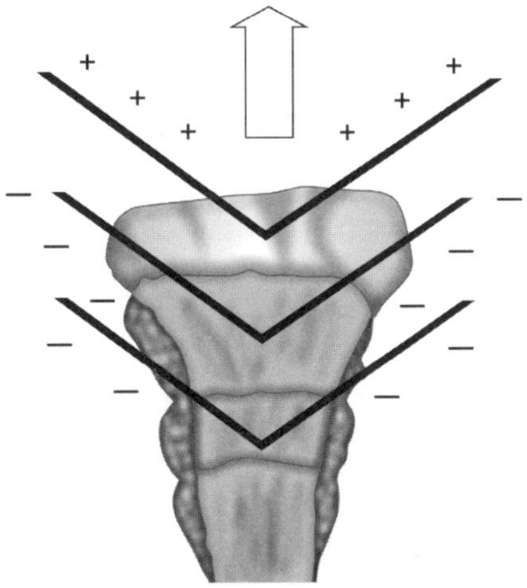

Fig. 2.8: Growth of condyle according to V principle

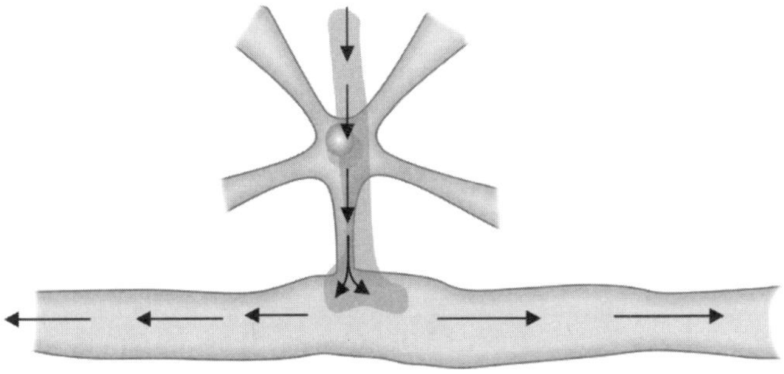

Fig. 2.9: Axoplasmic transport

keep the teeth closer to the midline then is either the rami or the coronoid processes.

In fact, the position of these lower teeth is virtually inviolate – orthodontists have met with little success in attempting to expand the lower arch.

Growth at the condyles also follows "V" principle. Each individual condyle is also remodeled according to the "V" principle (**Fig. 2.8**).

The condylar cartilage can be visualised as being situated on the inside of an ever-expanding "V" with its neck lengthened by reduction of the bone situated on the side of the 'V' away from the direction of growth.

Neurotrophic Theory of Growth (by Melvin Moss)

Interaction between nerves and other cells which initiates or control molecular modifications in other cells.

Neurotrophic functions are fundamental expression of neurocellular activitiy indicating that the nervous system is also concerned with the integrity of body structure.

These functions act homeostatistically to maintain and renew the structure and functional capacity of body parts.

Types of Neurotrophism

Depending upon target cells and tissues there are three types:

1. Neuromuscular
2. Neuroepithelial
3. Neurovisceral.

Axoplasmic Transport

Definition: It is the presumed by means of which neurotrophic substances passes by utilizing the processes of axoplasmic transport, from thin sites of origin in the neural cell body to the innervated tissues (**Fig. 2.9**).

Neuromuscular Trophism: Muscle development: Embryonic myogenesis, in vivo and in vitro, is independent of neural innervation, and hence of trophic control. Approximately at the myoblast stage of differentiation, the neural innervation is established without which further myogenesis usually cannot continue.

Neuroepithelial trophism: According to experiments done by Frank and Karli who electrolytically destroyed the trigeminal sensory gangalion in the adult rat, the subsequent epithelial changes include lingual ulcers, a sclero-hyperplastic lesion on check, and atrophy of palatal epithelium; apparently the homeostasis of this epithelium was lost following afferent deprivation.

Neurovisceral trophism: In the orofacial region, salivary glands among other splanchocranial viscera are trophically regulated at least partially.

Question 2

What are the features of growth?

Answer

Normal features of growth and development are:

- Differential growth
- Normality
- Variability
- Timing, rate and direction.

Differential Growth

- Not all tissue systems of the body grow at the same rate. Different tissues and in term different organs grow at different sides. This process is called "differential growth"
- Neural tissue grows early completing their maturation by 6–7 years of age
- Lymphoid tissue growth is completed in late childhood and growth of general tissue accelerates at the same time
- General body tissue follows an "S"-shaped curve with a definite slowing of the rate of growth during childhood and acceleration at puberty

- Maxilla and mandible follow the general body growth, the mandible slightly slower than maxilla initially but catches up later **(Fig. 2.10)**.

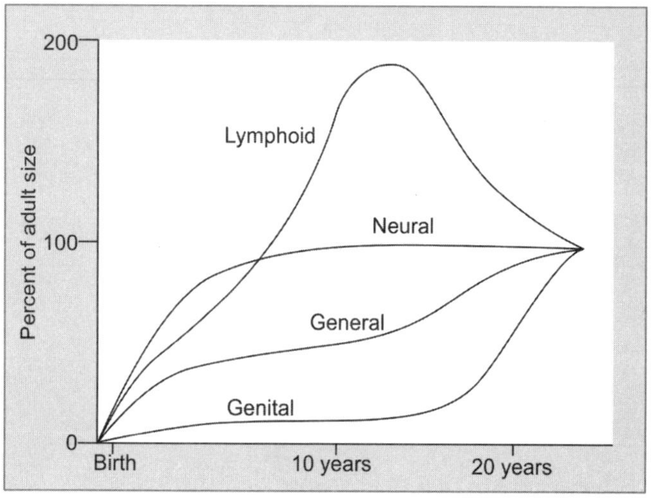

Fig. 2.10: This graph describes the growth of various tissue of body and is termed as "*Scammon's curve*"

Cephalocaudal Gradient of Growth

- Represents the changes in overall body proportions during normal growth and development **(Fig. 2.11A)**
- In fetal life, at about the third month of intrauterine development, the head takes up almost 50% of the total body length. At this stage, the cranium is large relative to the face and represents more than half the total head
- In contrast, the limbs are still rudimentary and the trunk is underdeveloped. By the time of birth, the trunk and limbs have grown faster than the head and face, so that the proportion of the entire body devoted to the head has decreased to about 30%.

The overall pattern of growth thereafter follows this course, with a progressive reduction of the relative size of the head to about 12% the adult.

Thus "Cephalocaudal gradient of growth". This simply means that there is an axis of increased growth extending from the head towards the feet.

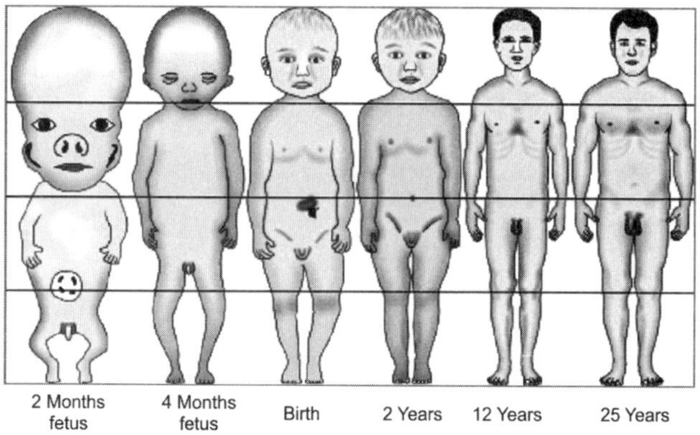

Fig. 2.11(A) Cephalocaudal Gradient in respect to whole body

Changes in Overall Body Proportions

At 3 month of intrauterine life the human fetus is almost 50% of the total body length. For this particular time, this is normal.

- At birth the trunk and limbs, which were earlier rudimentary have grown faster than the head and therefore the proportion of head size to the rest of the body length is 25–30%. Eventually at adulthood the head size is just 13%
- Changes in proportions of craniofacial region. At birth the face and jaws are relatively underdeveloped compared to their extent in adult. The mandible which is further away from brain tends to grow more and faster than the maxilla, which is closer **(Fig. 2.11B)**
- **Normality:** Normality usually refers to that which usually expected is ordinarily seen or typical
- Normals refers to a range, standard derivation is a way of depicting spread of values around the mean.

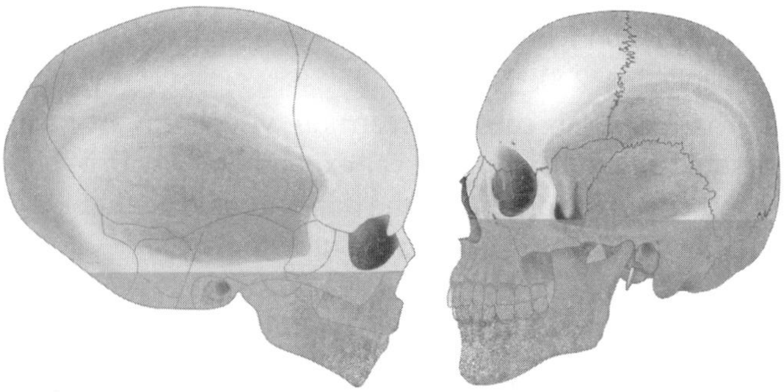

Fig. 2.11(B) Cephalocaudal gradient in respect to human skull

Variability

Variability quantitatively is categorised in terms of deviations from the usual patterns which is done using standard growth charts are useful in two ways:

1. Location of an individual relative to the peer gap established
2. Growth charts can be used to follow a clue overtime to evaluate whether there is an unexpected change in greater patterns.

Growth Spurts

- Refers to sudden increase in growth of general body
- Woodside in his study of Burlington Group showed.

	Girls	Boys
Just after birth	3 years	3 years
Juvenile growth Spurt	6–7 years	7–9 years
Pubertal growth spurt	10–12 years	12–15 years

Importance of Growth Spurts

Pubertal increments offer best time for large number of cases for the orthodontic and orthopaedic treatment. It also helps in determining the predictability, growth direction, patient management and total treatment time.

Orthopaedic correction of maxilla and mandible can be carried out.

Understanding the growth, predictability of future growth of maxilla, mandible and alveolar process helps in diagnosing and achieving excellent results of the mal-occlusion.

Growth spurts serve as excellent indicators for timing of orthodontic treatment.

SHORT ESSAYS

Question 1

Describe the methods of studying growth?

Answer

- Experimental approach
- Measurement approach.
  - Longitudinal study
  - Cross sectional study
  - Semilongitudinal study.

Longitudinal Study

These studies are carried over long period of time having the same sample.

Advantages

- Temporary temporal problems smoothen with time
- Variability in development within a group is put in proper perspective
- Serial comparison makes study of specific developmental pattern of individual possible.

Disadvantages

- Time consuming
- Expensive
- Sample loss or attrition.

Cross-Sectional Studies

These are measurements made of different samples or different individuals and studied at different periods.

Advantages

- Quicker, less expensive, statistical treatment of data is easier
- Studies can be readily repeated
- Method can be used in archaeological data.

Disadvantages

- It must be assumed that groups being measured and compared are similar
- Cross-sectional group averages tend to obscure individual variations.

Semilongitudinal Studies

Longitudinal and cross-sectional studies can be combined to seek the advantages of both in this way one might compress 15 years of study into 3 years of gathering growth data.

Implant Studies

Craniometry

- Involves measurements of skull found among human skeletal remains
- It was originally used to study the Neanderthal and Cro-magnon skull
- It can give information of extinct population and pattern of growth.

Advantages

Precise measurements can be made.

Disadvantages

All growth data must be cross sectional.

Anthropometry

- It includes measurements using soft tissue points overlying bony landmarks in living individuals
- It can also be done on dried skulls but variation in soft tissue thickness would produce different results
- Possible to follow the growth of an individual directly by making the same measurements repeatedly at different times thus producing longitudinal data.

Cephalometric Radiography

It allows direct measurement of bony skeletal dimensions and also allows the same individual to be followed over time.

Disadvantages

- Depends upon precise orientation of head before taking radiographs
- Requires precise control of magnification
- Since, it is a 2D representation of 3D structure all measurements are not possible.

Radioisotope

- Radioisotopes of certain elements or compounds are often used as in vivo markers for studying bone growth
- Such labelled material is injected and after some time located within the growing bone by means of autoradiographic techniques.
- Commonly used markers are :
  - Technetium 99
  - Calcium 45
  - Potassium 32.

Autoradiography

In this method radioactive precursors for structural and metabolic materials are detected within tissue by coating histological sections with a nuclear track emulsion.

Localisation of radioactive disintegration reveals the location of the precursors.

The commonly used autoradiographic labels are:

- 3 H thymidine
- 3 H proline
- Bromodeoxyuridine.

Quantitative and qualitative assessment of the label uptake is a physiologic index of cell activity.

Vital Staning

- First reported by Belchier in 1796 and also by John Hunter
- They attributed their finding to alizarin dye. injection of alizarin forms a thin coloured line on all active surfaces of bone growth during the period in which the dye is in the bloodstream, hence subsequent depositions are not coloured.
- The method reveals manner in which bone is laid down, the sites of bone growth, the direction and amount of growth, and the timing and relative duration of growth at different sites
- Alizarin, tetracycline and procion are dyes which are used extensively in vital staining in bone research.

Natural Marker

- The persistence of certain developmental features has led to their use as natural markers by means of serial radiograph
- *Example*: Trabaculae, nutrient canals and lines of arrested growth can be used for reference to study deposition, resorption and remodelling.

Implant Markers Bjork devised a method of implanting tiny bits of tantalum or biologically inert alloys into growing bone which served as radiographic reference markers for serial cephalometric study. The method allows precise orientation of serial cephalograms and information on the amount and sites of bone growth.

Finite Element Modelling (FEM)

It is an analytical method for calculating stresses and strain within mechanically loaded structures by breaking the structure down into group of small elements of known mechanical behaviour so that the response of the entire structure to loading is estimated.

Question 2

What are the mechanisms of bone growth?

Answer

Mechanisms of bone growth:

- Modelling
- Remodelling
- Displacement
- Cortical drift.

Modelling

- Bone modelling involves independent sites of resorption and formation that change the size and shape of a bone
- Bone modelling is a dominant process in growth as well as in adaptation to applied loads produced with headgear rapid palatal expansion, functional appliances, etc.

Remodelling

- A process involving deposition and resorption occurring in opposite ends
- It is a process of reshaping and resizing within a growing bone as it is relocated sequentially into a succession of new areas **(Fig. 2.12)**
- It is defined as a process of adding new bone tissue on one side of a bony cortex and taking it away from the other side
- The surface facing towards the direction of progressive growth receives new bone deposition (+). The surface facing away undergoes resorption (–)
- It produces a direct growth movement of any given area of a bone.

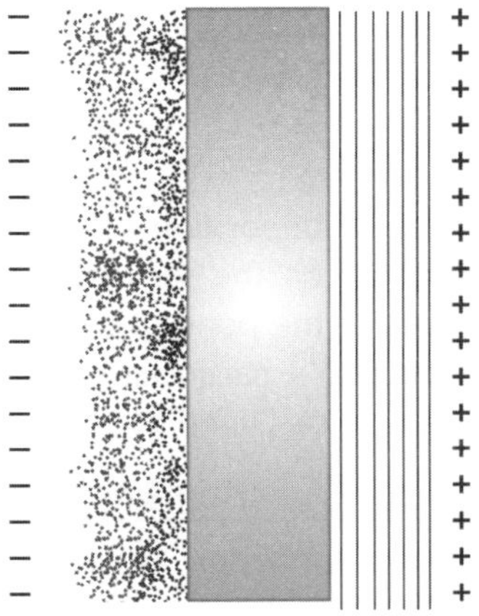

Fig. 2.12: Remodeling of bone with "-" depicting resorption and "+" depiction deposition

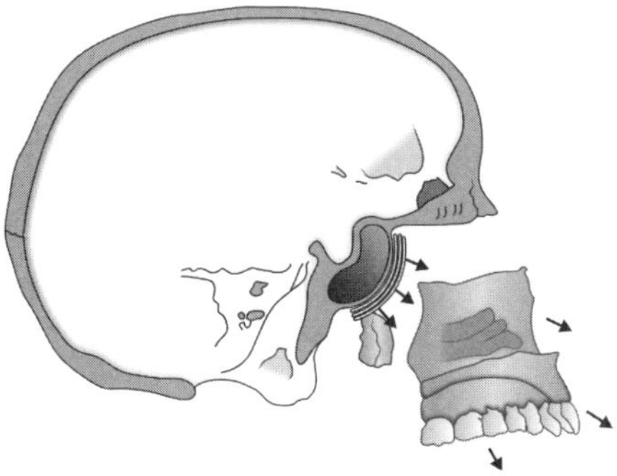

Fig. 2.13: Growth of maxilla due to displacement

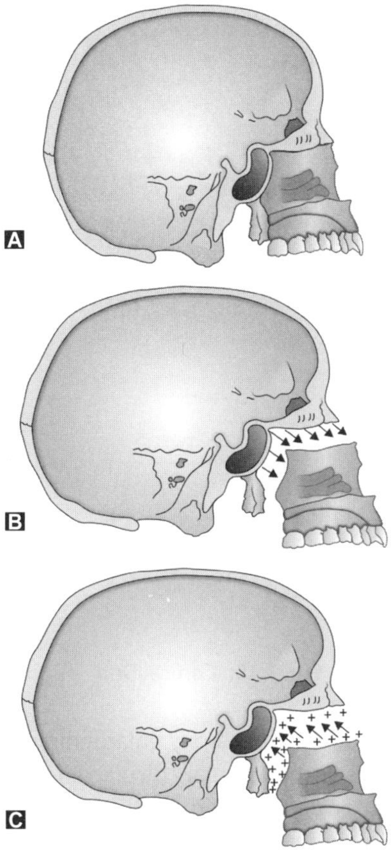

Fig. 2.14: (A) Diagram showing skull and maxilla; (B) Secondary displacement of maxilla in downward and forward direction because of bone deposition at cranial base; (C) Primary displacement of maxilla in downward and forward direction because of bone deposition on superior aspect of maxilla

Four Different Kinds of Remodelling Occur in Bone Tissues

- Biochemical remodelling, taking place at the molecular level. This involves the constant deposition and removal of ions to maintain blood calcium levels and carry out other mineral homeostasis functions
- Secondary reconstruction of bone by haversian systems and also the rebuilding of cancellous trabeculae
- Regeneration and reconstruction of bone during or following pathology and trauma
- Growth remodelling-remodelling process in facial growth.

Function of Growth Remodelling

- Progressively create the changing size of each whole bone
- Sequentially relocate each of the component regions of the whole bone to allow for overall enlargement
- Progressively shape the bone to accommodate its various functions
- Progressive fine-tune fitting of all the separate bones to each other to their contiguous, growing, functioning soft tissues; and
- Carry out continuous structural adjustments to adapt to the intrinsic and extrinsic changes in conditions.

Displacement

- Displacement is the movement of whole bone by some physical force that carries it, in toto, away from its contacts with other bones, which are also growing and increasing overall size at the same time
- This two-phase remodelling-displacement process takes place virtually simultaneously
- The displacement movement is presently believed by many researchers to be the pacemaking change with the rate and direction of the bone growth representing the transformative or secondary response **(Fig. 2.13)**
- It is of two types – primary and secondary displacement.

Primary Displacement

- As a bone enlarges, it is simultaneously carried away from other bones in direct contact with it. This creates

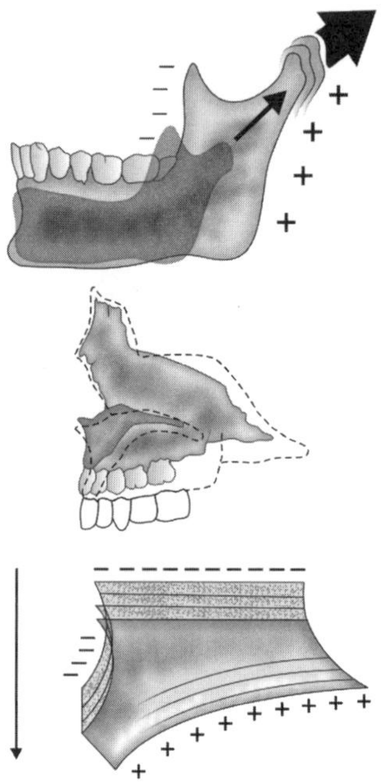

Fig. 2.15: Cortical Drift

the "space" within which bony enlargement takes place. The process is termed primary displacement (sometimes also called "translation") **(Fig. 2.14C)**

- The bone is carried away by the expansive force of all the growing soft tissues surrounding it. As this takes place, new bone is added immediately onto the contact surface, and the two separate bones thereby remain in constant articular junction
- As this takes place, new bone is added immediately onto the contact surface, and the two separate bones thereby remain in constant articular junction
- Primary displacement is associated with a bone's own enlargement, and it always takes place in the direction opposite to the vector of bone growth.

Secondary Displacement

- Secondary displacement is the movement of a whole bone caused by the separate enlargement of other bones, which may be nearby or quite distant **(Fig. 2.14B)**
- The secondary displacement is not associated with growth of the bone itself but initiated by enlargement of adjacent bones and soft structures and transferred to adjacent bones.

Cortical Drift

During the process of deposition of new bone on one surface and resorption on the surface (remodelling), the various components of the bone gets relocated to a new position with respect to a particular reference point. This process is called as Cortical Drift **(Fig. 2.15)**.

Question 3

Mechanism of bone formation or endochondral bone formation or intramembranous bone formation?

Answer

Bone formation occurs by two methods.

1. Intramembranous bone formation
2. Endochordal bone formation.

Intramembranous Bone Formation

- Occurs in areas exposed to tension **(Flowchart 2.2)**
- It differs from endochondral bone formation by formation of bone directly from mesenchymal tissues
- Seen in areas like:
  - Cranial vault
  - Maxilla
  - Mandible.

Flowchart 2.2: Intramembranous Bone Formation

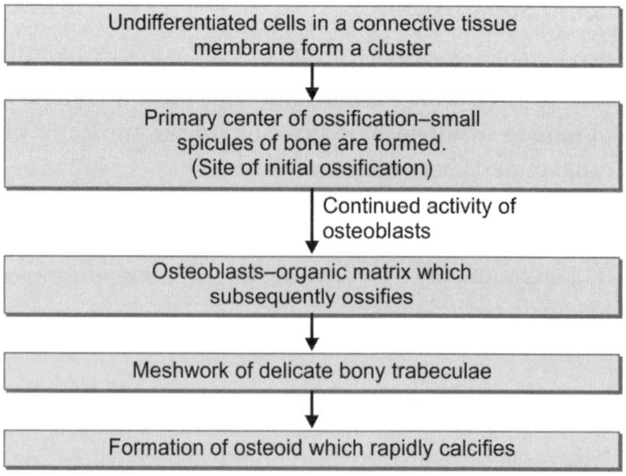

Endochondral Bone Formation

- Occurs in regions exposed to high levels of compression **(Flowchart 2.3)**
- Cartilages are of two types:
  1. Primary cartilage: Sphenooccipital synchodrosis nasal septal cartilage
  2. Secondary cartilage: Condylar, coronoid, angular.

In primary cartilages, cartilaginous matrix seems to isolate the dividing chondroblasts from local factors. In secondary cartilages local factors seem to modulate the growth rate due to absence of cartilaginous matrix.

In primary cartilage—chondroblasts divide and secrete intercellular matrix.

In secondary cartilage—prechondroblasts are the dividing cells and not surrounded by intercellular matrix.

Flowchart 2.3: Endochondral Bone Formation

Begins within cartilage tissue which is surrounded by its perichondrium

↓

Within the primary ossification center, the chondrocytes hypertrophy

↓

The matrix between these cells becomes calcified and small blood vessels from the perichondrium erode into this area

↓

Spontaneous resorption occurs in the old calcified matrix occurs and the lacuna spaces are created in this zone

↓

Connective tissue accompanying the blood vessels is osteogenic–cells differentiate into osteoblasts and produce osteoid tissue directly on the cartilage spicules

↓

A thin crust of bone is formed when the matrix becomes calcified

SHORT NOTES

Question 1

What is Growth centre vs Growth site?

Answer

Growth Sites

- The remodelling of a bone is actually carried out by the osteogenic membranes and the surrounding tissues, rather than by the hard part of the bone
- This blanket of resorptive and depository areas surrounding the bone are called as Growth fields
- Fields that have some significant role in the growth process are often termed growth sites.

Growth Centres

- Some growth sites are called "growth centers"
- They are considered to be areas that somehow control the overall growth of the bone
- This term also implies that the "force", "energy" or "motor" for a bone resides primarily or solely within its growth centre.

CHAPTER 3 Growth and Development: Cranial and Facial Structures

LONG ESSAYS

Question 1

Describe the pre-natal development of cranial base?

Answer

Cranium can be divided into two parts:

1. Neurocranium: It protects and supports the brain and sense organs.
2. Viscerocranium: It is related with alimentary, respiratory tracts, face, maxilla and mandible.

Basicranium or cranial base is related to the both neural and visceral components. At cellular level, bones of cranial base developed in the following processes:

- Hyperplasia (Prominent feature of all forms of growth)
- Hypertrophy
- Accretion (excretion of extracellular material).

Chondrification

- The earliest evidence of cartilage formation of cranial base is seen in the late somite period, i.e. 4th week of intra-uterine (IU) life
- Mesenchyme derived from paraxial mesoderm and neural crest condenses between the developing brain and foregut to form the base of the "ectomeningeal capsule"
- This condensation indicates the earliest evidence of skull formation
- During this period, the occipital sclerotomal mesenchyme concentrates around the notochord underlying the developing hindbrain
- From this region the mesenchymal concentration extends cephalically, forming the floor of the brain
- Approximately 40th day of IU life, mesenchyme starts converting into cartilage. Chondrification centres form the following cartilages:
  - Parachordal cartilage
  - Hypophyseal cartilage
  - Otic cartilage
  - Nasal cartilage.

Parachordal Cartilages

- Chondrification centres forming around the cranial end of the notochord are appropriately called the parachordal cartilages
- Parachordal cartilages fuse with the sclerotomes arising from occipital somites surrounding the neural lube
- The sclerotome cartilage is considered to be the first part of the skull to develop and it forms the boundaries of foramen magnum, providing the anlagen for basilar and condylar parts of the occipital bone.

Hypophyseal Cartilages

- Oro-pharyngeal membrane closes off the stomodeum. Just cranial to this membrane, the hypophyseal pouch (Rathke's pouch) arises from the stomodeum
- This pouch gives rise to the anterior lobe of pituitary gland (adenohypophysis)
- Two hypophyseal cartilages develop on either side of the hypophyseal stem and fuse to form the basisphenoid or post-sphenoid cartilage
- This contains the hypophysis, and will later give rise to the sella turcica and posterior part of the body of the sphenoid bone
- Cranial to the pituitary gland, fusion of the two pre-sphenoid or trabecular cartilages forms precursor to the pre-sphenoid bone that will form the anterior part of the body of the sphenoid bone
- Laterally the chondrification centres of the orbito-sphenoid (lesser wing) and alisphenoid (greater wing) contribute to the wings of sphenoid bone.

Otic Capsule

It chondrifies and fuses with the parachordal cartilages to ossify later as the mastoid and petrous portions of the temporal bones. Otic capsule does not chondrify in humans.

Nasal Capsule

- Nasal capsule chondrifies in the 2nd month of IU life to form a box of cartilage with a roof and lateral walls divided by a median cartilage septum
- The capsules surrounding the nasal, otic sense organs chondrify and fuse to the cartilages of the cranial base
- The median nasal septum remains cartilaginous except posteroinferiorly, where in the membrane on each side of the septum, intramembraneous ossification centres forms the vomer bone, which is initially a paired bone, and its two halves unite before birth.

Chondrocranial Ossification

- Approximately 110 ossification centres appear in the embryonic human skull
- Many of these centres fuse to produce 45 bones in the neonatal skull, but in the young adult, 22 skull bones are recognised
- Unossified chondrocranial remnants persist at birth as the alae and septum of the nose, spheno-occipital and spheno-petrous junctions, and the apex of the petrous bone and between the separate parts of occipital bone.

Occipital Bone

- Derived from both the basicranial cartilage, contributed by the occipital sclerotomes and the desmocranial membrane, the occipital bone ossifies from 7 centres, which are 2 intra-membranous and 5 endochondral around the medulla oblongata, which determines the foramen magnum
- The squamous portion above the superior nuchal line ossifies from a pair of intra-membranous ossification centres in the 8th week of IU life
- Infranuchally, the squamous portion ossifies from a pair of endochondral ossification, centres at the 10th week
- The single median basicranial endochondral ossification centre appears at the 11th week from the basioccipital bone anterior to the foramen magnum and the anterior one-third of the occipital condyles
- A pair of endochondral ossification centres appears at the 12th week from the exoccipital bones, lateral to the foramen magnum, including posterior two-thirds of the occipital condyles
- The occipital squame starts to fuse with the exoccipital at the posterior intraoccipital synchondrosis during 2nd or 3rd year post-natally
- The exoccipitals join the basioccipital at the anterior intraoccipital synchondrosis and it disappears during the 3rd or 4th year, by the age of 7, the squamous, exoccipital and basilar portions have united into a single occipital bone.

Temporal Bone

- The squamous and tympanic components of this bone ossify in membrane, whereas the petrosal and styloid elements ossify endochondrally from about 21-ossification centres
- The squamous portion ossifies intra-membranously from a single centre appearing in the 8th week, the zygomatic process extends from this ossification centre
- The tympanic ring surrounding the external acoustic meatus ossifies from 4 intra-membranous centres starting in the 3rd month of Intra uterine life(IU)
- The petrosal part ossifies endochondrally in the otic capsule from about 14 centres, these centres start to appear in the 16th week and fuse during the 6th month IU when the contained inner ear labyrinth has reached its final size
- Styloid process ossifies from two centres in the hyoid (2nd) branchial arch cartilage; the upper centre appears just before birth and the lower centre just after birth
- At 22 weeks of IU the petrous and tympanic ring fuse incompletely, leaving the petrotympanic fissure. At birth, the tympanic ring fuses incompletely with the squamous part of temporal bone
- The petrous, squamous and proximal styloid process-parts fuse during the 1st year of life. The mandibular (glenoid) fossa is only a shallow depression at birth, deepening with development of articular eminance.

Ethmoid Bone

Endochondral bone, which forms the median floor of the anterior cranial fossa and parts of the roof, lateral walls and median septum of the nasal cavity, ossifies from three centres.

1. A single median centre in the mesethmoid cartilage forms the perpendicular plate and crista galli, just before birth
2. A pair of centres for the lateral labyrinths appears in the nasal capsular cartilages at the 4th month of IU
3. At 2 years of age the perpendicular plate unites with the labyrinths through fusion of the cribriform plate to form a single ethmoid bone.

Inferior Nasal Choncha

This purely endochondral bone ossifies in the cartilage of the lateral part of the nasal capsule from a single centre that appears in the 5th month of IU and it detaches from the ethmoid to become the independent bone.

Sphenoid Bone

- Sphenoid bone has up to 19 intra-membranous and endochondral ossification centres

- Its central body (basisphenoid), derives from the basicranial cartilage, whereas its wings and pterygoid plates have both cartilaginous and intramembranous ossification centres
- Sphenoid body derives from pre-sphenoid and post-sphenoid centres. A single median and 2 paired pre-sphenoid ossification centres arise in the 4th month of IU in the mesethmoid portion of basicranial cartilage to form the pre-sphenoid bone anterior to the tuberculum sellae
- The post-sphenoid bone arising from two sets of paired centres in the basisphenoid cartilage on either side of the upwardly projecting hypophyseal pouch (Rathke's) during the 4th month of IU forms the sella turcica, the dorsum sellae and basisphenoid
- Endochondral ossification centres for the greater wings of the sphenoid appear in the alisphenoid cartilages, and for the lesser wings in the orbito-sphenoid cartilages
- Also intra-membranous ossification centres appear in the 8th week for some parts of greater wings and for the medial and lateral pterygoid plates
- The mid-sphenoidal synchondrosis between the pre- and post-sphenoid fuses shortly before birth
- In most mammals other than man, this synchondrosis fuses late post-natally or not at all
- Basisphenoid and alisphenoids are still separated at birth by mixed cartilaginous/ligamentous articulations
- The spheno-occipital synchondrosis fuses in adolescence.

Question 2

Discuss the post-natal growth of cranial base?

Answer

Expansion of the cranial base takes place as a result of two processes:

1. Growth of the cartilage remnants of the chondrocranium that persists between the basicranial bones
2. Expansive forces emanating from the growing brain displaces the bones at the suture lines (capsular functional matrix).

- Cranial base has a potent role in the development of structure, dimensions, angles and placement of various facial parts
- Floor of the cranium is a template from which face develops. Any difference in the development of basicranium will be reflected in the facial growth
- Endocranial surface of cranial floor has a different mode of development when compared with the calvaria or roof of the cranium because of its complex structure and curvature
- Remodelling is required to accommodate the massively enlarged human brain
- Remodelling process provides for the direct expansion of the various endocranial fossae in conjunction with sutural growth and growth at synchondrosis
- Various endocranial compartments are separated from one another by elevated bony portions.
    - Middle and posterior fossae are divided by the petrous elevation
    - The olfactory fossae are separated by crista galli
    - Right and left middle cranial fossae are separated by the longitudinal midline sphenoidal elevation
    - Right and left anterior and posterior cranial fossae are divided by a longitudinal midline bony ridge.
- All these elevated partitions, unlike the remainder of the cranial floor are depository in nature
- The reason is that as fossa expands outwards by resorption, the partitions between them must enlarge inwards by deposition to maintain the proportions
- The mid-ventral segments of cranial floor grow more slowly than the floor of the laterally located fossae
- This accommodates the slower development of the medulla, pons, hypothalamus, optic chiasma in contrast to the massive rapid expansion of the hemispheres **(Fig. 3.1)**
- The process of remodelling growth in the basicranium provides for the changing stability of these nerves and vascular passageways
- The foramen moves by deposition and resorption keeping pace with compensating movement of nerve/vessel
- The foramen enclosing each cranial nerve and major blood vessel undergoes drift process to constantly maintain the proper position (relocation)
- Growth in the posterior cranial fossa is more when compared with growth of the spinal cord and foramen magnum
- Differential remodelling process maintains the proportionate placement of spinal cord, even though the floor of the posterior cranial fossa, which surrounds the spinal cord expands to a considerably greater extent than the circumference of the foramen magnum.

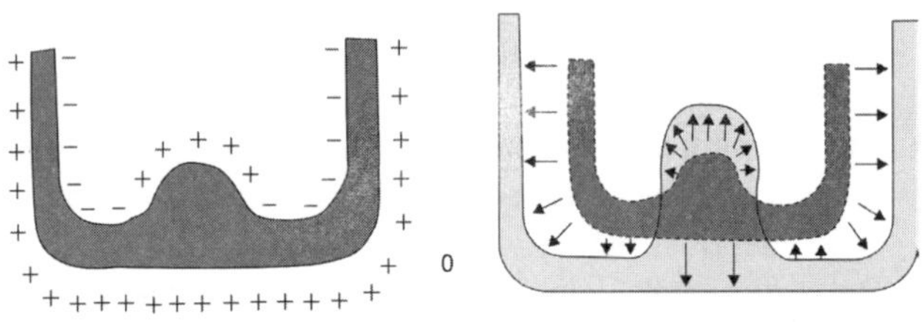

Fig. 3.1: Growth at cranial base with "+" depicting bone deposition and "-" depicting bone resorption and "↑" the direction of growth

Synchondrosis

Different synchondrosis are seen in cranial base. These are:

- Spheno-frontal synchondrosis
- Fronto-ethmoidal synchondrosis
- Spheno-ethmoidal synchondrosis
- Spheno-occipital synchondrosis
- Intersphenoidal synchondrosis.

Fronto-ethmoidal and spheno-ethmoidal synchondrosis: It ceases contributing the antero-posterior elongation after the age of 7 years. Further growth of anterior cranial base is associated with expansion of the developing frontal air sinuses.

Spheno-occipital synchondrosis: It is a major contributor in the post-natal growth of the cranial base. This is the last of all synchondrosis to fuse and starts fusing at 12-13 years of age in girls and 14-15 years of age in boys and completes its ossification of the external aspect by 20 years of age. This prolonged growth period allows for continued posterior expansion of the maxilla to accommodate last erupting molar teeth and provides space for growing nasopharynx **(Fig. 3.2)**.

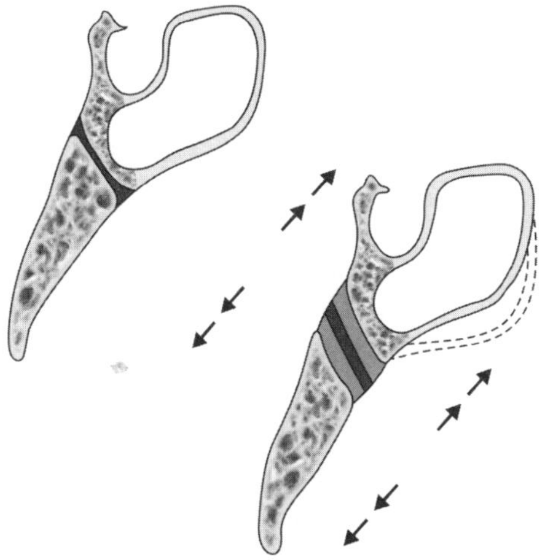

Fig. 3.2: Growth at synchondrosis with "↑" depicting the growth

- The interior of the sphenoid bone eventually becomes hollowed to form the sizable sphenoidal sinus. Sphenoidal sinus expansion does not push the maxilla. The sinus secondarily grows as the body of the sphenoid bone expands around it, keeping constant junction with the moving nasomaxillary complex
- The cranial cartilages have been regarded as autonomous growth units that develops in conjunction with brain, and somehow independent of it
- The size, shape and characteristics of cranial floor have evolved in direct phylogenetic association with the brain it supports, but the basicranium itself has presumably developed a genetic capacity of its own growth that is somehow independent of the brain
- The expansion of the middle cranial fossa and its neural contents has a major secondary displacement effect on the anterior cranial floor, the underlying nasomaxillary complex suspended from the latter, and the mandible
- At about 5 years of age, frontal lobe growth and anterior cranial fossae expansion are largely complete
- The temporal and middle cranial fossa, however continue to enlarge for several more years and the expansion of each temporal lobe continues to displace the frontal lobe forwards and this inturn, causes tension in the osteogenic suture systems between these two areas
- The anterior fossae and the maxillary complex are carried anteriorly by the frontal lobes, which are moved forward because of temporal lobe enlarging behind it **(Fig. 3.3)**

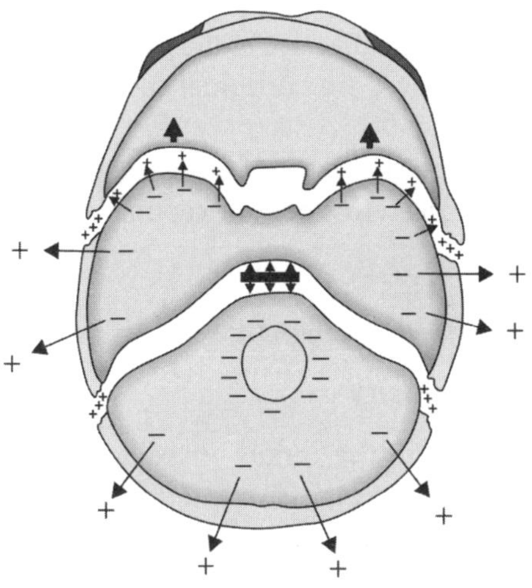

Fig. 3.3: Growth of cranium

- The resorption occurs from the lining side of the forward walls of the middle cranial fossa
- Deposition occurs on the orbital face of the sphenoid and in the spheno-frontal suture
- Forward displacement of the anterior cranial fossae as the frontal lobes are displaced anteriorly
- The petrous elevation increases by deposition on the endocranial surface
- The foramen magnum is progressively lowered by resorption on the endocranial surface and deposition on the ectocranial side
- Endocranial fossa enlarges by a combination of endocranial resorption and ectocranial deposition.

Question 3

Describe the pre- and post-natal growth of maxilla?

Answer

Pre-natal Growth of Maxilla

- Maxilla develops from a centre of ossification in mesenchyme of maxillary process of 1st arch, which is associated closely with cartilage of nasal capsule
- At the end of 3rd week of IU life, this process grows downwards to meet the maxillary processes of the first branchial arch, which grow forwards
- These processes unite at the end of the 4th week of IU to form the maxillary jaw
- In the 7½ week of IU, the lamella begins to grow forwards, backwards and downwards to form the frontal process and alveolar wall
- After the 3rd month of IU, there is generalised enlargement of the face in all directions
- In the 8th week of IU, bilaterally located bony centres in the anterior palate give rise to the premaxilla and maxilla
- The palatal shelves are horizontal and grow towards the midline
- At 9 weeks, the shelves are in near contact and the pre-maxillary–maxillary ossification centres appear **(Figs. 3.4 to 3.7)**.

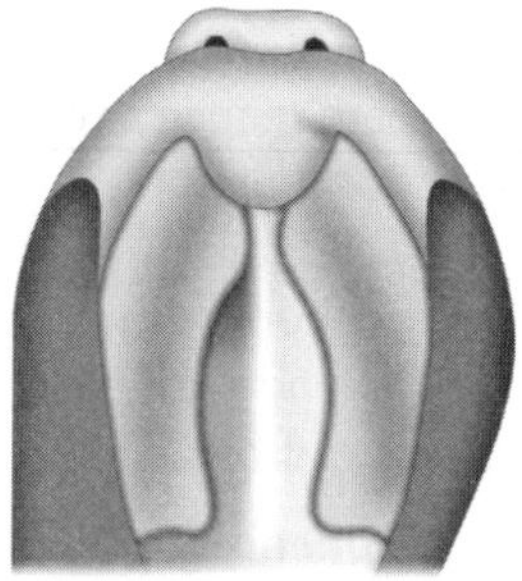

Fig. 3.4: At 9 weeks, the shelves are in near contact and the premaxillary–maxillary ossification centres appear

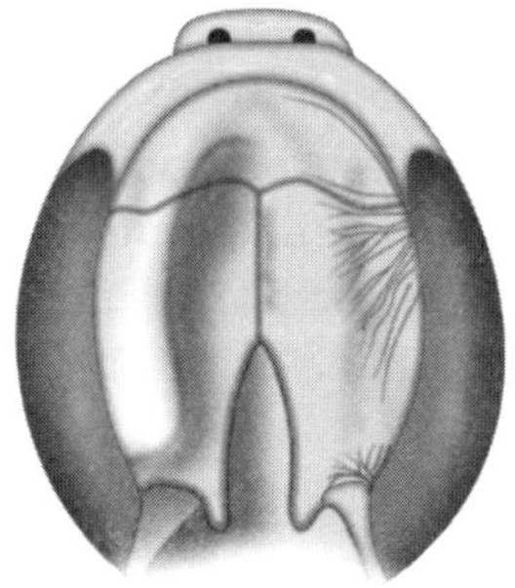

Fig. 3.5: At 10 weeks, the soft tissue of the palate has fused and ossification centres of the pre–maxilla-maxilla grow medially

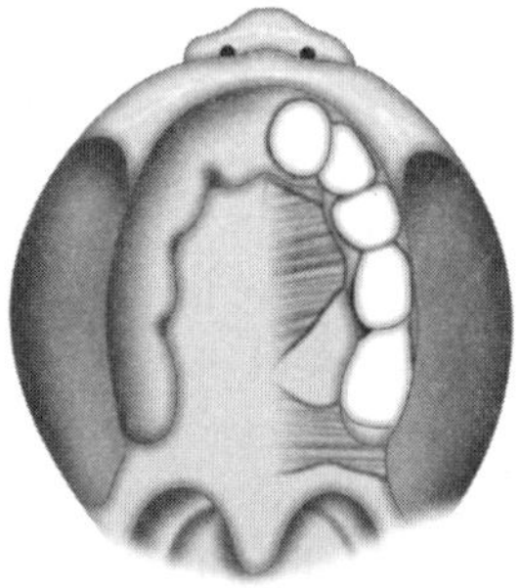

Fig. 3.6: At 14 weeks, the premaxillary bone supports the incisors and the maxillary bone supports the cuspids and first molars. The palatine bone supports the second molars

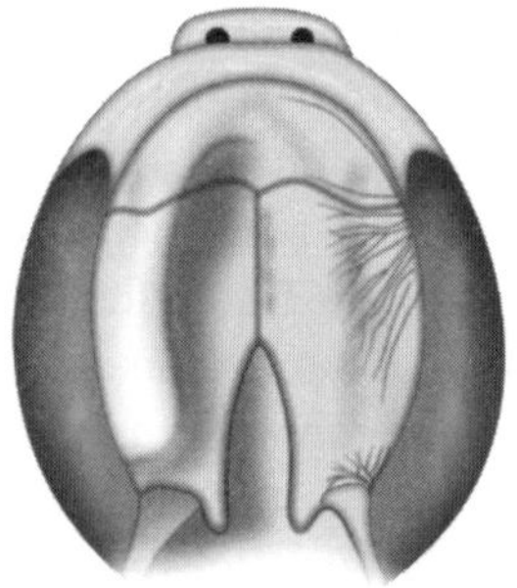

Fig. 3.7: A midline suture extends the length between the premaxillary, maxillary and palatine bones. A bilateral suture also appears between the palatal aspects of the premaxilla and maxilla

Post-natal Growth of Maxilla

Maxillary Tuberosity

- During growth, the entire maxilla is moved and repositioned in a progressive anterior direction
- As this takes place, apposition occurs on periosteal surfaces of the maxillary tuberosity
- Since this surface faces posteriorly and laterally, bone deposition here causes growth in corresponding directions
- This produces lengthening and slight widening of the maxillary arch at its posterior end
- Thus, growth at the tuberosity increases the longitudinal dimensions of the maxilla, and also lengthens the dental arch as the teeth increase in number
- Also, growth of the middle cranial fossa causes secondary displacement of the maxilla in a downwards and forwards direction **(Figs. 3.8A and B)**.

Zygomatic Process of Maxilla

- Apposition occurs on the posterior surface of the zygomatic process with simultaneous resorption on its anterior or facial surface
- This region moves in a posterior direction towards the base of the skull as the entire maxillary bone increases in size

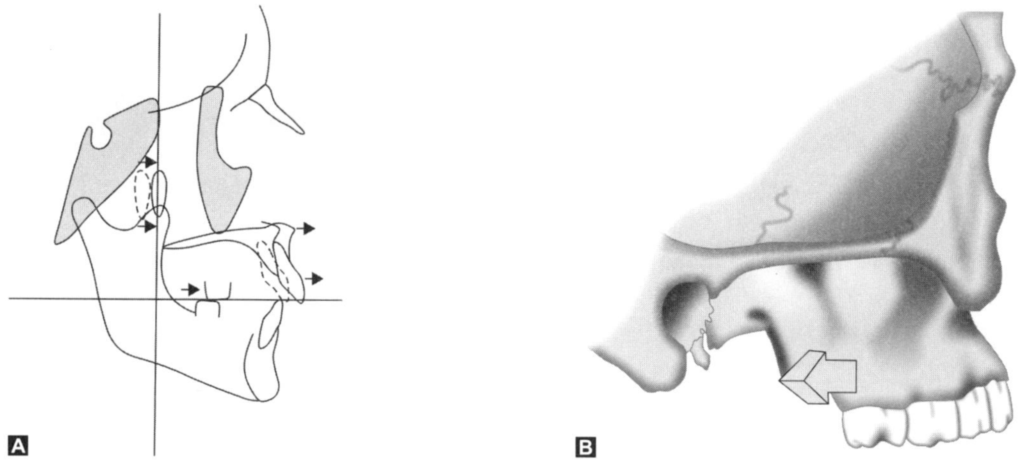

Figs. 3.8A and B: Growth of maxilla due to bone deposition at maxillary tuberosity

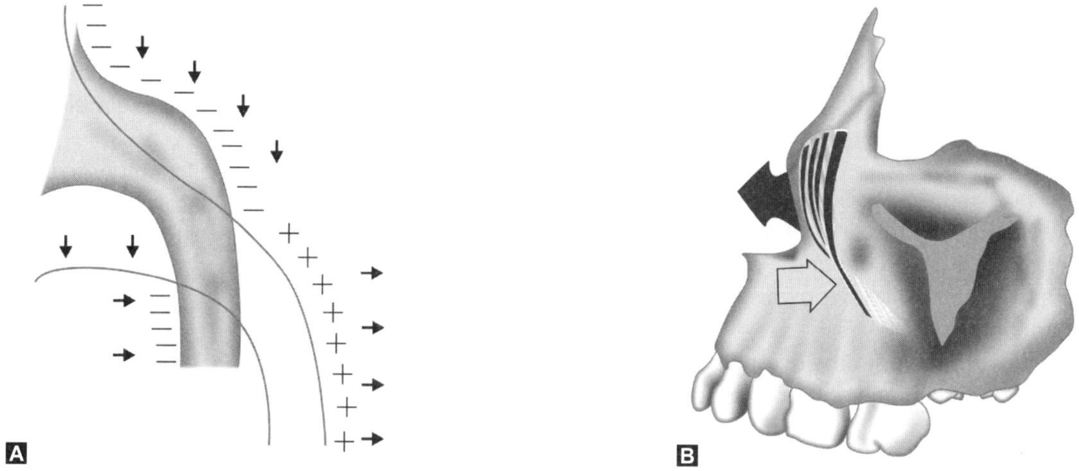

Figs. 3.9A and B: Growth of maxilla due to bone deposition at zygomatic process

- Thus, the anterior surface of the zygomatic process of maxilla and the facial surface of the maxillary body are relocated in a continuous posterior direction in order to maintain their constant relative positions in the growing maxilla as a whole
- The orbital side of the frontal process, anterior face of zygomatic bone and lateral rim of the orbit are all resorptive and grow posteriorly
- Thus, the zygomatic bone is relocated posteriorly, corresponding to the posterior growth of the maxillary tuberosity and the zygomatic processes
- Simultaneously with these movements, the zygomatic arch also increases in general size by apposition on its lateral surface and resorption from the medial side **(Figs. 3.9A and B)**.

Maxillary Arch

- The dominant area of growth occurs at the posterior margin of the arch on the maxillary tuberosity
- Along with this, bone deposition takes place along the entire inner or palatal side of the arch, with contralateral resorption from the labial and buccal sides by V principle
- As the maxilla grows in a posterior direction, the entire bone is 'thrust' anteriorly
- The width of the dental arch increases by apposition on the lateral (buccal) surface of the tuberosity in the molar area posterior to the zygomatic process **(Fig. 3.10)**.

Palatine Processes of the Maxilla

- Growth in this region corresponds to the V-principle

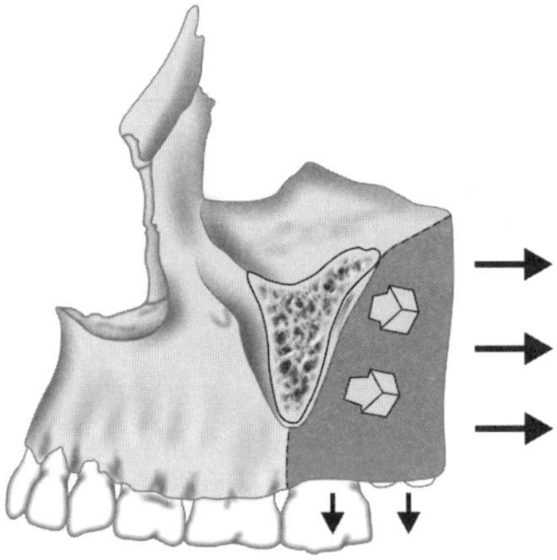

Fig. 3.10: Growth of maxilla in backward and downward direction

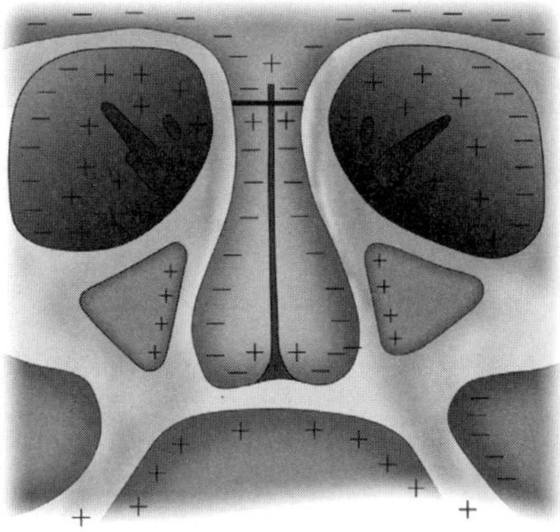

Fig. 3.11: Growth of maxilla due to deposition and resorption at palatine processes of the maxilla, premaxilla, orbit, maxillary sinus, nasal region and forehead

- Apposition occurs on the oral surface, with corresponding proportionate removal from the nasal surface
- The palatal arch thus, increases in size and undergoes a downward movement **(Fig. 3.11)**.

Premaxilla

- The labial surface of the cortex in the premaxillary region is resorptive in nature; the lingual side of the cortex receives periosteal deposits of bone
- This relocates the premaxilla in a downwards, and slightly posterior direction
- The nasal spine also moves in the downwards direction, with apposition on its inferior surface and contralateral resorption from the nasal side **(Fig. 3.11)**.

Orbit

- The orbital surface of the maxillary bone faces in three directions— laterally, anteriorly and superiorly
- Deposition of bone on these surfaces brings about an increase in size and corresponding growth movement in each of these directions
- The medial walls of the orbits move farther apart, thus increasing the width of the nasal bridge and the underlying nasal cavities
- Apposition on the inner floor of the orbital cavity relocates it anteriorly and laterally, while maintaining the internal dimensions of the orbit in constant proportion **(Fig. 3.11)**.

Maxillary Sinus

- The inner cortical lining of the sinus is resorptive in nature
- This contributes to enlargement of the sinus during maxillary growth by resorption from the inside and regional deposition on the various outer surfaces **(Fig. 3.11)**.

Nasal Region

- The lateral wall of the nasal cavity (frontal process of maxilla) is oriented in three directions—lateral, anterior and superior
- Appositional bone growth causes simultaneous growth in these directions
- Inner or mucosal side of the frontal process is resorptive which enlarges breadth of nasal cavities
- The adjacent nasal bones also serve to increase the dimensions of the nasal cavity by bone deposition on their facial surface and resorption from their inner (mucosal) surface **(Fig. 3.11)**.

Forehead

- Inner table of the forehead drifts anteriorly as long as the frontal lobe of the cerebrum grows. This ceases by 6–7 years of age
- The outer table continues to drift anteriorly, leading to separation of the two tables leading to enlargement of frontal sinus **(Fig. 3.11)**
- Vertical lengthening of the nasomaxillary complex involves:
  - Remodelling growth
  - Displacement.

Question 4

Describe the pre-natal and post-natal development of mandible?

Answer

Pre-natal Development of Mandible

- At about the 4th week of IU life, six pharyngeal arches are laid out, but the fifth one usually disappears as soon as it is formed, leaving only five

- The first arch is called the mandibular arch and second is the hyoid arch
- Each of these five arches contain:
  - A central cartilage rod that forms the skeleton of the arch
  - A muscular component termed as branchiomere
  - A vascular component
  - A neural element.
- The first structure to develop in the primordium of the lower jaw is the mandibular division of trigeminal nerve that precedes the mesenchymal condensation forming the first (mandibular) arch
- At around 36–38 days of IU life, there is ectomesenchymal condensation
- Some mesenchymal cells enlarge, acquire a basophilic cytoplasm and form osteoblasts
- These osteoblasts secrete a gelatinous matrix called osteoid and result in ossification of an osteogenic membrane
- The resulting intra-membranous bone lies lateral to meckel's cartilage of 1st (mandibular) arch
- In the 6th week of the IU life, a single ossification centre for each half of the mandible arises in the bifurcation of inferior alveolar nerve into mental and incisive branches
- During 7th week of IU life bone begins to develop lateral to meckel's cartilage and continues until the posterior aspect is covered with bone **(Fig. 3.12)**
- Between 8th and 12th week of IU life, mandibular growth accelerate, as a result mandibular length increases
- Ossification stops at a piont, which later become mandibular lingula, the remaining part of meckel's cartilage continues to form sphenomandibular ligament and spinous process of sphenoid
- Secondary accessory cartilage appears between tenth and fourteenth week of IU life to form head of condyle, part of coronoid process and mental protuberance **(Fig. 3.13)**.

Endrocondral Bone Formation

It is seen in three areas of mandible:

1. Condylar process
2. Coronoid process
3. Mental process.

Condylar Process

- At 5th week of IU life, an area of mesenchymal condensation is seen above the ventral part of developing mandible
- At about 10th week, it develops in cone-shaped cartilage
- It migrates inferior and fuses with mandibular ramus at about 4 months
- This cone-shaped cartilage is replaced by bone but its upper end persists acting as growth cartilage and articular cartilage **(Fig. 3.14)**.

Coronoid Process

- Secondary accessory cartilage appears in region of coronoid process at about 10-14 weeks of IU life
- This cartilage becomes incorporated into expanding intra-membranous bone of ramus and disappears before birth.

Mental Region

- In mental region, on either side of symphysis, one or two small cartilages appear and ossify in 7th week of IU life to become mental ossicles
- These ossicles become incorporated into intra-membranous bone when symphysis ossify completely.

Post-natal Development of Mandible

- At birth the two rami of the mandible are short, condylar development is minimum and there is no articular eminence in glenoid fossa

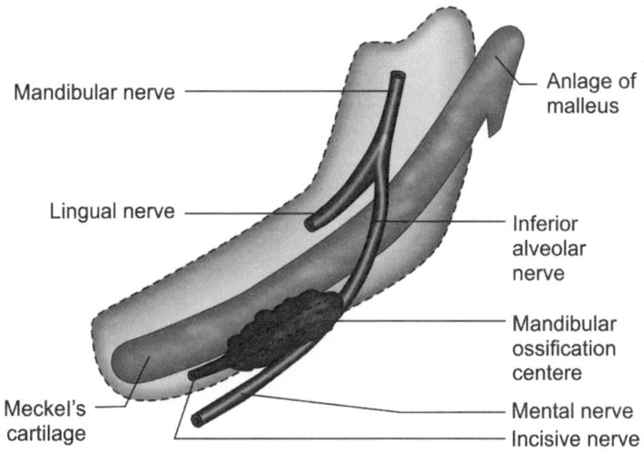

Fig. 3.12: Pre-natal development of mandible

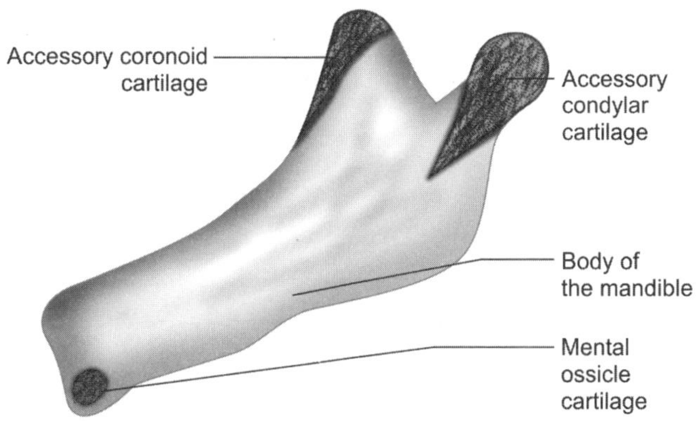

Fig. 3.13: Fetal mandible

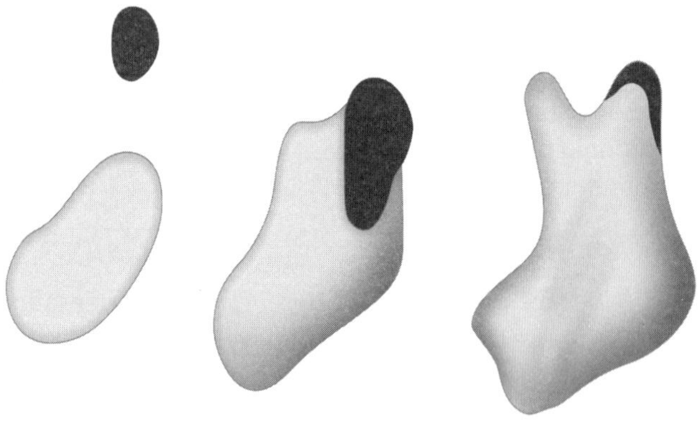

Fig. 3.14: Development of condylar process

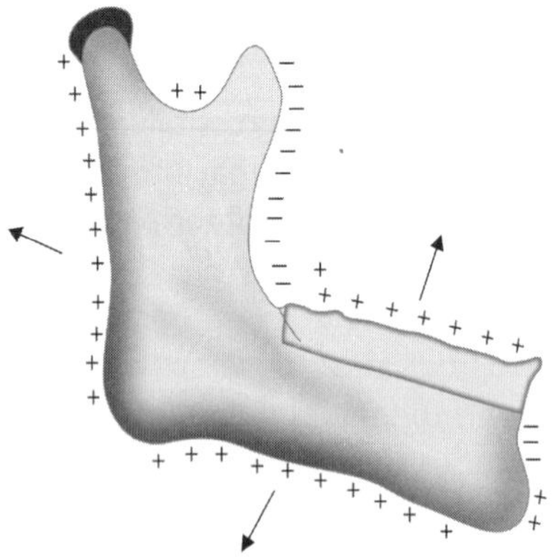

Fig. 3.15: Post-natal growth of mandible

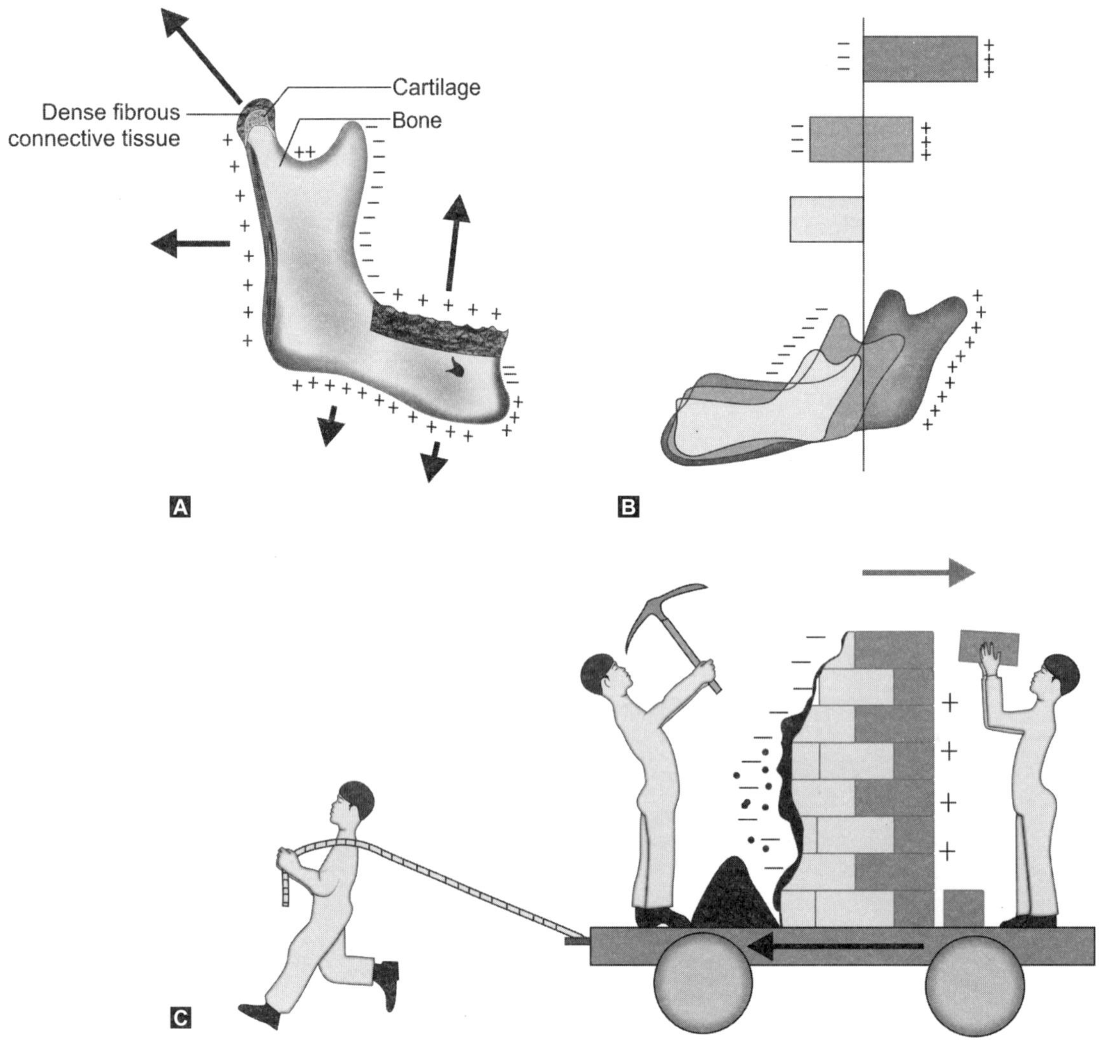

Figs. 3.16A to C: Growth of mandible

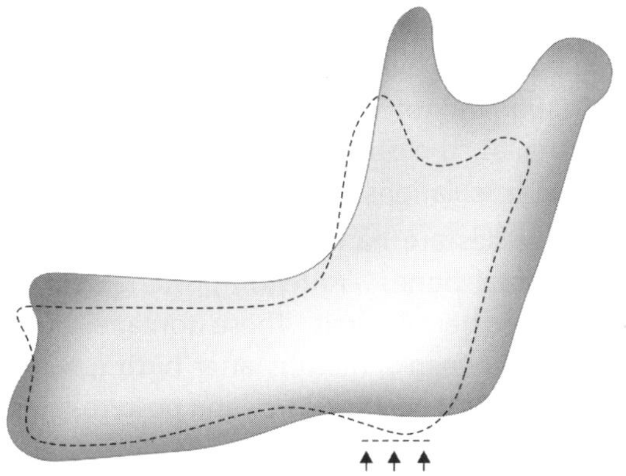

Fig. 3.17: Change in gonial angle after little muscle activity

- A thin layer of fibrocartilage and connective tissue exists at the midline of symphysis to separate right and left mandibular bodies
- At 4th month of age and end of first year, symphysial cartilage is replaced by bone
- During first year of life, appositional growth is active at alveolar border, at distal and superior surfaces of the ramus, at the condyle, along the lower border of mandible and on its lateral surface **(Fig. 3.15)**.

After first year of life, these changes occur **(Figs. 3.16A to C)**:

- Mandibular growth become more selective, condyle shows considerable activities, mandible moves and grows downwards and forwards
- Appositional growth occurs on posterior border of the ramus and on the alveolar process
- Resorption occurs along the anterior border of ramus lengthening the alveolar border and maintaining the anterior-posterior dimension of ramus **(Fig. 3.16B)**
- Gonial angle changes after little muscle activity **(Fig. 3.17)**
- The two rami also diverge outwards from below to above so that additive growth is at coronoid notch, coronoid process and condyle also increases the superior inter-ramus dimension **(Fig. 3.18)**

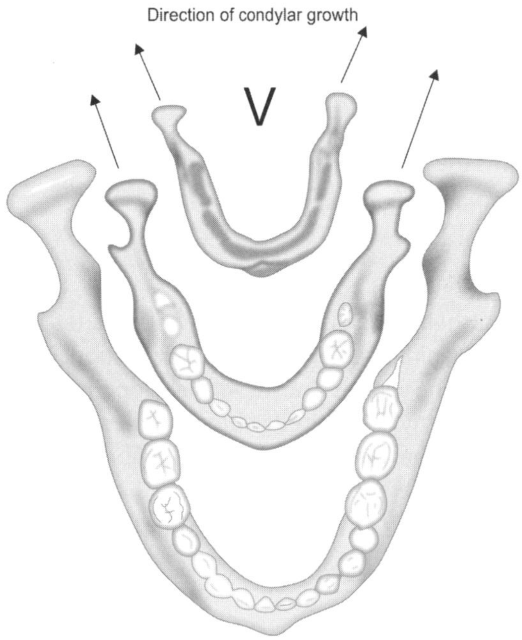

Fig. 3.18: Transverse dimension is mainly due to growth at posterior border in an expanding V pattern

- Alveolar process of mandible grows upwards and outwards on an expanding arc. This permit dental arc to accommodate the larger permanent teeth **(Fig. 3.16A)**.

Chin

- In males, the apposition of the bone at symphysis seems to be about the last change in shape during the growing period
- This change is much less apparent in the females
- On lingual surface, behind the chin heavy periosteal growth occurs with the dense lamellar bone merging and overlapping on the labial side of the chin.

SHORT ESSAYS

Question 1

Describe the pre-natal growth of cranial vault?

Answer

The cranial vault is a derivative of the mesenchyme, which is initially arranged in the form of a capsular membrane around the developing brain.

The membrane has two parts:

1. Endomeninx—derived from neural crest cells
2. Ectomeninx—derived from neural crest cells and paraxial mesoderm.

The ectomeninx differentiates into:

- Inner dura mater
- Outer superficial membrane with osteogenic properties.

The part of the superficial membrane which is over the dome of the brain ossifies intra-membranously and forms the vault.

The part that is below the brain, ossifies endochondrally and forms the *cranial base*.

The endomeninx differentiates into:

- Piamater
- Arachnoid.

During their development, the two layers (ectomeninx and endomeninx) remain in close apposition, except in areas where the venous sinuses will develop. The duramater shows distinctly organised fibre bundles, which later develop into the various folds—falx cerebri, falx cerebelli and tentorium cerebelli.

These bands also, to an extent, control the shape of the brain, which would expand as a perfect sphere if it were not for them.

Endomeninx gives rise to the following bones:

- Mesoderm: Frontal, parietal, sphenoid, petrous temporal and occipital
- Neural crest: Lacrimal, nasal, squamous temporal, zygomatic, maxilla and mandible.

The individual bones form from various primary and secondary ossification centres.

Frontal Bone

- Single primary centre in the region of the superciliary arch. This appears in the 8th week of IU life
- Three secondary ossification centres appear in the zygomatic process, nasal spine and trochlear fossae.

Parietal Bone

One primary centre each in the region of parietal eminence. These do not fuse with each other, and a sagittal fontanelle remains between them, at birth.

Occipital Bone

Squamous portion ossifies intra-membranously— primary centre appearing just above the supranuchal lines.

Temporal Bone

- Squamous part of temporal bone: Single ossification centre appearing at the root of the zygoma
- Tympanic ring of the temporal bone: Four centres on the lateral wall of the tympanum.

Also, the development of sutural bones occurs if any unusual ossification sites develop. Most centres of ossification appear during the 7th or 8th week of IU, but ossification is not complete until after birth. Apart from fontanelles, the sutures themselves are wide, with syndesmotic articulations.

The fontanelles are named according to their relation with the parietal bones—Anterior, posterior, two antero-laterals, two postero-laterals. These fontanelles close at varied times between 2 months after birth (postero- and antero-lateral) and 2 years (antero- and postero-lateral).

Question 2

Describe the post-natal growth of cranial vault?

Answer

Growth of the cranial vault is directly influenced by pressure from the neurocranial capsule **(Fig. 3.19)**.

As the brain expands the cranial vault bones are separated, at the sutures and the resulting space is closed by proliferation of connective tissue at the suture, and its subsequent ossification. But the bones are *not pushed* outwards **(Figs. 3.20A to C)**.

Each bone is enmeshed in a *stroma*, which is continuous with the meninges and skin. Hence, as the brain grows, this connective tissue stroma separates the bones at the sutures.

Another change taking place is periosteal growth. In general, deposition occurs both, at the inner table and outer table of the bones of the vault, and resorption occurs at the endosteal surface. The effect is two fold:

- To flatten the bones
  - At birth, the bones are quite curved
  - The remodelling serves to flatten the bones and hence, arrange them along a bigger arch
  - There may be certain areas of reversal of the resorption-deposition pattern mentioned earlier, in order to achieve this **(Fig. 3.21)**.

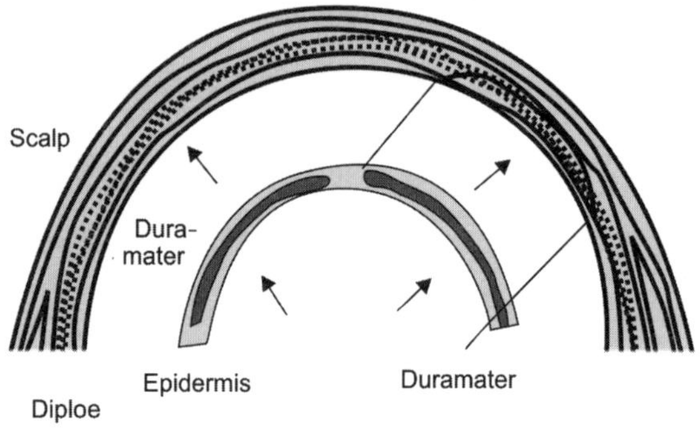

Fig. 3.19: Neurocranial capsule

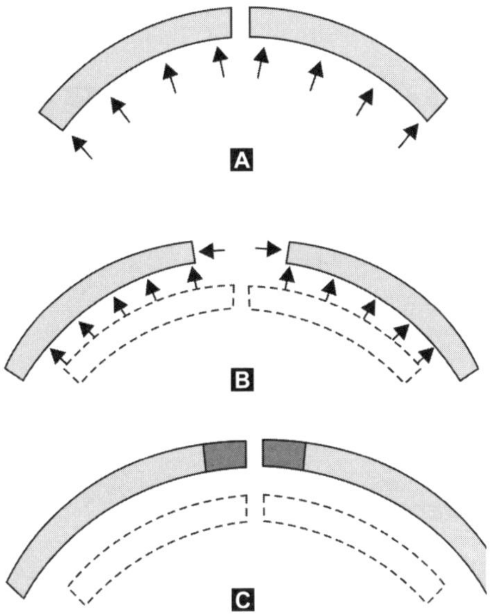

Figs. 3.20A to C: (A) Outward pressure on cranial vault by developing brain; (B) Vault expands at sutures; (C) Bone at sutures gets deposited to approximate the gap created due to expansion of cranial vault

- This also helps to increase the thickness of the bones
  - At birth, the bones are thin and lack the spongy diploë between the inner and outer tables
  - According to Sicher, the thickening is not uniform, as the inner table is influenced by the growth of the brain, while the outer table is influenced by mechanical force, especially of muscles in the supraorbital, otic and mastoid regions
  - Another response to functional stresses is the development of the frontal sinus (Benninghoff)
  - As the thickness of the bone increases, the supraorbital ridges develop due to more thickening of the outer table
  - Then, the spongy bone between the inner and outer table is slowly filled in by the developing sinus
  - Ninety percent of the cranial vault growth is completed by the age of 5–6 year, as has been shown by Davenport
  - This is in accordance with Scammons curve for brain growth as well as the cephalocaudal gradient.

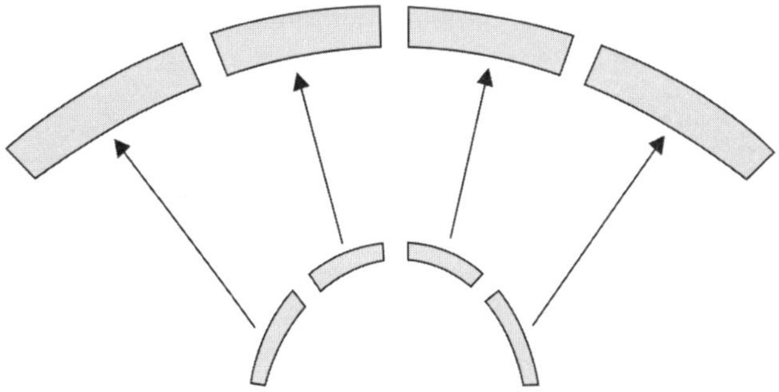

Fig. 3.21: Curved bone become flat with growth and increasing age

CHAPTER 4 Development of Dentition and Occlusion

LONG ESSAYS

Question 1

Explain in detail the periods of occlusal development?

Answer

The occlusal development can be divided into four periods:

1. Pre-dental period
2. Deciduous dentition period
3. Mixed dentition period
4. Permanent dentition period.

Pre-dental Period

- The period from birth till 6 months of age
- The child does not have teeth during this period.

Gum Pads

- Gum pads are the alveolar processes at the time of birth
- They are pink, firm and covered by a fibrous periosteum
- These have horse shoe shape and develop in two parts, viz, the lingual part and the labio-buccal part
- Groove known as dental groove separate the two portions of gum pads from each arch
- Transverse grooves divide the gum pads in 10 segments
- A developing deciduous tooth sac is present in each of these segments
- Gum pad is separated from the palate and floor of the mouth by gingival groove
- Lateral sulcus is a transverse groove between canine and deciduos molars
- The upper gum pad is wider as well as longer than the mandibular gum pad
- Upper and lower gum pads contact in the first molar region and spacing is present between the anterior regions. This spacing is normal and helps the infant in suckling.

Status of Dentition

- For 6 months post birth, the child does not have any teeth as the gum pads are not wide enough to accomodate the teeth
- During first year of life, the gum pads grow rapidly allowing the incisors to erupt in good alignment
- If teeth are present at the time of birth, they are referred to as natal teeth
- If teeth erupt during the first month of age, they are referred to as neonatal teeth
- They both are present in the mandibular incisor region and show a familial tendency.

Deciduous Dentition Period

- The deciduous or primary teeth begin to erupt at the age of about 6 months
- Eruption of deciduous teeth is over by 2.5–3.5 years of age.

Eruption Age and Sequence of Deciduous Dentition

- Mandibular central incisors are the first teeth to appear in oral cavity erupting aroung 6-7 months of age
- A variation of 3 months in the tooth eruption from the mean age, is considered normal
- The sequence in which deciduous dentition erupt is A – B – D – C – E
- The deciduous dentition generally establishes by 3 years of age
- Between 3 and 6 years of age, very few changes are seen.

Spacing in Deciduous Dentition

- There are spaces present between the deciduous teeth which are known as *physiological spaces or developmental spaces*
- Spaces in primary dentition are important for the normal development of the permanent dentition

- If spaces are absent in the primary dentition, it indicates that crowding of teeth can occur upon eruption of large permanent teeth
- Spacing is commonly present mesial to the maxillary canines and distal to the mandibular canines
- These spaces are known as *primate spaces or simian spaces or anthropoid spaces* **(Fig. 4.1)**. These spaces aid in placement of the canine cusps of the opposing arch.

Flush Terminal Plane

- Terminal plane is the mesio distal relatioship between the distal surface of maxillary and mandibular second primary molar
- Normally the distal surfaces of the upper and lower second deciduous molar are in the same vertical plane and is called as Flush terminal plane

Deep-bite

- Deep-bite is generally seen in the early stages of development
- This deep bite appears more accentuated since the deciduous incisors are more upright than their successor
- The deep-bite reduces with age due to following factors :
    - Eruption of deciduous molars
    - Attrition of incisors
    - Forward movement of the mandible due to growth.

Mixed Dentition Period

- Mixed dentition period begins as about 6 yrs of age
- This period is called mixed dentition period since both primary as well as permanent teeth are present in the oral cavity
- Permanent first molars are the first teeth to erupt during this period along with the replacement of deciduous incisors with permanent incisors.
- Mixed dentition can be classified into three phases.
    1. First transitional period
    2. Intertransitional period
    3. Second transitional period.

First Transitional Period

In this period, first permanent molars erupt, the primary incisors are replaced with permanent incisors.

Emergence of First Permanent Molars

- It erupts at around 6 years of age
- Distal surface of the second deciduous molar act as a guide to establish position and location of first permanent molars
- The mesio-distal relation between the distal surfaces of the upper and lower second deciduous molars can be of three types:

1. **Flush terminal plane:** When the distal surface of the upper and lower second deciduous molars are in same vertical plane, **(Fig. 4.2)**
    - It is a regular and normal feature of deciduous dentition
    - When the erupting permanent 1st molars are in flush terminal, it is called as end- on molar relation
    - To convert into Class I molar relation from end- on molar relation, lower molar has to move forward by 3- 5 mm relative to upper molar
    - This is possible by the utilisation of the physiologic spaces and leeway space in the lower arch and by the forward growth of the mandible as compared to maxilla
    - This shift in lower molar from a flush terminal plane to a class I relation occur in either of the two ways, i.e., early shift and late shift
        - Early shift: It takes place during early mixed dentition period **(Fig. 4.3)**.

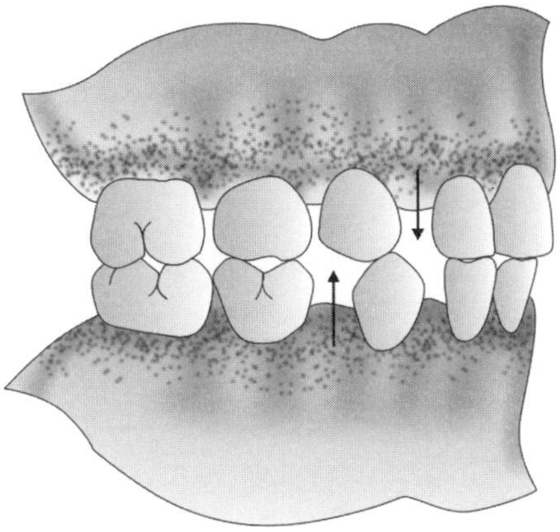

Fig. 4.1: Primate spaces

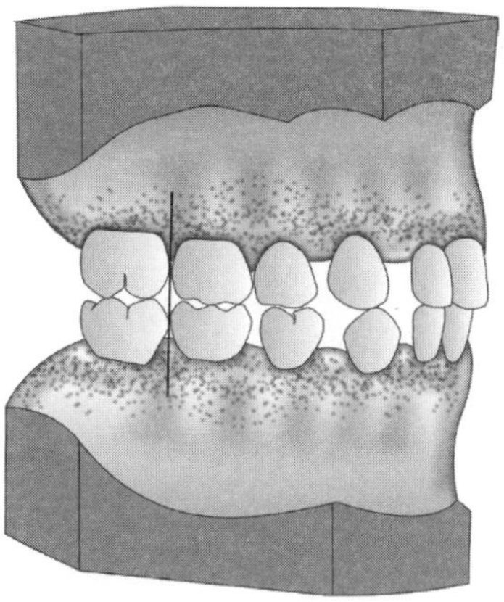

Fig. 4.2: Flush terminal plane

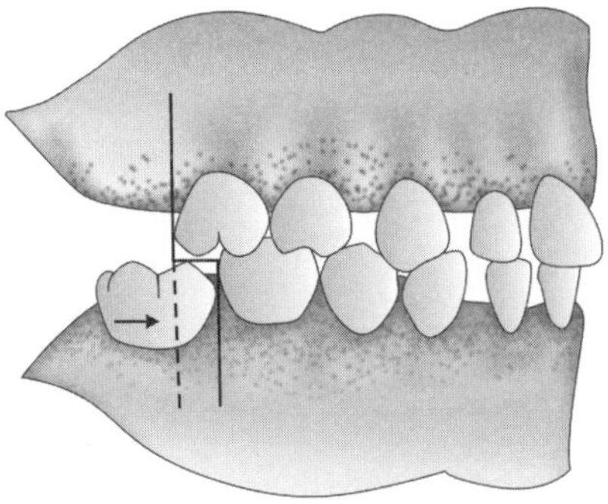

Fig. 4.3: Early shift of the erupting first permanent molars moving utilizing the primate spaces

- » The force exerted by the eruption of first permanent molar pushes the primary 1st and 2nd molar forward to close the primate spaces and thus establishing a Class I molar relationship.
- ➤ Late shift: Many children lack the primate space and therefore the erupting permanent molars are unable to move forward in class I relationship **(Fig. 4.4)**.
  - » In such cases, the Class I molar relationship is established by drifting of mandibular molar in mesial direction in space created after the shedding of deciduous 2nd molar.

2. **Mesial step terminal plane:** In this the distal surface of mandibular 2nd deciduous molar is in more mesial position then that of maxillary molar **(Fig. 4.5)**
   - Therefore, the permanent molars erupt directly into Angle's class I occlusion
   - This type of relationship is seen when thereis early forward growth of mandible
   - If the differential growth of the mandible in a forward direction persists, it can lead to an angles class III molar relation. If the forward mandibular growth is less, it leads to class I molar relationship.
3. **Distal step terminal plane:** In this, the distal surface of the mandibular 2nd primary molar is more distal to that of the maxillary 2nd primary molar **(Fig. 4.6)**.
   - Therefore the erupting permanent molar may be in Angle's class II occlusion.

Exchange of Incisors

- The deciduous incisors are replaced by the permanent incisors, during the first transitional period
- The mandibular central incisors are generally first to erupt
- The permanent incisors are considerably larger than the deciduous teeth
- The difference between the amount of space needed for the accommodation of the permanent incisors and the amount of space available for this is known as incisal liability.

Incisal Liability

- It is about 7 mm in the maxillary arch and around 5 mm in the mandibular arch
- The factors that overcome the incisal liability are as follows:
  - Utilisation of interdental spaces i.e., the physiologic or the developmental spaces . seen in primary dentition
  - Increase in inter-canine width
    - ➤ During the transition from the deciduous incisors to the permanent incisors, an increase in inter canine width is seen in both maxillary and mandibular arch. This increase of inter-canine width increases the perimeter of the upper and lower arch, thus providing space for the accomodation of permanent incisors.
  - Change in incisors inclination : Permanent incisors are more inclined then primary incisors, thus they require less space in the arch.

Inter-transitional Period

During this period, deciduous molars and canines are seen between the permanent incisors and the first permanent molars

This phase during the mixed dentition period is relatively stable and no changes are seen. Second Transitional Period

- During this period, the deciduous molars and the canines are replaced by premolars and permanent canines
- The total mesio-distal width of the permanent canines and premolars are usually less than that of the deciduous canines and molars

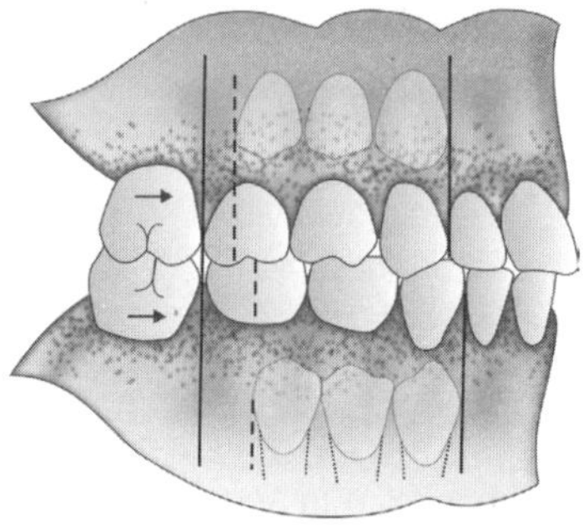

Fig. 4.4: Late shift by utilization of the leeway space

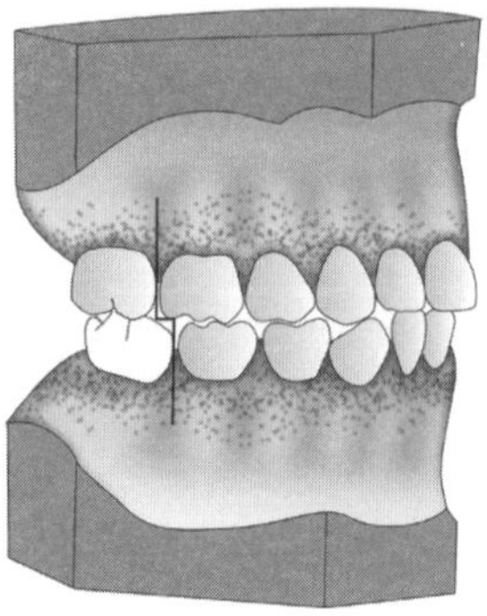

Fig. 4.5: Mesial step terminal plane

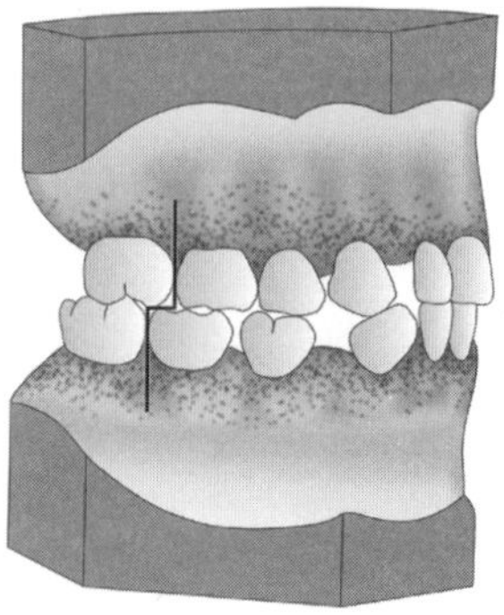

Fig. 4.6: Distal step terminal plane

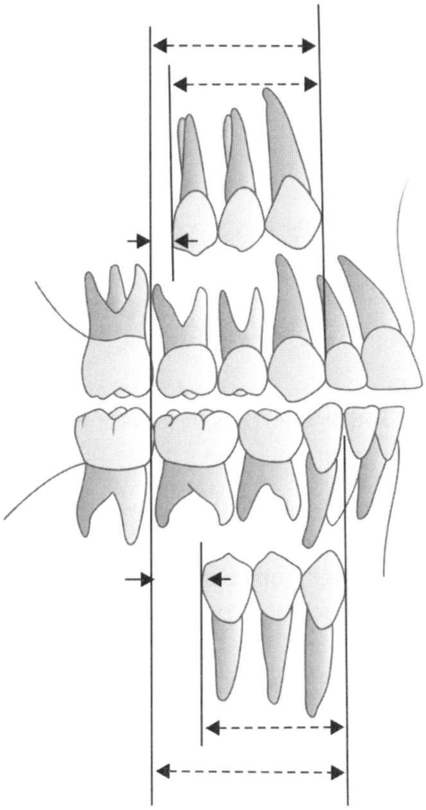

Fig. 4.7: Leeway space of Nance

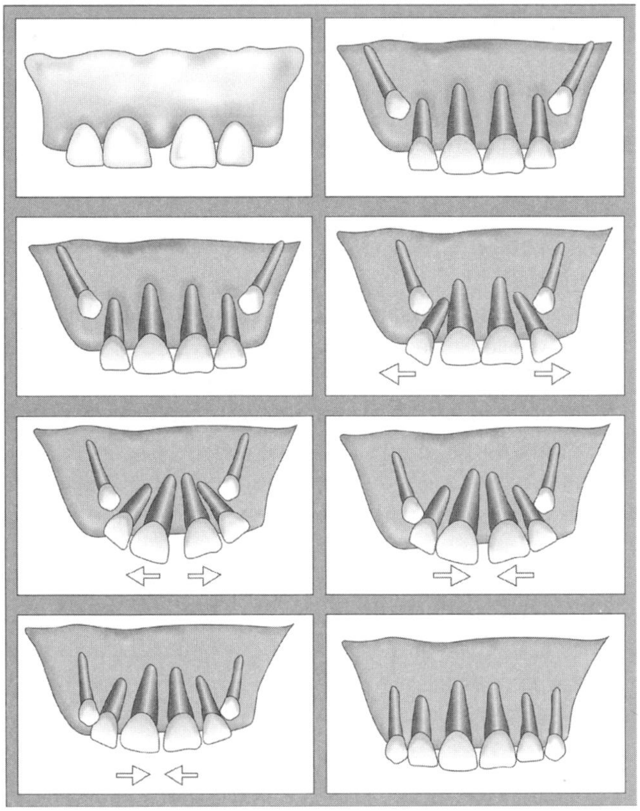

Fig. 4.8: Ugly ducking stage in the development of dentition

- This surplus space is known as leeway space of Nance **(Fig. 4.7)**
- The leeway space of Nance is greater than in mandibular arch as compared to maxillary arch
- It is around 3.4 mm, i.e., 1.7 mm on each side of the arch in the mandibular arch, and around 1.8 mm, i.e., 0.9 mm on each side of the maxillary arch
- This excess space, is utilised for the mesial drift of the mandibular molars to establish class I molar relationship.

Ugly Duckling Stage

- It is a self correcting or a transient malocclusion seen in the maxillary incisor region between 8 and 9 years of age
- It is seen during the eruption of the permanent canines
- The roots of the lateral incisors are in a mesial direction, when the developing permanent canines erupt
- This leads in transmitting the force on to the root of the central incisors, which also gets displaced mesially
- Because of this there is a distal tipping of the two central incisors which causes a midline diastema
- This situation is known as ugly duckling stage **(Fig. 4.8)**
- This situation does not require any treatment, as it is a self correcting situation as the canines erupt and the pressure is transferred from the root to the coronal area of the incisors.

Permanent Dentition Period

- After the birth, the secondary dentition forms within the jaws except the first permanent molar which are formed before birth
- The permanent incisors develop lingual or palatal to the deciduous incisors, and move labially as they erupt
- The premolars develop below the diverging roots of the deciduous molar.
- The eruption sequence in maximally arch are:
  6 – 1 – 2 – 4 – 3 – 5 – 7 or
  6 – 1 – 2 – 3 – 4 – 5 – 7
- In mandibular arch:
  6 – 1 – 2 – 3 – 4 – 5 – 7 or
  6 – 1 – 2 – 4 – 3 – 5 – 7.

SHORT ESSAYS

Question 1

Write a short-note on gum pads?

Answer

- Gum pads are the alveolar processes at the time of birth **(Fig. 4.9)**
- They are pink, firm and covered by a fibrous periosteum
- These have horse shoe shape and develop in two parts, viz, the lingual part and the labio-buccal part
- Groove known as dental groove separate the two portions of gum pads from each arch
- Transverse grooves divide the gum pads in 10 segments
- A developing deciduous tooth sac is present in each of these segments
- Gum pad is separated from the palate and floor of the mouth by gingival groove
- Lateral sulcus is a transverse groove between canine and deciduos molars

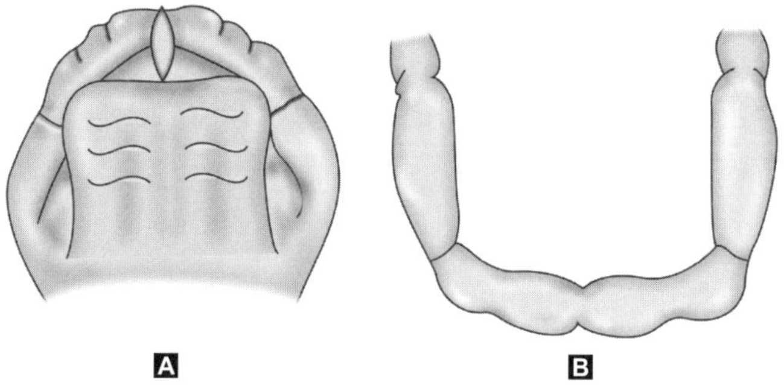

Fig. 4.9A and B: Gum pads (A) Maxillary (B) Mandibular

- The upper gum pad is wider as well as longer than the mandibular gum pad
- Upper and lower gum pads contact in the first molar region and spacing is present between the anterior regions
- This spacing is normal and helps the infant in suckling.

CHAPTER 5 Functional Development

SHORT ESSAYS

Question 1

What are the stages of Mastication?

Answer

In Infants

- Food is taken in by the infant, first by suckling
- According to Bosma, in a new born, the classic suckle position shows that the head is in an extended position, tongue lies low on to the floor the mouth, in an elongated position, with both maxillary and mandibular jaws lying apart with lips pursed around the nipple
- As the infant learns to ingest food, reduced activity of lips and extent of mandibular thrust is seen however, activity of most of the muscles of cheek, floor of mouth and tongue still persists. The tongue helps in mixing of food with saliva
- As the bolus mixes with saliva, it is forced between the gum pads/occlusal surfaces of the erupting teeth
- Simultaneously along with the above process, the bolus mashes against the hard palate, because the muscles of the cheek forces the food backwards towards the tongue
- The mandible is then forcibly closed, once the bolus of the food has been adjusted between the occlusal surfaces.

In Adults (6 Stages by Murphy)

1. The preparatory phase:
   - During this phase the food is ingested and positioned with the help of tongue within the oral cavity and the mandible moves towards the chewing side.
2. Food contact:
   - During this phase there is a momentary pause in movement
   - This pause is caused due to the sensory receptors concerning the apparent viscosity of the food.
3. The crushing phase:
   - This phase begins with high intensity but slows down as the food is crushed into small pieces and packed.
4. Tooth contact:
   - Accompalished by a small change in direction without any delay.
5. The grinding phase:
   - This phase coincides with transgression of the mandibular molars across there maxillary counterparts.
6. Centric occlusion:
   - Centric occlusion is achieved when movement of the teeth comes to a definitive stop at a single terminal point from which the preparatory phase of next stroke begins.

Question 2

What is Degluitation/Stages of Degluitation/Infantile Swallow/Swallowing?

Answer

Infantile (Visceral) Swallow

According to Moyers following are the characteristics of the infantile swallow (**Fig. 5.1**):

- The jaws are held apart with tongue lying between the gum pads
- The mandible is stabilized due to the VII cranial nerves muscle contraction and the tongue
- Sensory interchange between the lips and the tongue guides and controls the process of swallow.

The intrinsic and rhythmic peristaltic activity of the superior, middle and the inferior pharyngeal constrictors, guides the liquid or bolus of food back into the pharynx past the epiglottis into the esophagus.

The glottis closes off the pharynx as the posterior peripheral portion are forced backward against the superior constrictor ring.

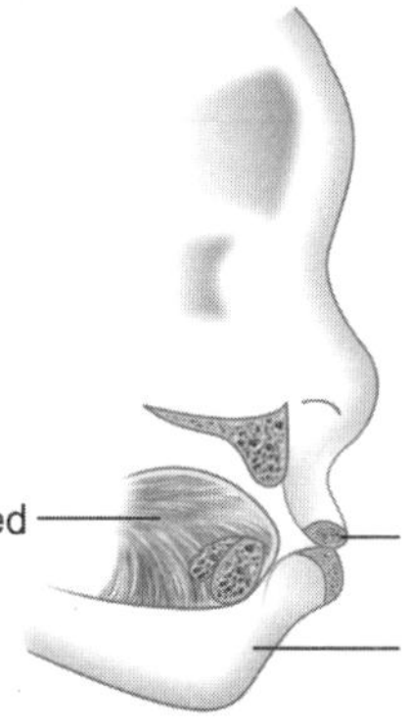

Fig. 5.1: Infantile swallow

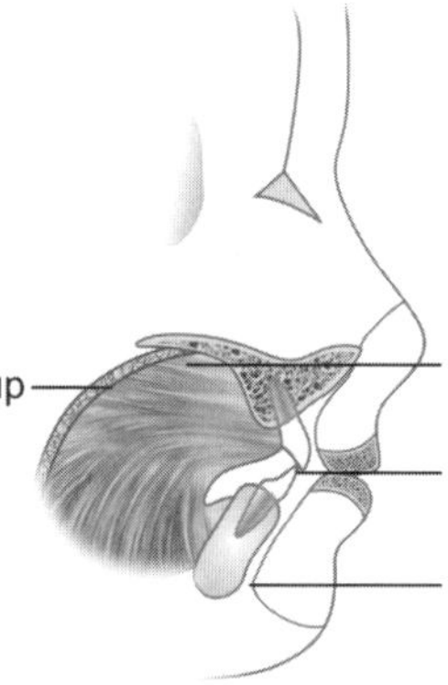

Fig. 5.2: Mature swallow

Mature (Somatic) Swallow

Pattern of swallowing changes with the eruption of dentition and introduction of semi- solid and solid food in the diet **(Fig. 5.2)**.

The mature swallow characteristics given by Moyers, usually by 18th months of age are as follows:

- The teeth are held together
- The mandible is stabilized, by the contraction of the mandibular elevators
- The tip of the tongue is placed against the palate, above and behind the incisors
- During the mature swallow, there is minimal contraction of the lips.

Phases of Deglutition

According to Fletcher, the deglutition cycle is divided into four phases.

1. Preparatory
2. Oral phase
3. Pharyngeal phase
4. Esophageal phase.

Preparatory

This phase begins once the solid food has been masticated or liquid is ingested. The bolus of liquid is placed on the dorsum of the tongue while the oral cavity is sealed by lips and tongue.

Oral Phase

In this phase the tongue drops downwards and backwards while the soft palate moves in upward direction, simultaneously the larynx and hyoid bone also move upward. This combination of movements creates a path for the bolus/ liquid.

The solid food is pushed by the wave like rippling action of tongue, the liquid flows with the help of lingual constrictions. Masticatory muscles stabilizes the oral cavity and also maintain and anterior and lateral lip seal during this process.

The Pharyngeal Phase

The pharyngeal phase starts once the bolus passes the fauces. During this phase the whole pharyngeal tube rises upwards alongwith the closure of soft palate along the posterior pharyngeal wall which seals off the nasopharynx. Pharynx and tongue continue the peristaltic movement to push the bolus of the food. Hyoid and tongue move forward.

The Esophageal Phase

Once the bolus passes the cricopharyngeal sphincter, into the esophagus, the hyoid bone, soft palate and the tongue return to their original positions.

Question 3

What are Trajectories of Forces?

Answer

- The trajectorial theory of force states that the " lines of orientation of the bony trabeculae corresponds to the pathways of maximal pressure and tension and that the bony trabeculae are thicker when the stress is greater"
- The trabeculae do not all cross each other at 90° but at varying angles and they do not form predominantly straight lines
- Many of the trajectories are irregular and wavy varying from bone to bone
- Changes in functional forces produce measurable changes in bony architecture and are within the limits of inherent morphogenetic pattern

- Benninghoff studied extensively the architecture of cranial and facial skeletal and stress trajectories by piercing holes. These trajectories involve both compact and spongy bone.

The head is Composed of two Units

1. Craniofacial unit / maxilla
2. Mandible / movable unit.

Maxilla consists of vertical and horizontal pillars / buttresses.

Vertical Pillars

- All these pillars arise from the alveolar processes and ends in the base of the skull
- The maxilla provides a maximum strength with minimum of material
- The maxillary bones are supported by strong buttress that strengthen the facial frame
- These buttresses consist of 3 columns of bone on each side of the face
- These bear the main stress of mastication.

Canine Pillar (Frontonasal Buttress)

The trajectorial lines runs superiorly by the sides of piriform aperture and the crest of nasal bone to the frontal bone. Anteriorly the fronto nasal buttress is for the transmission of forces from the region of incisors, canines and first premolars.

Zygomatic Pillar (Malar Zygomatic Buttress)

The trajectorial I lines arises from the alveolar process of teeth on the buccal segment. Runs superiorly and in the malar area divides into 3 branches.

- 1st Branch: Runs inferiorly to the orbital cavity and joins the frontonasal buttress
- 2nd Branch: Running superiorly along the lateral wall of orbit to join the frontal bone
- 3rd Branch: Running along the zygomatic arch.

Laterally, the malar zygomatic buttress transmits stress from the buccal group of teeth. Also stresses from the masseter are received by the malar bone and zygomatic arch.

Pterygoid Pillar (Pterygoid Buttress)

Posteriorly the pterygoid pillar forms a curved support which passes to the strong middle portion of base of the skull.

Horizontal Pillars

Are the reinforcing units for the vertical buttresses. These include:

- Trajectories running superiority and inferiority to the orbital cavity
- Trajectorial lines of the hard palate.

Along with these, some of the auxiliary buttresses are:

- The walls of orbits
- The zygomatic arches
- Lesser wings of sphenoid.

Mandible

- Mandible being a unit by itself and a movable bone, the trabecular pattern is different from that of maxilla
- Trabecular column radiate from beneath the teeth in the alveolar process and join together in a common stress pillar or trajectory system that terminates in the mandible condyle
- The mandibular canal and nerve are protected at the same time by this concentration of trabeculae, demonstrating the "Unloaded nerve concept"
- The thick cortical layer of compact bone along the lower border of the mandible offers the greatest resistance to the bending forces
- Others trajectory patterns are seen at the symphysis, at the gonial angle and leading downward from the coronoid process into the ramus and body of the mandible
- These accessory trajectories are mainly due to the direct effect of attachment of muscles of mastication.

CHAPTER 6 Occlusion: Basic Concepts

LONG ESSAYS

Question 1

Discuss Curve of Spee, Curve of Wilson, Monson's Curve, Centric Relation and Centric Occlusion?

Answer

Curve of Spee

It is defined as the anatomical curve established by the occlusal alignment of the teeth, as projected onto the median plane, beginning with the cusp tip of the mandibular canine and following the buccal cusp tips of the premolar and molar teeth, continuing through the anterior border of the mandibular ramus, ending with the anterior most portion of the mandibular condyle.

Also called as "anteroposterior curve" (Glossary of Prosthodontic terms; Volume 94 number 1) (**Fig. 6.1**).

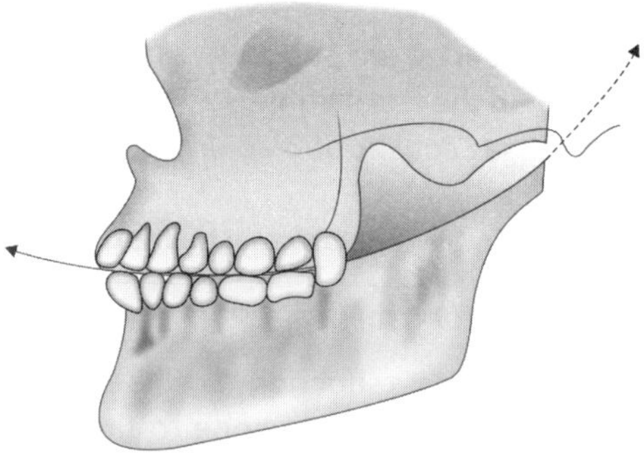

Fig. 6.1: Curve of Spee

Curve of Wilson

According to Wilson, in theory that occlusion should be spherical, the curvature of the cusps as projected on the frontal plane expressed in both arches; the curve in the lower arch being concave and the one in the upper arch being convex.

The curvature in the lower arch is affected by an equal lingual inclination of the right and left molars so that the tip points of the corresponding cross-aligned cusps can be placed into the circumferences of a circle.

The transverse cuspal curvature of the upper teeth is affected by the equal buccal inclinations of their long axis (Glossary of Prosthodontic terms; Volume 94 number 1) (**Fig. 6.2**).

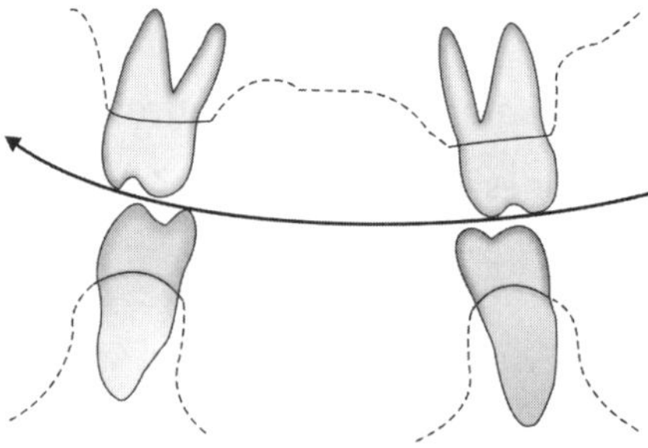

Fig. 6.2: Curve of Wilson

Monson's Curve

It is an ideal curve of occlusion in which each cusp and incisal edge touches or conforms to a segment of the surface of a

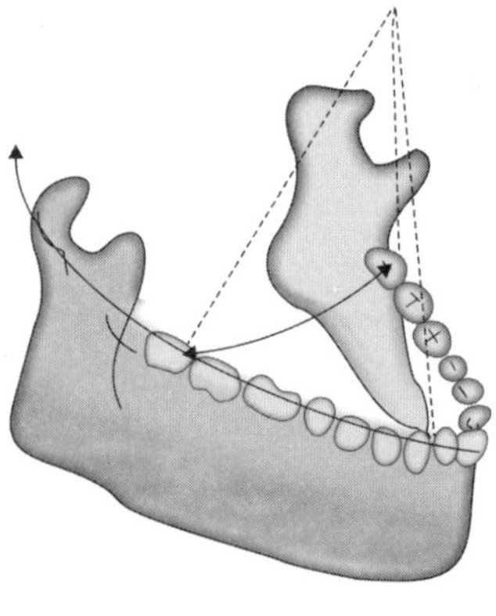

Fig. 6.3: Monson's curve

sphere 8 inches in diameter with its center in the region of the glabella (Glossary of Prosthodontic terms; Volume 94 number 1) **(Fig. 6.3)**

Centric Relation

It is the maxillomandibular relationship in which the condyles articulate with the avascular portion of their respective disks with the complex in the anterior-superior position against the shapes of the articular eminencies.

This position is independent of tooth contact. This position is clinically discernible when the mandible is directed superior and anteriorly.

It is restricted to a purely rotary movement about the transverse horizontal axis (Glossary of Prosthodontic terms; Volume 94 number 1).

Centric Occlusion

It is the occlusion of opposing teeth when the mandible is in centric relation. This may or may not coincide with the maximal intercuspal position(Glossary of Prosthodontic terms; Volume 94 number 1).

Question 2

What are Andrew's 6 keys of occlusion?

Answer

Andrews proposed six keys of normal occlusion:

- Key 1—Interarch relationship
  - The mesiobuccal cusp of permanent maxillary first molar occludes in the groove between buccal groove of the mandibular first molar
  - The distal marginal ridge of the maxillary first molar occludes with the mesial marginal ridge of the mandibular second molar
  - The mesiolingual cusp of the maxillary first molar occludes in the central fossa of the mandibular first molar **(Fig. 6.4)**.
- Key 2—Crown angulation (Tip)
  - The gingival portion of crowns of all teeth is distal to incisal portion along the long axis of the tooth
  - The degree of crown tip is the angle between the long axis of crown and a line perpendicular to the occlusal plane **(Fig. 6.5)**
  - When the gingival portion of the long axis of crown is distal to the incisal portion it is designated with a "+" reading, while a "–" reading is denoted when the gingival portion of the long axis of crown is mesial to the incisal portion.

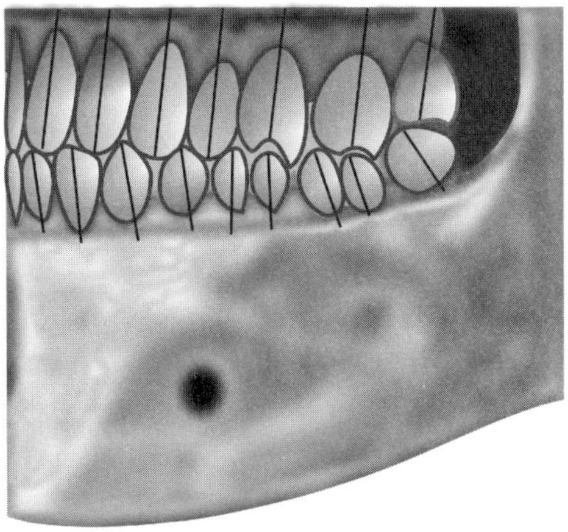

Fig. 6.4: Occlusion of maxillary first molar in the central fossa

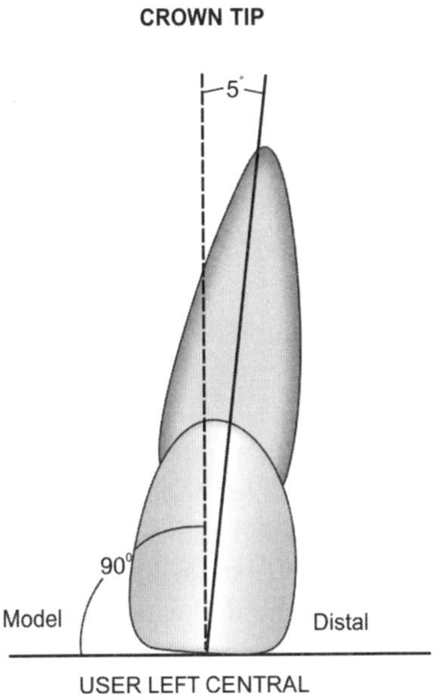

Fig. 6.5: The degree of crown tip

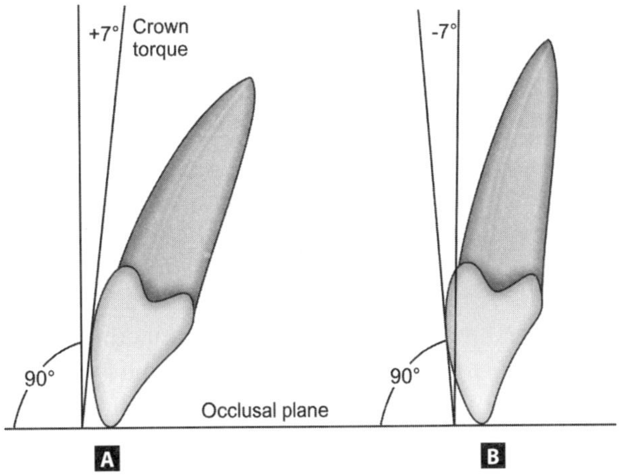

Figs. 6.6A and B: Diatal view—upper left central

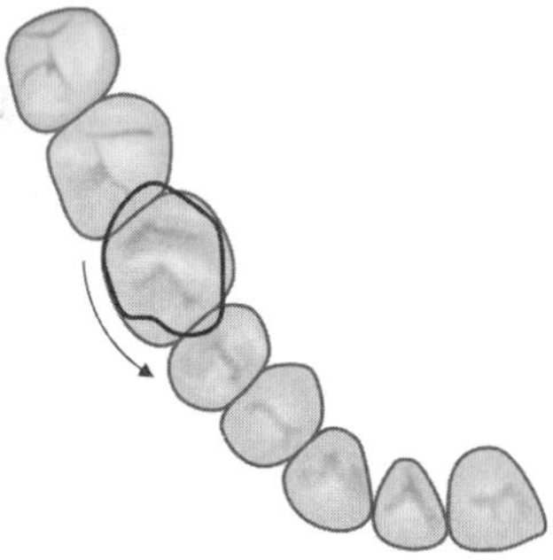

Fig. 6.7: The fourth key to normal occlusion

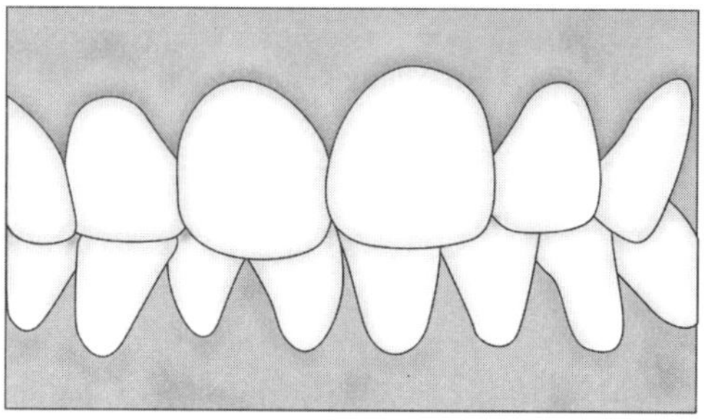

Fig. 6.8: Tight contacts

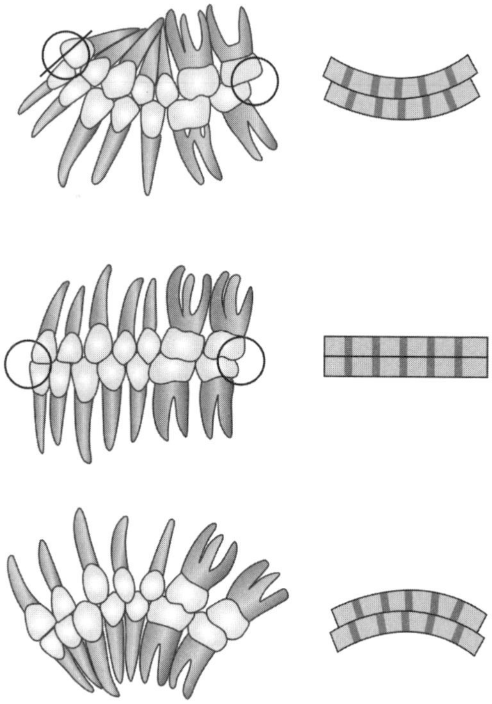

Fig. 6.9: The planes of occlusion

- Key 3—Crown inclination (**Fig. 6.6**):
  - It represents the angle formed by a line which is perpendicular to the occlusal plane and a line that is tangent to the bracket sight
  - This is expressed in plus or minus degrees
  - A "+" reading is given if the gingival portion of the tangent line is lingual to the incisal portion (**Fig. 6.6A**)
  - A "–" reading is recorded when the gingival portion of the tangent line is labial to the incisal portion (**Fig. 6.6B**).
- Key 4—Rotations: In normal occlusion, teeth should not have any rotations (**Fig. 6.7**).
- Key 5—Tight contacts: Contact points between the teeth should be tight (without any spaces) (**Fig. 6.8**).
- Key 6—Occlusal plane (**Fig. 6.9**):
  - Flat plane should be the treatment goal as a form of over treatment since there is natural tendency for the curve of spee to deepen with time
  - A deep curve of spee results in a more contained area for the upper teeth, making normal occlusion impossible
  - A reverse curve of spee is an extreme form of over-treatment, allowing excessive space for each tooth to be intercuspally placed.

SHORT NOTES

Question 1

Define canine guided occlusion?

Answer

During lateral movements of mandible, only the maxillary and mandibular canines of working side come into contact and all the posterior teeth come into disclusion both on working and balancing side.

The canine teeth is best suited for this kind of guidance because of the following:

- The canine has a good crown root ratio thus it is capable of tolerating heavy occlusal and masticatory forces
- The canine root has a greater surface area then adjacent teeth, therefore it offers greater proprioception
- Palatal surface of the upper canine is concave and thus, is better suited for guiding lateral movement.

CHAPTER 7

Classification of Malocclusion

LONG ESSAYS

Question 1

Define and describe Angle's classification of malocclusion?

Answer

According to WHO, malocclusion can be defined as "an anomaly which causes disfigurement or which impedes function, and requires treatment if the disfigurement or functional defect was likely to be an obstacle to the patient's physical or emotional well-being".

Types of Malocclusions

Malocclusion can be broadly divided into:

- Individual tooth malposition or intra arch malocclusion
- Maxillo-mandibular malocclusions or inter arch malocclusion.

Individual Tooth Malpositions

Abnormal relationship of a tooth with its neighboring teeth, is termed as individual tooth malposition. Some of the commonly seen individual tooth malpositions are:

- *Distal inclination or distal tipping*: This refers to a condition where the crown of the tooth is tilted or inclined distally
- *Mesial inclination or mesial tipping*: This is a condition where the crown of the tooth is tilted or inclined mesially
- *Lingual inclination or lingual tipping*: This is an abnormal lingual or palatal tilting of the tooth. This condition is also called retroclination
- *Buccal inclination or buccal tipping*: This refers to labial or buccal tilting of the tooth. This condition is also called proclination
- *Mesial displacement*: This refers to a tooth that is bodily moved in a mesial direction towards the midline
- *Distal displacement*: This refers to a tooth that is bodily moved in a distal direction away from the midline
- *Lingual displacement*: Is a condition where the entire tooth is displaced in a lingual direction
- *Buccal displacement*: Is a condition in which the tooth is displaced bodily in a labial or buccal direction
- *Infraversion or infraocclusion*: Refer to a tooth that has not erupted enough compared to other teeth in the arch
- *Supraversion or supra occlusion*: Refers to a tooth that has overerupted compared to other teeth in the arch
- *Rotations*: Refers to tooth movements around its long axis
- *Disto lingual or mesio buccal rotation*: Describes a tooth which has moved around it long axis so that the distal aspect is more lingually placed
- *Mesio lingual or disto buccal rotation*: This is a condition where the tooth has rotated around its long axis so that the mesial aspect is more lingually placed
- *Transposition*: this term describes a condition where two teeth have exchanged places.

Inter Arch Malocclusions

These malocclusion involves an abnormal relationship of between a set of teeth of one arch relative to other arch i.e., maxilla and mandible. These can occur in sagittal, transverse or vertical plane.

Sagital Plane Malocclusions

- *Pre-normal occlusion*: It is a condition in which the lower arch is more forwardly placed when the patient bites in centric occlusion
- *Post-normal occlusion*: It is a condition in which the lower arch is more distally positioned when the patient bites in centric occlusion.

Vertical Plane Malocclusions

- *Deep bite or increased over bite*: This refers to a condition where there is an increased vertical overlap between the maxillary and the mandibular anterior teeth
- *Open bite*: Is a condition when there is no vertical overlap between upper and lower teeth. Therefore a space may

present between the maxillary and mandibular teeth when the patient is in centric occlusion.

Transverse Plane Malocclusions

- They include various types of cross bites, and scissor bite
- The term crossbite refers to abnormal transverse relationship between upper and lower arches
- Scissor bite refers to a condition in which the mandibular arch is contained within the maxillary arch.

Angle's Classification

Angle (1898) gave his classification of occlusion based on the mesial-distal relations of the teeth, dental arches and jaws **(Fig. 7.1)**.

- Normal occlusion
- Class I (neutroclusion)
- Class II (distoclusion)
- Class III (mesioclusion).

Basis for Angle's Classification

- Most common irregularity of teeth is seen in antero-posterior direction of teeth and jaws
- Curvature and line of occlusion is unique to each individual.
  - Angle believed that all the teeth are important, however keeping function and influence in mind, some of the teeth play more important role, with first permanent molars being the most important, especially maxillary 1st permanent molars
  - Angle called maxillary 1st permanent molars as Keys to Occlusion based on following factors:
    - They are the largest teeth along with good anchorage support
    - Their position in the arch maintains the function of mastication
    - They establish the vertical distance of upper and lower jaws, esthetics and dental height
    - They play an important role in the positioning of other permanent teeth as they erupt 1st in the oral cavity.

Class I Normal Occlusion

- Normal (class I) molar relation, in this a smooth curve of line of occlusion is seen passing through the central fossa of each maxillary molar and the cingulum of the maxillary canine and incisor teeth **(Fig. 7.2)**
- In mandibular arch the same curve passes along the buccal cusps of molars and incisal edges of anterior teeth.
  - The mesiobuccal cusp of the mandibular first molar occludes in the embrasure area between the maxillary second premolar and first molar **(Fig. 7.3)**
  - The mesiobuccal cusp of the maxillary first molar is aligned directly over the buccal groove of the mandibular first molar **(Fig. 7.3)**
  - The mesiolingual cusp of the maxillary first molar is situated in the central fossa area of mandibular first molar **(Fig. 7.3)**.

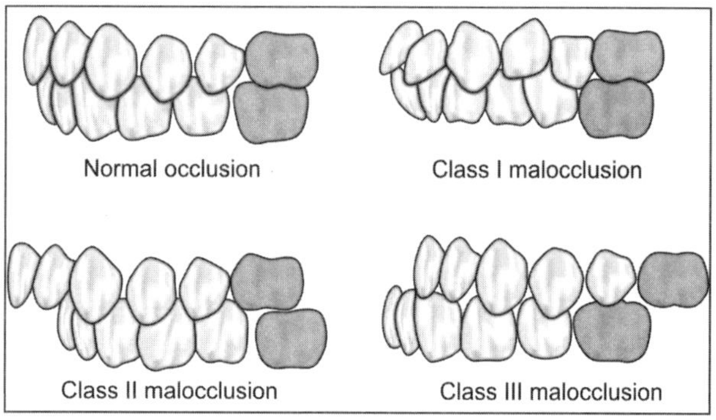

Fig. 7.1: Sub-divisions of Angle's classification

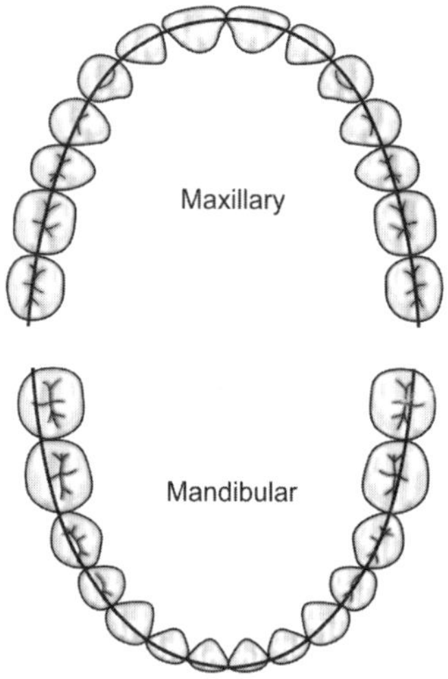

Fig. 7.2: Normal occlusion—curve passing through the central fossa of each upper molar and across the cingulum of the upper canine and incisor teeth and along the buccal cusps and incisal edges of the lower arch

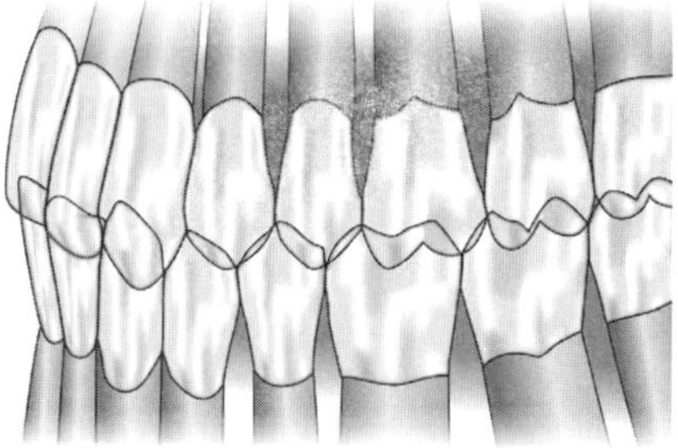

Fig. 7.3: The mesio-buccal cusp

Angle's Class I Malocclusion

- Normal anteroposterior relationship between maxilla and mandible
- Normal class I molar relation
- Normal muscle function
- Line of occlusion is incorrect because of malposed teeth, rotations or other causes
- The mesiobuccal cusp of maxillary permanent first molar occludes in the buccal groove of the mandibular permanent first molar and the mesiolingual cusp of maxillary permanent first molar occludes with the occlusal fossa of the mandibular permanent first molar when the jaws are at rest and the teeth are approximated in centric occlusion (**Fig. 7.4**).

Angle's Class II Malocclusion

- Lower dental arch is in a distal relationship to the upper dental arch
- Class II molar relation
- Line of occlusion not specified
- The mesiobuccal cusp of the mandibular first molar occludes in the central fossa area of the maxillary first molar
- The mesiobuccal cusp of the mandibular first molar is aligned with the buccal groove of the maxillary first molar
- The distolingual cusp of the maxillary first molar occludes in the central fossa area of the mandibular first molar
- There are 2 divisions in class II malocclusions (**Fig. 7.5**).

Class II Division 1

A Class II malocclusion in which the maxillary incisor teeth are in labioversion, resulting in an increased overjet.

- Proclined upper incisors
- 'V' shaped maxillary arch
- Supraversion of the lower anteriors
- Abnormal muscle activity.

Class II Division 2

A Class II malocclusion in which the maxillary incisor teeth are not in labioversion. This is typically with the maxillary central incisors are tipped palatally,with a short anterior lower facial height and an excessive overbite.

Different types of Class II Division 2 malocclusion are seen based on differences in the spatial conditions in the maxillary dental arch:

- Type A: maxillary central and lateral incisors of are tipped palatally, without the occurrence of crowding
- Type B: the maxillary central incisors are tipped palatally while the laterals are tipped labially
- Type C: maxillary central and lateral incisors are tipped palatally, with the canines labially positioned.

Differences between Class II Division 1 and Class II Division 2 Malocclusion

Class II Subdivision

When the class II molar relationship occurs on one side of the dental arch only, the malocclusion is referred to as a subdivision of its division (**Table 7.1**).

It can be:

- Class II div.1 subdivision
- Class II div.2 subdivision.

Class III

The mandibular dental arch and the body of the mandible are in bilateral mesial relationship to the maxillary arch (**Fig. 7.6**).

- The mesiobuccal cusp of the maxillary first molar is situated over the embrasure between the mandibular first and second molar
- The distobuccal cusp of the mandibular first molar is situated in the embrasure between the maxillary second premolar and first molar

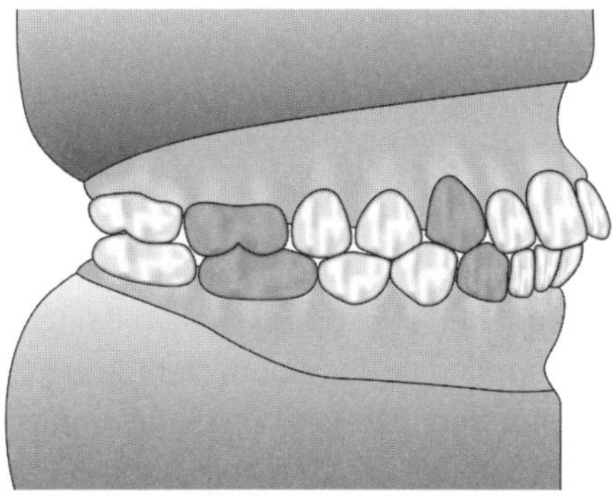

Fig. 7.4: Class I malocclusion

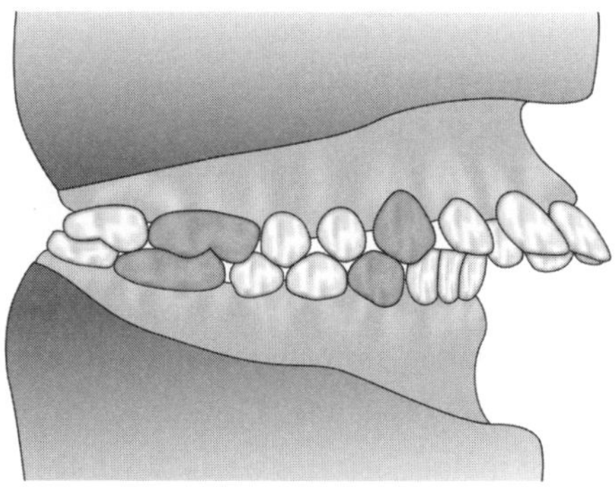

Fig. 7.5: Class II malocclusion

Table 7.1: Difference between Class II division 1 and Class II division 2

Features	Class II division 1	Class II division 2
Profile	Convex	Straight to mild convexity
Lips Upper Lower Competency	 Short Everted Incompetent	 Normal Normal Competent
Mentolabial sulcus	Deep	Deep or normal
Mentalis muscle	Hyperactive	-
Malar process	Not prominent	Prominent
Lower facial height	Normal or increased	Decreased
Arch form	"V" shaped	Square, "U" shaped
Palate	Deep	Normal
Incisors	Proclined	Centrals are retroclined
Overjet	Increased	Decreased
Overbite	Deep overbite	Closed bite
Crown root	Normal angulation	Axis of crown and root are bent and is referred to as collum angle
Path of closure	Normal	Backward
Interocclusal clearance	Normal/ increased/ decreased	Increased

- The Mesio-lingual cusp of the maxillary first molar is situated in the mesial pit of the mandibular second molar.

Class III Malocclusion can be classified into:

- True Class III
- Pseudo Class III.

True Class III

This is a skeletal Class III malocclusion of genetic origin that can occur due to the following causes:

- When mandible is excessively large
- Mandible is forwardly placed
- Smaller than normal maxilla
- Maxilla is retropositioned
- Combination of the above causes.

Pseudo Class III

In this situation, to avoid premature contact of incisors or canines, the mandible is protruded a little during the final stages of closure.

This type of malocclusion is also known as 'postural' or 'habitual' Class III malocclusion.

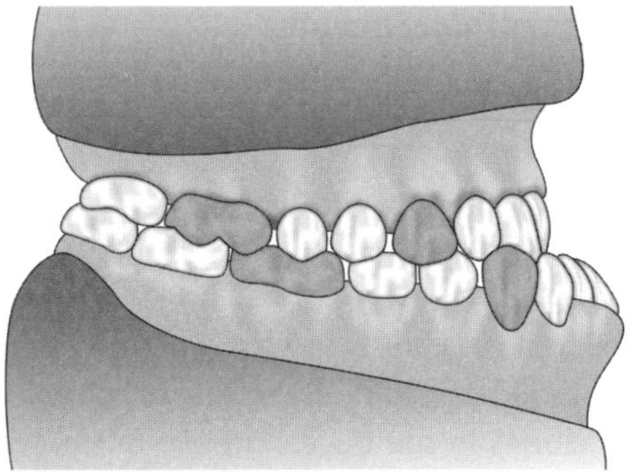

Fig. 7.6: Class III malocclusion

The following are some of the reasons for pseudo Class III malocclusion:

- Occlusal prematurities
- In cases when the child loses deciduous posterior teeth prematurely, the child tends to move the mandible forward in order to establish contact in the anterior region
- Child having enlarged adenoids tends to move the mandible in a forward direction in order to prevent the tongue from contacting the adenoids.

Clinical Differentiation of True and Pseudo Class III malocclusion

- In pseudo class III, profile improves as mandible drops from occlusal contact to postural rest position
- Translation of mandible forward from rest to occlusal position can be elicited by placing fingertips on TMJ. True class III has an even pattern of closure
- Molar relationship in pseudo class III shifts from class I to class III as mandible closes. In true class III the molar relationship remains class III in both positions. Mandible is manipulated posteriorly to ascertain if it is possible to assume a normal relationship with maxilla.

Class III Subdivision

Class III molar relation on one side and Class I on the other.

Drawbacks of Angle's Classification

- Considered Anteroposterior relationship, not vertical and transverse
- First permanent molars are not fixed points
- Cannot be applied if first molars are missing
- Cannot be applied to deciduous dentition
- No differentiation between skeletal and dental mal-occlusion
- Classification does not highlight etiology.

SHORT ESSAYS

Question 1

Discuss Simon's classification?

Answer

Growth of the face and jaws occurs in the three planes of space-height, width and depth, abnormalities also occur in any one or more of the foregoing planes. Simon's classification relates the denture to the face and cranium in the three planes of space, i.e., (1) The Frankfort horizontal (2) The Orbital plane and (3) The raphe or median sagital plane.

1. The Frankfort horizontal plane or the eye-ear plane is determined by drawing a straight line through the margin of the bony orbit directly under the pupil of the eye, to the upper margin of the auditory meatus (the notch above the tragus of the ear). This plane helps in determining the deviations in the height of the dental arches and teeth in relation to the face and cranium.
2. The orbital plane is a perpendicular at right angles to the eye-ear plane at the margin of the bony orbit directly under the pupil of the eye. This plane determines the sagital deviations of the dental arches and the axial inclination of the teeth to the face and the cranium.
3. The raphe or median sagital plane is determined by points approximately 1.5 cm apart on the median raphe of the palate. The raphe or median plane passes through these two points at right angles to the Frankfort horizontal plane. This plane determines the deviations in the general form and width of the dental arches and the axial inclination of the teeth in relation to the midline of the palate and the head.

In normal arch relationship, according to Simon, the orbital plane passes through the distal axial aspect of the canine. This is known as "The law of the canine".

The Simon classification is based on the following:

- Deviation from the raphe or median saggital plane. Arch form and inclination of tooth axis are determined from this plane
    - Contraction: a part or all of the dental arch is contracted toward the raphe median plane. The abnormality may be mandibular, alveolar, dental, anterior, posterior, unilateral or bilateral
    - Distraction: a part or all of the dental arch is wider than usual from the raphe median plane.
- Deviations from the Frankfort horizontal plane: the angle between the Frankfort horizontal and the occlusal plane, the form of the occlusal curve, and the inclination of the teeth axis are determined from this plane
    - Attraction: the distance between the occlusal plane and the Frankfort horizontal is comparatively shorter than normal. This distance is as a rule normally shorter in the young than in older persons and in some ethnic groups
    - Abstraction: the distance between the occlusal plane and the Frankfort horizontal is comparatively longer than normal.
- Deviations from the Orbital plane: sagital symmetry and inclination of the axis of the teeth are determined from this plane.
    - Protraction: the teeth, one or both dental arches, and or jaws are too far forward. Normally the orbital plane passes through the distal incline of the canine
    - Retraction: the teeth, one or both dental arches and or jaws are too far retruded. The orbital plane passes too far anteriorly to the canines.

  Deviations of the dental arches in relation to the orbital plane, according to Simon, may occur as follows:
    - Both the jaws in normal relation to each other
    - Upper jaw normal, lower jaw distal
    - Upper jaw normal, lower jaw mesial
    - Lower jaw normal, upper jaw mesial
    - Lower jaw normal, upper jaw distal
    - Upper jaw mesial, lower jaw distal
    - Upper jaw distal, lower jaw mesial.

In addition to the foregoing differential diagnostic information, the relation of the vault of the palate to the face and the cranium also may be determined by means of the three planes of face.

Question 2

Discuss Ackermann-Proffit's Classification of Malocclusion?

Answer

- In 1969 Ackermann and Proffit proposed a diagrammatic classification of malocclusion, in which characteristics and their inter relationships are assessed **(Fig. 7.7)**
- Common factor in all dentitions is the symmetry of teeth and dental alignment in the dental arches. This is represented as the universe (Group 1)
- Many malocclusion alter the profile of the patient. Thus Profile forms Group 2
- Antero Posterior(sagittal), Vertical and lateral (Tranverse) and their interrelationships (Groups 3 to 9) are represented by three interlocking subsets within the profile set.

This classification system can most easily be described by outlining the method of application. There are five steps in this classification:

- Step 1: In this step, the alignment and symmetry of the teeth in the dental arches are analyzed. Alignment is the key word of Group 1; among the possibilities are ideal, crowding (arch-length deficiency), spacing, and mutilated. Ideal occlusion and Angle Class I malocclusions, fall into Group 1
- Step 2 is done by looking at patient's profile. In the profile view, in this the anterior divergence (mandible prominent) or posterior divergence (mandible recessive) of face is seen and the lips are described as convex (prominent), straight, or concave relative to the nose and chin
- In Step 3 the dental arches are viewed in transverse plane, and the buccolingual relationships of the posterior teeth are noted. The term type is used to describe the various kinds of cross-bite. It is determined whether the malocclusion is skeletal, dento- alveolar or combination of both
- In Step 4 the patient and dental arches are viewed in the saggital plane (anteroposterior direction). In this, the Angle classification is used and along with skeletal, dentoalveolar, or a combination is mentioned

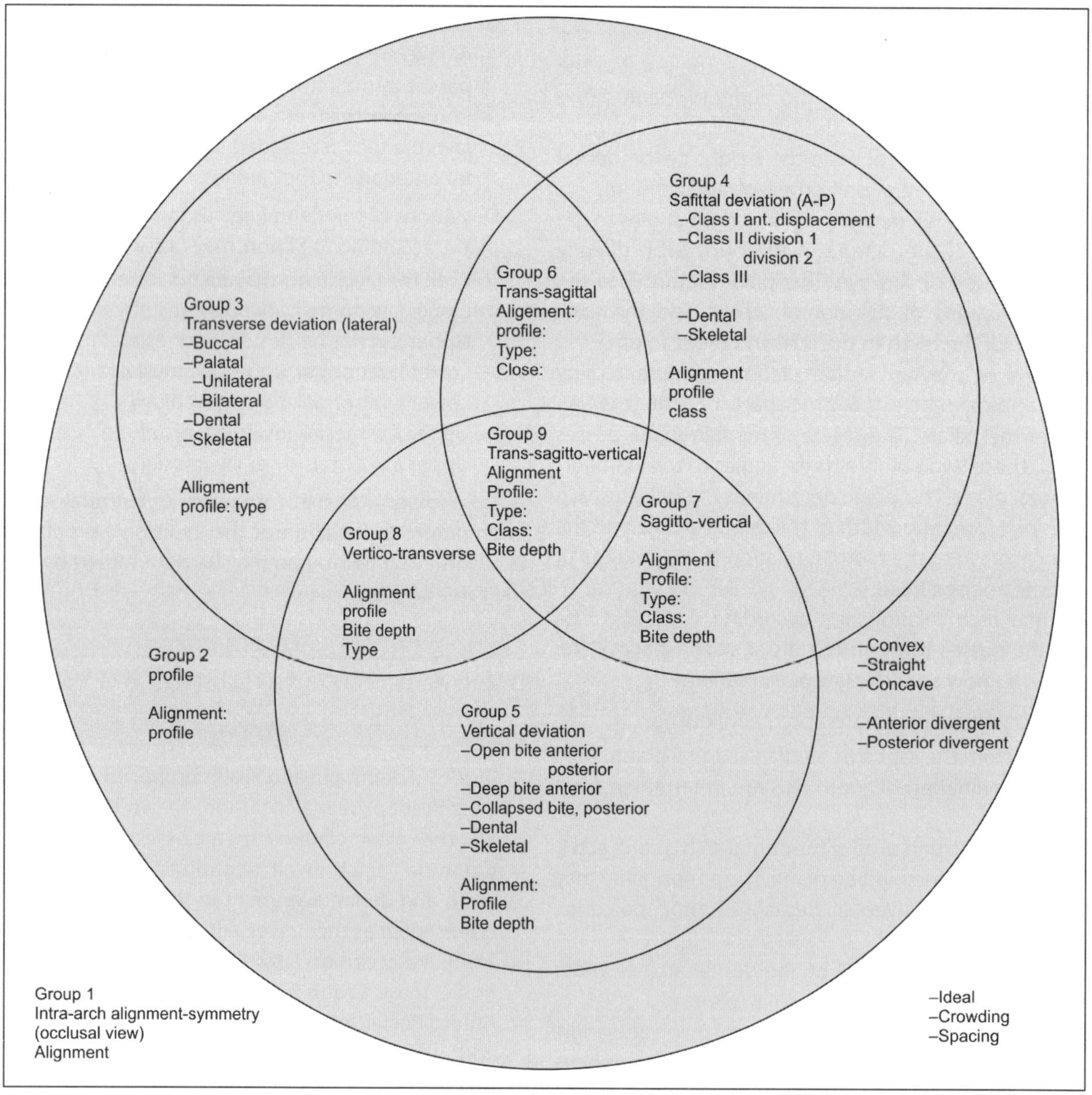

Fig. 7.7: Ackermann-Proffit classification

- In Step 5 the patient and the dentition are viewed with regard to the vertical dimension i.e., anterior open-bite, anterior deep-bite, posterior open-bite, or posterior collapsed bite. Skeletal or dento alveolar or both origin of problem is determined.

This approach defines nine groups of malocclusions. The higher the group no., higher will be the complexity of the problem. Thus, a Group 9 malocclusion is the most complicated, since in that there is an alignment problem, profile problem, and also problems in the lateral, vertical and anteroposterior dimensions.

SHORT NOTES

Question 1

Describe Lischer's Classification?

Answer

Lischer's Classification

Lischer gave the following terminologies:

- **Neutro-occlusion**: Normal relation of dental arches. It is synonymous with Angle's Class I malocclusion
- **Disto-occlusion**: Synonymous with Angle's Class II, used to describe all cases of post-normal occlusion
- **Mesio-occlusion**: Synonymous with Angle's Class III and describes all cases of prenormal occlusion

The suffix "version" was added to describe the wrong position of individual teeth as follows:

- Linguo version: lingually placed teeth/tooth **(Fig. 7.8)**
- Labio version: Labially placed tooth/teeth **(Fig. 7.9)**
- Mesio version: tooth/teeth mesial to normal position **(Fig. 7.10)**
- Disto version: tooth/teeth distal to normal position **(Fig. 7.11)**
- Infra version: infraerupted tooth/teeth **(Fig. 7.12)**
- Supra version: supraerupted tooth/teeth **(Fig. 7.13)**
- Torsiversion: rotated teeth **(Fig. 7.14)**
- Axioversion: out of the alignment **(Fig. 7.15)**
- Transversion or wrong sequential order **(Fig. 7.16)**.

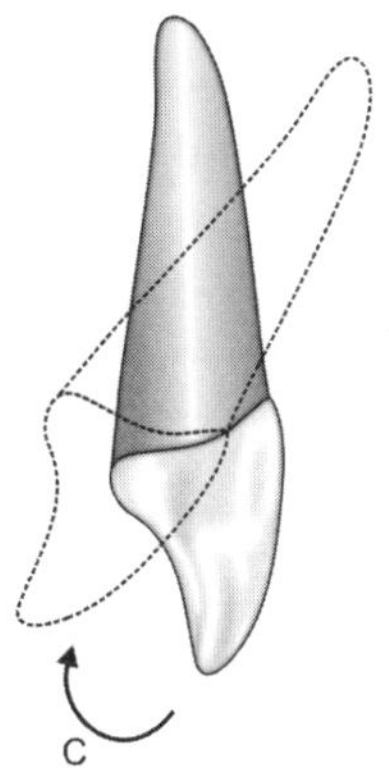

Fig. 7.8: Linguo-version

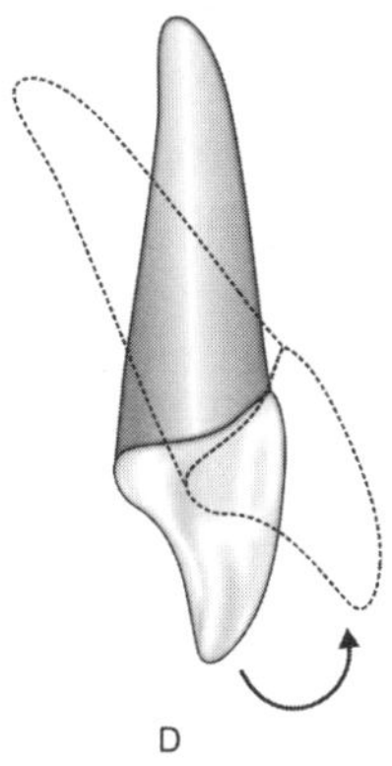

Fig. 7.9: Labio-version

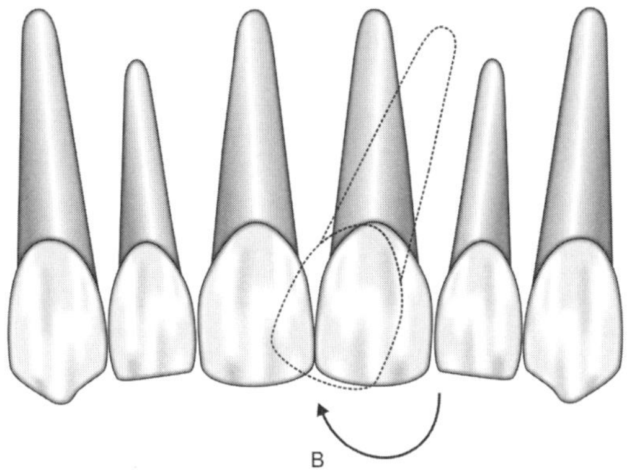

Fig. 7.10: Mesio-version

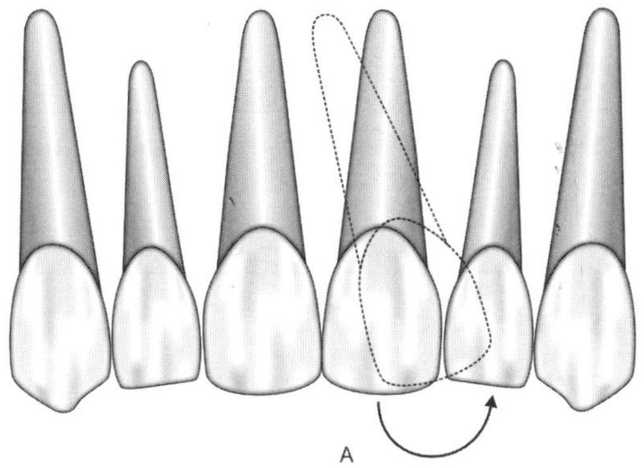

Fig. 7.11: Disto-version

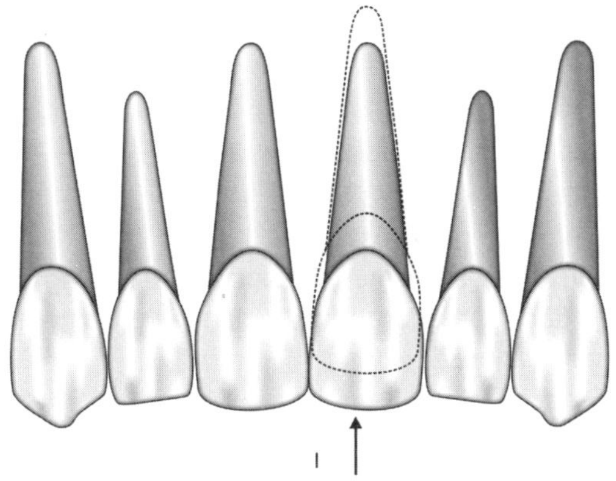

Fig. 7.12: Infra-version

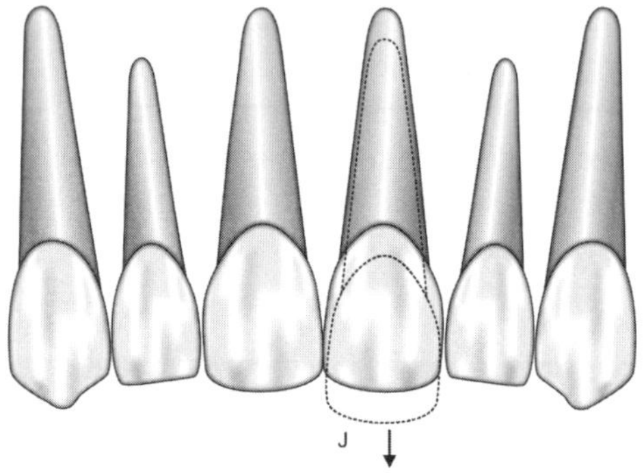

Fig. 7.13: Supra-version

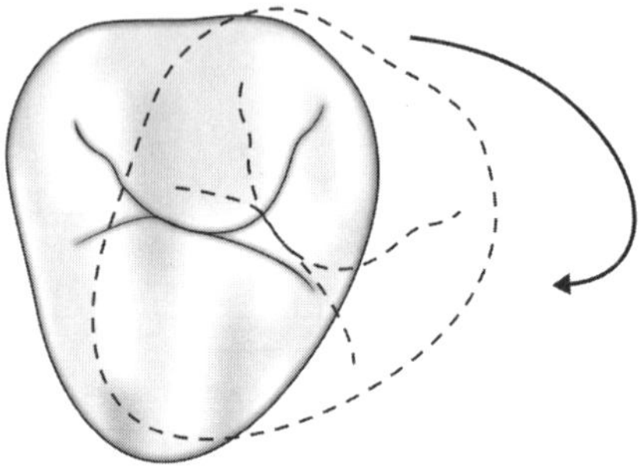

Fig. 7.14: Torsi-version

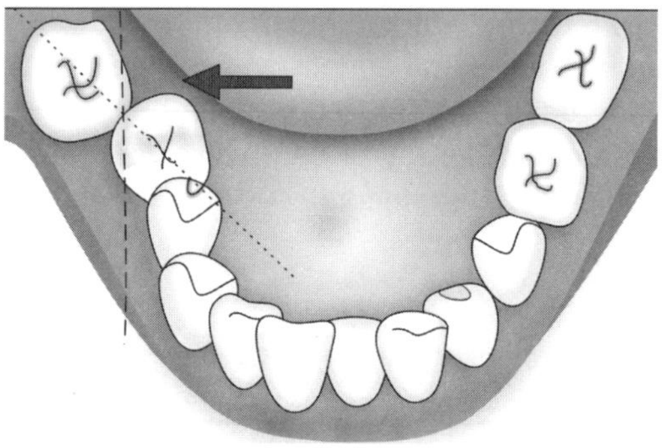

Fig. 7.15: Axio-version

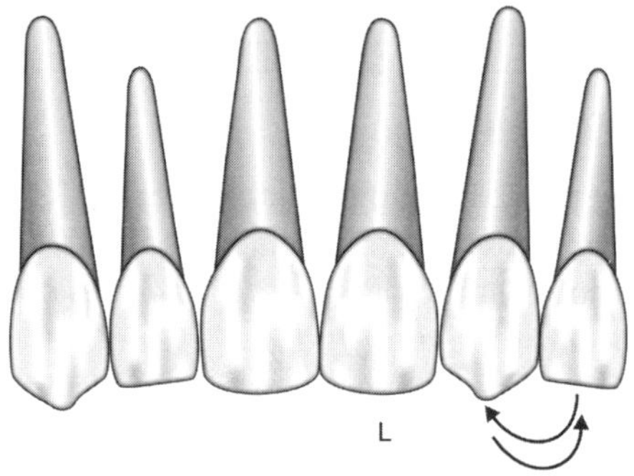

Fig. 7.16: Trans-version

Question 2

Discuss Dewey's Classification/ modification of Angle's Classification?

Answer

Dewey's Classification

Dewey classification is a modification of the Angle's classification of malocclusion. He divided the Angle's class I into five types and Angle's Class III into three types. There were no modifications for Class II. He considered the same molar relationship as in Angle's classification.

Modifications of Class I are

- **Type I**: Crowded anterior teeth
- **Type II**: Maxillary incisors in labio version
- **Type III**: Anterior Cross bite
- **Type IV**: Posterior Cross bite
- **Type V**: Molars are in mesioversion due to shifting following loss of tooth anterior to first molars, all other teeth are in normal relationship.

Modifications for Class III are

- **Type I**: Normal incisal overlapping present
- **Type II**: Edge to edge incisor relationship
- **Type III**: Incisors are in cross bite.

Question 3

Discuss Bennett's Classification/Classification of Malocclusion based on etiology?

Answer

Bennett introduced a classification of abnormalities of occlusion which was based on their etiology. Briefly the classification is as follows:

- **Class I**: One or more teeth are positioned abnormally due to local causes
- **Class II**: Abnormal formation of a part or whole of either arch due to developmental defects of bone
- **Class III**: Abnormal relationship between upper and lower arches, and between either arch and facial contour and correlated abnormal formation of either arch.

Question 4

Discuss Ballard's classification?

Answer

This classification is used to determine skeletal relationships of maxilla and mandible with each other. It is used more accurately at the chair side. According to this the different skeletal classes are:

- **Skeletal Class I**: The teeth are inclined normally and the dental base relationship is also normal. The upward projections of the axis of the lower incisors would pass through the crowns of the upper incisors
- **Skeletal Class II**: the mandible appears to be placed backwards relative to the maxilla. The lower incisor axis would pass palatally to the upper incisor crown
- **Skeletal Class III**: The mandibular apical base is placed relatively too far forward. The projections of the lower incisor axis would pass labial to upper incisor crowns.

Assumptions made in this classification:

- Inclinations of the incisor teeth within each arch are normal
- However, it frequently occurs that this is not so and a mental correction of the incisor inclinations has to be made
- This is done so that the axis of the lower central will make an angle of about 90° with the mandibular plane (tangent on the inferior border of the mandible), and that of the upper centrals at an angle of 110° to the Frankfort horizontal plane. (orbitale to porion).

Question 5

Discuss Incisor classification?

Answer

Incisor Classification

- **Class I**: The lower incisor edges occlude with or lie directly below the cingulum plateau of the upper central incisors. If the overbite is incomplete the lower incisors are repositioned along their long axis until they meet the upper incisors **(Fig. 7.17A)**.
- **Class II**: The lower incisor edges lie posterior to the cingulum plateau of the upper central incisors. There are two divisions of Class II:
  - Division 1: the upper central incisors are of average inclination or are proclined. The overjet is thus increased **(Fig. 7.17B)**
  - Division 2: the upper central incisors are retroclined; the overjet is usually within normal limits but the overbite is often increased **(Fig. 7.17C)**.

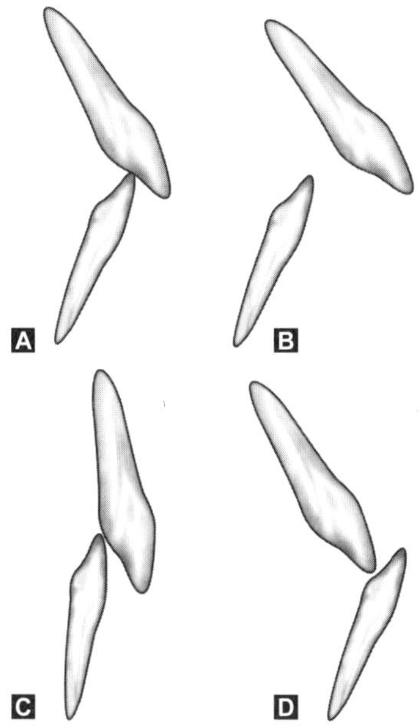

Fig. 7.17: Incisor classification

- **Class III**: The lower incisor edges lie anterior to the cingulum plateau of the upper central incisors **(Fig. 7.17D)**.

Question 6

Discuss Canine classification?

Answer

- **Class I canine relationship**: The upper permanent canine occludes in the embrasure between the lower permanent canine and first premolar.
- **Class II canine relationship**: The upper canine occludes a whole tooth width further anteriorly and lies in the embrasure between the lower canine and lateral incisor.
- **Class III canine relationship**: The upper canine occlude a whole tooth width further posteriorly than normal and occludes in the embrasure between the lower first and second premolars.

Chapter 8 Aetiology of Malocclusion

LONG ESSAYS

Question 1

What are the various classification of aetiology of malocclusion? Explain in detail the Graber's classification?

Answer

Graber's Classification

- General factors
- Local factors.

General Factors

- Hereditary
- Congenital
- Environmental.
  - Pre-natal (trauma, maternal diet, German measles, maternal metabolism, etc.)
  - Post-natal [birth injury, cerebral palsy, temporomandibular joint (TMJ) injury].
- Pre-disposing metabolic climate and disease
  - Endocrine imbalance
  - Metabolic disturbance
  - Infectious diseases
  - Dietary problems (nutritional deficiency).
- Abnormal pressure habits and functional aberrations
  - Abnormal sucking
  - Thumb and finger sucking
  - Tongue thrust and tongue sucking
  - Lip and nail biting
  - Abnormal swallowing habit (improper deglutition)
  - Speech defects
  - Respiratory abnormalities (mouth breathing, etc.)
  - Tonsils and adenoids
  - Psychogenetics and bruxism.
- Posture
- Trauma and accident
- Local Factors.
  - Anomalies of number: Supernumerary teeth, missing teeth (congenital absence or loss due to accidents, caries, etc.)
  - Anomalies of tooth size
  - Anomalies of tooth shape
  - Abnormal labial frenum: Mucosal barriers
  - Premature loss of deciduous teeth
  - Prolonged retention of deciduous teeth
  - Delayed eruption of permanent teeth
  - Abnormal eruptive path
  - Ankylosis.

Moyer's Classification

- Heredity
  - Neuromuscular system
  - Bone
  - Teeth
  - Soft parts.
- Developmental defects of unknown origin
- Trauma
  - Pre-natal trauma and birth injuries
  - Post-natal trauma.
- Physical agents
  - Premature extraction of primary teeth
  - Nature of food.
- Habits
  - Thumb sucking and finger sucking
  - Tongue thrusting
  - Lip sucking and lip biting
  - Posture
  - Nail biting
  - Other habits.
- Diseases.
  - Systemic diseases
  - Endocrine disorders

- Local diseases.
  - Nasopharyngeal diseases and disturbed respiratory function
  - Gingival and periodontal disease
  - Tumours
  - Caries
  - Malnutrition.

White and Gardiner's Classification

- Dental base abnormalities
  - Antero-posterior malrelationship
  - Vertical malrelationship
  - Lateral malrelationship
  - Disproportion of size between teeth and basal bone.
- Pre-eruption Abnormalities
  - Abnormalities in position of developing tooth germ
  - Missing teeth
  - Supernumerary teeth and teeth abnormal in form
  - Prolonged retention of deciduous teeth
  - Large labial frenum
  - Traumatic injury.
- Post-eruption Abnormalities.
  - Muscular
    - Active muscle force
    - Rest position of musculature
    - Sucking habits
    - Abnormalities in path of closure.
  - Premature loss of deciduous teeth
  - Extraction of permanent teeth.

GRABER'S CLASSIFICATION

Graber has classified the aetiological factors as local and general factors:

- The general factors affect the body as a whole and have a major effect on the greater part of the dento-facial structures
- On the other hand, local factors produce a localised effect confined to one or more adjacent or opposing teeth.

Heredity

- It is a major causes of malocclusion
- A child may inherit conflicting traits from both the parents leading to abnormalities in the dento-facial region
- Consanguineous marriages is another example of genetic cause for malocclusion, which may lead to uncoordinated inheritance of teeth and jaws
- According to Lundstrom, following human traits can be influenced by gene:
  - Tooth size: Microdontia and macrodontia a
  - Arch dimensions: Dental arch length and width.
  - Crowding/spacing: They are presumed to be a result of inheritance of arch length and tooth material
  - Abnormalities of tooth shape: Peg shaped lateral incisors shows high genetic predisposition
  - Abnormalities of tooth number: Anodontia and oligodontia
  - Overjet: It is believed to be genetically influenced
  - Interarch variations: Difference in the transverse, sagittal and vertical planes between the upper and lower jaws
  - Frenum: Size, position and shape of the frenum can be genetically influenced.

Congenital Defects

- These are also called as developmental defects, and are the malformations present at the time of the birth
- They can occur due to factors like genetic, radiologic, chemical, endocrine, infections and mechanical
- Congenital anomalies can be classified as general and local congenital abnormalities
- General congenital factors are as follows:
  - Malnutrition
  - Metabolic, nutritional and structure
  - Accidental traumatization of the foetus by internal forces
  - Endocrinopathies
  - Infectious diseases
  - Stressful pregnancy
  - Intrauterine pressure
  - Accidents during pregnancy and child birth.
- Local congenital factors are as follows:
  - Cleidocranial dysostosis
  - Macro and microglossia
  - Clefts of the face and palate
  - Abnormalities of jaw development due to intrauterine position.

Frequently encountered congenital conditions are as follows:

- Clefts of the lip and palate
- Congenital syphilis
  - It can be transmitted from infected mother to the child
  - Following features can be seen in the child with congenital syphilis:
    - Maxilla may be smaller in size relative to the mandible
    - Extensive dental decay
    - Mulberry molars
    - Enamel deficiencies
    - Hutchinsons incisors
    - Anterior crossbites.

- Maternal rubella infections: During pregnancy, maternal rubella infections can cause the following:
  - Extensive caries
  - Retarded eruption of teeth
  - Dental hypoplasia
- Cleidocranial dysostosis
  - It is a congenital condition
  - There is absence of clavicle i.e., either unilateral or bilateral, partial or complete
  - Following features can be seen in the patient:
    - Presence of short and thin roots
    - Presence of supernumerary teeth
    - Over retained deciduous teeth and retarded eruption of permanent teeth
    - Maxillary retrusion and mandibular protrusion.
- Cerebral Palsy
  - There is a lack of muscular coordination
  - It is caused due to birth injuries
  - Malocclusion occurs because of uncontrolled and aberrant muscle activity which upsets the muscle balances.
- Environment: There are several pre-natal and post-natal environmental factors that can cause malocclusion.
  - Pre-natal factors:
    - There may be asymmetric development of face in cases with abnormal foetal posture during gestation period
    - Most of these deformities are temporary and disappear with age
    - Maternal fibroids, amniotic lesions, maternal diet and metabolism also come under pre natal factors
    - Drug Thalidomide usage during pregnancy, and maternal infection like German measles can lead to congenital deformities.
  - Post-natal factors:
    - Forceps delivery can cause injury to the TMJ which can undergo ankylosis. There is may be deficient mandibular growth
    - Cerebral palsy can occur due to injuries sustained during birth
    - Malocclusions due to lack of muscular balance
    - Condylar fractures can result from traumatic injuries which causes retardation in growth, further resulting in facial asymmetry
    - Presence of scar tissues like burns or cleft lip surgery may produce malocclusion due to their restrictive influences on growth
    - Milwaukee braces are used for the treatment of scoliosis. These braces derive support from the mandible. Prolonged use of these braces can cause marked mandibular growth retardation.

Local Factors

- Anomalies of number of teeth:
  - Normal number of teeth should be present to achieve good occlusion
  - Malocclusion can be caused due to presence or absence of one or more teeth.
- Supernumerary teeth:
  - Supernumerary teeth are the teeth that are present extra besides the normal complement
  - These teeth do not resemble normal teeth and have abnormal morphology
  - If these teeth resemble normal teeth then they are termed as supplemental teeth
  - Mesiodens is a commonly seen supernumerary tooth which occurs in the maxillary midline
  - Unerupted mesiodens is one of the cause of midline diastema
  - Supernumerary teeth can also be seen in the premolar or third molar regions
  - Supplemental teeth are most commonly seen in the premolar and lateral incisor area
  - The supernumerary and supplemental teeth can cause non-eruption of adjacent teeth and can lead to ectopic eruption of normal teeth
  - These teeth also occupy arch length leading to crowding and rotation of adjacent teeth.
- Missing teeth: Congenitally missing teeth are more commonly seen as compared to supernumerary teeth and can be seen in either of the jaws. Following teeth are commonly missing in decreasing order:
  - Third molars
  - Maxillary lateral incisor
  - Mandibular second premolar
  - Mandibular incisor
  - Maxillary second premolars.
- Anomalies of tooth size
  - There should be harmony between the tooth and arch length and between maxillary and mandibular tooth size to have normal occlusion
  - In case of arch length toomaterial discrepancy, spacing (greater arch length) or crowding (greater tooth material) may occur
  - Presence of small sized maxillary lateral incisor is commonly seen
  - Fusion between two adjacent teeth or between supernumerary tooth, and a normal tooth predispose to malocclusion
  - Variations in size of tooth can occur along with variation of shape.

- Anomalies of tooth shape
  - Anomalies of tooth size and shape are inter-related
  - Malocclusion can occur due to abnormally shaped teeth
  - Frequently seen tooth shape anomalies are as follows:
    - Peg shaped maxillary lateral incisor is accompanied by spacing
    - Abnormally large cingulum on maxillary incisor
    - There may be an additional lingual cusp on mandibular second premolar.
  - In patient with congenital syphilis, peg shaped laterals and mulberry molars are classical features
  - in developmental defect like amelogenesis imperfecta, hypoplasia of teeth, fusion and gemmination, are examples of anomalies of shape
  - Dilaceration is a condition in which there is abnormal angulation between the crown and root of a tooth.
- Abnormal labial frenum
  - Maxillary midline diastema is often related to large or highly placed maxillary frenum
  - A blanch test is performed to diagnose this condition which is performed by stretching the upper lip for a period of time, after which a blanching occurs over the interdental papilla
- Premature loss of deciduous teeth
  - When there is a loss of tooth before its permanent successor is sufficiently advanced in development and eruption to occupy its place, it is referred to as premature loss of deciduous teeth
  - This leads to migration of adjacent teeth into the space and thus can prevent the eruption of the permanent successor in its normal place or may prevent their eruption
  - Early loss of anteriors most often do not produce any malocclusion.
- Prolonged retention of deciduous teeth
  - When there is over retention of deciduous teeth, beyond the usual eruption age of their permanent succession, it is inferred to as prolonged retention of deciduous teeth
  - This prevents the normal eruption of permanent successor
  - This condition usually results in lingual or palatal eruption of their permanent successor
  - The casues for the prolonged retention of deciduous teeth are as follows:
    - Absence of underlying permanent teeth
    - Endocrinal disturbance such as hypothyroidism
    - Ankylosed deciduous teeth that fail to resorb
    - Non-vital deciduous teeth that do not resorbs.
- Delayed eruption of permanent teeth: Various reasons for delay in the eruption of permanent teeth are as follows:
  - Presence of supernumerary teeth blocking the errupting permanent tooth
  - A heavy mucosal barrier
  - Endocrinal disorders such as hypothyroidism
  - Presence of deciduous root fragment that are not resorbed
  - Abnormal eruption path
  - Maxillary canines develop almost near the floor of the orbit and travel down to their final position in the oral cavity
  - Therefore, they are most often found erupting in an abnormal position
  - Ankylosis: When a part or whole root surface is directly fused to the bone with the absence of intervening periodontal ligament, it is referred to as ankylosis
  - Generally occurs due to trauma to the tooth which perforates the periodontal ligament
  - Ankylosis can also be seen with certain infections, endocrinal disorders and congenital disorders such as dysostosis
  - Dental caries: Dental caries can cause premature loss of deciduous or permanent teeth thereby causing migration of adjacent teeth
  - A substantial loss of arch length can be expected if several adjacent teeth are involved by proximal caries and they remain unrestored
  - Improper dental restorations: Premature contacts can be caused due to over controlled occlusal restorations, which can lead to functional shift of the mandible during foreclosure
  - Under contoured occlusal restorations can permit the opposing dentition to supra-erupt.

Pre-disposing Metabolic Climate and Disease

Malocclusion can be caused due to a number of endocrinal disorders, infections conditions and metabolic disturbances.

- Endocrine imbalance:
  - Hypothyroidism: It has one or more of the following features:
    - Retardation due to lost of calcium deposits in bones and teeth
    - Delay in tooth bud formation and eruption of teeth
    - Delayed carpel and epiphyseal calcification
    - Deciduous teeth are often over-retained and the permanent teeth are slow to erupt
    - Abnormal root resorption
    - Irregularity in tooth arrangement.

- Hyperthyroidism: It is accompanied with premature erruption of deciduous, tooth, disturbed root resorption of deciduous teeth and early eruption of permanent teeth.
- Hypoparathyroidism: It is associated with calcium metabolic changes
  - Delay in tooth eruption, altered tooth morphology, delayed eruption of deciduous and permanent teeth, and hypoplastic teeth
  - Increase in blood calcium levels
  - There is an interruption of tooth development in growing children
  - Mobility of teeth may be seen because of loss of cortical bone and resorption of the alveolar process.

- Metabolic Disturbances:
  - In acute febrile disease reduction of speed of growth and development is commonly observed
  - Disturbance in tooth eruption and shedding is seen which lead to malocclusion
  - Dietary deficiency during growth may result in abnormal development causing malocclusion
  - Example, rickett leads tomalocclusion and disturbs the dental development.
- Posture: Malocclusion can also be caused due to poor posture habit
- Accident and Trauma: Children are prone to injuries of the dento-facial region during early years of life which lead to development of malocclusion esppecially from the injuries which go unnoticed.

CHAPTER 9

Habits

LONG ESSAYS

Question 1

Define habits classify habits. Discuss in detail aetiology, phases of development, effect, diagnosis and management of thumb sucking?

Answer

A habit can be defined as the tendency towards an act that has become a repeated performance, relatively fixed, consistent and easy to perform by an individual.

Classification

I. Useful Habits and Harmful Habits

Useful Habits

These includes habits which are considered essential for normal function such as proper positioning of the tongue, respiration and normal deglutition.

Harmful Habits

These includes habits that have a deleterious effect on the teeth and their supporting structures such as thumb sucking, tongue thrusting, etc.

II. Empty and Meaningful Habits

Empty Habits

They are habits that are not associated with any deep rooted psychological problems.

Meaningful Habits

They are habits that have a psychological bearing

III. Pressure, Non-pressure and Biting Habits

Pressure Habits

These include sucking habits such as thumb sucking, finger sucking and also tongue thrusting.

Non-pressure Habits

Habits which do not apply a direct force on or its supporting structure are known as non-pressure habits. Example: Mouth breathing.

Biting Habits

Example: Nail biting, pencil biting, and lip biting.

IV. Compulsive and Non-compulsive Habits

Compulsive Habits

They are deep seated habits which have an acquired fixation in the child. The child tends to suffer increased anxiety when attempts are made to rectify the habit.

Non-compulsive Habits

They are habits that are easily adapted and dropped as the child gains maturity.

Thumb Sucking

It is defined as placement of the thumb or one or more fingers in varying depth into the mouth

Etiology

Many theories are given for thumb sucking. They are as following:

- Freudian theory: It was given by Sigmund Freud
  - According to him "as a child passes through various distinct phases of psychological development of which the oral and the anal phases are seen in the first 3 years of life"
  - Oral phase: In this phase the mouth is believed to be an oro-erotic zone. The child has the tendency to place his fingers or any other object into the oral cavity
  - Stoppage of this habit may cause serious emotional effects to the child and also lead to child develop other habits.

- Oral drive theory of Sears and Wise: It was given by Sears and Wise in 1950: They said that suckling can lead to thumb sucking
- Benjamin's theory: It was put forward by Benjamin. According to this theory thumb sucking occurs from rooting or placing reflex seen in all mammalian infants
- Psychological aspect: Children deprived of parental love, are believed to develop habits due to a insecurity feeling
- Learned pattern: According to this theory, thumb sucking can be a learned pattern with no underlying cause.

Phase of Development

Phase I: (Normal and Sub-clinically Significant)

- Seen during the 0-3 years of life
- Thumb sucking during the phase is normal which usually terminates at the end of this phase.

Phase II: (Clinically Significant Sucking)

- Seen between 3 – 6 / 1/2 years of age
- The presence of sucking during this period indicates that the child is anxious
- Interception of habit should be initiated during this stage to solve the dental problems.

Phase III: (Intractable Sucking)

Underlying psychological aspect of the habit may be present if this habit persists even after fourth or fifth years of life.

Effect of Thumb Sucking

- Thumb sucking leads to lot of changes in the dental arch and the supporting structure
- The severity of the malocclusion due to this habit depends on the following factors like:
  - Duration: The amount of time spent in this habits
  - Frequency: how frequent is the habit is performed in a day
  - Intensity: The intensity with which the habit is performed.

Effects of thumb sucking are as follows:

- Labial tipping of the maxillary anterior teeth leadin to increase in proclination
- Anterior open bite can occur due to restriction of incisor eruption and supraeruption of the buccal teeth
- Development of tongue thrust habit as a result of the open bite is commonly seen
- Proclination of the maxillary anteriors leads to increase in overjet
- Hypotonic upper lip with hyperactive mentalis is seen
- Narrowing of maxillary arch due to conntraction of cheek muscles which inturn causes development of posterior crossbite.

Diagnosis

- Frequency and duration should be determined
- Child's emotional status should be determined by evaluating the following:
  - Feeding habits
  - Parental care of the child
  - Whether the parents are working
  - Intraoral clinical examination should be done which includes all the features like proclination, open bite etc
  - Fingers of the child should be examined
  - Presence of callus on fingers shows that child has a thumb sucking habit.

Management

Management can be done by 3 approaches i.e.,:

1. Psychological approach
2. Mechanical approach
3. Chemical approach.

Psychological Approach

Children who are deprived of parental love are resorted to this habit.

- Therefore a proper counselling of the parents should be done in order to provide the child with adequate love and aflection
- Child's attention: Should also be diverted to other activities like toys and playing
- The child should be motivated by the parents and the dentist
- Theory known or beta hypothesis by Dunlop says that if the habit is to be discontinued, then the habit should be consciously and purposefully repeated
- Child should be asked to sit front of a mirror and asked to suck his thumb observing himself as he indulges into the habit
- If the child is asked to do the same thing at a time when he is involved in some other activity, then this procedures proves to be very effective.

Mechanical Approach

- These are the appliances which help the child who is willing to quit the habit but is not able to do so because habit has entered a subconscious level.

- These appliances usually consists of crib placed palatal to the maxillary incisors
- These appliances can be of two types i.e.,
  - Removable habit breakers
  - Fixed habit breaker.
    - Removable habit breakers: These are passive removable appliances that consist of a crib and is anchored to the oral cavity by means of clasps on the posterior teeth
    - Fixed habit breakers: In these appliances, there is a heavy gangue stainless steel wire that can be designed to form a frame that can be soldered to bands on the molars.

Other aids include bandaging the thumb and bandaging the elbow.

Chemical Approach

In this approach bitter tasting or foul smelling products can be placed on the thumb.

The preperations which can be used are:

- Pepper dissolved in a volatile medium
- Quinine
- Asafetida.

Question 2

Define tongue Thrust. Give its classification, etiology, clinical features and its management?

Answer

Tongue thrust can be defined as a condition in which the tongue makes contact with any teeth anterior to the molars during swallowing.

Classification

Classification is given by James S. Braner and Holt

- Type I: Non-deforming tongue thrust
- Type II: Deforming anterior tongue thrust
  - Sub group 1: Anterior open bite
  - Sub group 2: Anterior proclination
  - Sub group 3: Posterior cross bite.
- Type III: Deforming lateral tongue thrust
  - Sub group 1: Posterior open bite
  - Sub group 2: Posterior cross bite
  - Sub group 3: Deep over bite.
- Type IV: Deforming anterior and lateral tongue thrust.
  - Sub group 1: Anterior and posterior open bite
  - Sub group 2: Proclination of anterior teeth
  - Sub group 3: Posterior crossbite.

Simple Classification of Tongue Thrust

- Simple tongue thrust
- Complex tongue thrust.

Simple Tongue Thrust

Following features can be observed:

- Presence of an anterior open bite
- Good intercusption of teeth
- Tongue is thrust forward during swallowing to establish an anterior lip seal
- Abnormal mentalis muscle activity is seen.

Complex Tongue Thrust

Following features can be observed

- Teeth apart swallow is characterstic of this type of tongue thrust
- The occlusion of teeth is poor
- During swallowing, contraction of circumoral muscles is seen
- Temporal muscle constriction is absent during swallowing
- The anterior open bite can be diffuse or absent.

Clinical Features

Clinical features are as follows:

- Proclined anterior teeth
- Bimaxillary protrusion
- Anterior open bite
- Posterior open bite in cases of lateral tongue thrust
- Posterior crossbite.

Management

It includes interception and treatment of malocclusion.

Habit Interception

- Tongue thrust can be intercepted by use of habit breakers as used for thumb sucking
- Both fixed and removable cribs or rakes are valuable aids in breaking the habit
- Child is taught the correct method of swallowing
- By practicing various muscle exercises of the tongue, can help in training to adapt to the new swallowing pattern.

Treatment of Malocclusion

Can be treated by either removable or fixed orthodontic appliances.

Question 3

What is mouth breathing habit. Give its classification, pathophysiology, clinical features, diagnosis and management?

Answer

Habit of breathing by mouth instead of nose is termed as mouth breathing habit.

- It is one of the causes for malocclusion
- Under physical exertion like exercise or sports activity, most of the people indulge is moth breathing.

Classification

It can be classified into 3 types:

1. Obstructive
2. Habitual
3. Anatomic.

Obstructive

Complete or partial obstruction of the nasal passage can cause in mouth breathing.

Following are the cause of nasal obstruction.

- Nasal polyp
- Chronic inflammation of nasal mucosa
- Deviated nasal septum
- Localized benign tumor
- Obstructive adenoids
- Congenital enlargement of nasal turbinates
- Allergic reaction of the nasal mucosa.

Habitual

A habitual mouth breather is the one who continues to breathe through his mouth even when the nasal obstruction has been removed.

Anatomic

The morphology of the lips does not allow complete closure of the mouth, for example, patient with short upper lip.

Pathophysiology

At the time of oral respiration, following three changes can be seen in posture.

1. Lowering of the mandible
2. Positioning the tongue downwards and forwards
3. Tipping back of the head:
   - Lowering of the tongue and mandible upsets the oro-facial equilibrium
   - There is an unrestricted buccinator muscle activity which effects the position of the teeth and jaw growth.

Clinical Features

Clinical feature are as following:

- Narrow nose and nasal passage
- Long and narrow face
- Short and flaccid upper lip
- An expressionless or blank face
- Contracted upper arch
- Anterior marginal gingivitis
- Increased overjet
- Anterior open bite may occur
- Dryness of mouth
- Caries.

Diagnosis

- Recording of complete and thorugh history of child and parents
- Thourough clinical examination
- Few tests such as mirror test or water test to diagnose mouth breathing
- Cephalometrics: Establishing the nasopharyngeal space, size of adenoids and in diagnosing the long face associated with mouth breathing.
  - Rhinomanometry: It is the study of nasal air flow characteristics using flow meters, and pressure gauge
  - These help in estimation of air flow through the nasal passage and nasal resistance.

Management of Mouth Breathing

- Removal of pharyngeal of nasal obstruction
- Interception of habit: Mouth breathing can be intercepted by use of a vestibular screen
  - Alternatively adhesive tapes can be used to establish lip seal.
- Rapid maxillary expansion: Patients who have narrow, constricted maxillary arches benefit from rapid palatal expansion procedures aimed at widening the arch.
  - Rapid maxillary expansion has been found to increase the nasal air flow and decrease the nasal air resistance.

Question 4

Define bruxism. What is its etiology, clinical features, diagnosis and treatment?

Answer

Bruxism can be defined as the grinding of teeth for non-functional purposes

Etiology

- Psychological and emotional stress
- Pericoronitis and periodontal pain can trigger bruxism in some individuals
- Occlusal interference or discrepancy can predispose to grinding.

Clinical Features

- Occlusal wear facts on the teeth
- Teeth and restorations fractures
- Tenderness and hypertrophy of masticatory muscles
- Teeth mobility
- Muscle pain when the patients make up the morning
- TMJ pain and discomfort might occur.

Diagnosis

- A proper history and clinical examination
- Articulating paper to diagnose occlusal prematurities
- Electro-myographic examination to check for hyperactivity of the muscles of mastication.

Treatment

- Proper psychological counselling should be done
- Hypnosis, relaxing exercises and massage can help in relieving muscle tension. For eliminating prematurities, occlusal adjustments should be done
- Night guards or other occlusal splint which cover the occlusal surfaces of teeth help in eliminating occlusal interferences, break the neuromuscular adaptation and prevent occlusal wear.

CHAPTER 10

Epidemiology of Malocclusion

SHORT ESSAYS

Question 1

What is handicapping labio-lingual deviation index (HLD index)?

Answer

Handicapping labio-lingual deviation index (HLD index) was developed by Harry L Draker in 1960.

- It was proposed to select subjects with severe or handicapping malocclusions and dentofacial anomalies
- Handicapping lingual deviation index scoring:

	Conditions Observed	HLD Score
1.	Cleft palate	Score 15
2.	Severe traumatic deviations	Score 15
3.	Overjet in mm	
4.	Overbite in mm	
5.	Mandibular protrusion in mm	× 5
6.	Open bite in mm	× 4
7	Ectopic eruption, anterior only each tooth	× 3
8.	Anterior crowding	
	Maxilla	
	Mandible	
	Total	

- A score of 13 and over 13 represents physical handicap
- Scoring:
  - O: condition absent
  - X: Condition present
  - M: Mixed dentition (if present)
  - A: Clinical approval
  - D: Clinical disapproval.

Question 2

What is orthodontic treatment priority index (TPI)?

Answer

Orthodontic treatment priority index (TPI) was developed by RM Grainger in 1967. Eleven weighted and defined measurements were taken:

- Upper anterior segment overjet
- Lower anterior segment overjet
- Overbite of upper anterior lower anterior
- Anterior open bite
- Congenital absence of incisors
- Distal molar relation
- Mesial molar relation
- Posterior crossbite (maxillary teeth buccal to normal)
- Posterior crossbite (maxillary teeth lingual to normal)
- Teeth displacement
- Gross anomalies.

TPI is based on a scale of "0–3", "4–6" and "6 and over 6".

The TPI tends to give more consistent percentage of prevalence relative to age. TPI scores can be exposure in range of:

- 0–2.5 = Less
- 2.5–4.5 = Middle
- And above 4.5 = High.

Seven malocclusion syndromes were defined:

- Maxillary expansion syndrome
- Overbite
- Retrognathism
- Open bite
- Prognathism
- Maxillary collapse syndrome
- Congenitally missing incisors.

CHAPTER 11 Orthodontic Diagnosis

LONG ESSAYS

Question 1

What is diagnosis? Explain in detail about orthodontic diagnosis?

Answer

Diagnosis: The determination of the nature of a disease or condition, by study and consideration of the patient's history, as well as the signs and symptoms and their manifestation.

Comprehensive orthodontic diagnosis is established by use of certain clinical implements called diagnostic aids.

Orthodontic diagnostic aids are of two types:

1. Essential diagnostic aids
2. Supplemental diagnostic aids.

Case History

- Case history involves eliciting and recording of relevant information from the patient and parent to aid in the overall diagnosis of the case
- **Name**: The patient's name should be recorded for the purpose of communication and identification. Addressing a patient by his or her name has a beneficial psychological effect as well
- **Age**: The patient's chronological age should be recorded. Age consideration help in diagnosis as well as treatment planning. There are certain transient conditions (ugly duckling stage) that occur during development are considered normal for that age. Thus, knowing the age helps in identifying and anticipating these conditions. In addition, there are certain treatment modalities that are best carried out during the growing age
- **Sex**: This is important in planning treatment as the timing of growth events such as growth spurts is different in males, and females. Females usually precede males in onset of growth spurts
- Puberty and termination of growth occurs in:
    - Girls: 10.5–15 year of age
    - Boys: 12–17 year of age.

Address and Occupation

- Communication
- Assessing socio-economic condition
- Patient coming from far places.

Chief Complaint

- Patient's own words
- To identify priorities and desires of the patient
- Treatment objectives.

Pre-natal History

- Nutritional disorders
- Disease and accidents to the mother during pregnancy
- The questions which relate to the birth including time of birth, fetal position at birth, teratogenic drugs like aminopterin, aspirin, thalidomide, dilantin intake during pregnancy and the type of delivery should be noted.

Post-natal History

- Manner of feeding
- Nutritional disturbances
- Regarding eruption of first deciduous tooth
- General development (initiation of talking, walking)
- Information regarding sucking and other 'bad habits'.

Medical and Dental History

- A careful medical and dental history is needed for orthodontic patients both to provide proper background for understanding the patients overall situation, and to evaluate specific orthodontically related concerns

- To note whether the patient is on long-term medication of any type, which helps in revealing systemic disease/ metabolic problems that the patient did not report
- Although chronic medical problems in adults or children do not contraindicate orthodontic treatment if the medical problem is under control, but special precautions may be necessary if orthodontic treatment is to be carried out.
  - Childhood and other generalised disease.
    - Diseases which affect the development of the jaws (for instances rickets, dysostosis)
    - All diseases which are important in influencing the type of breathing (cold, pneumonia, otitis, allergies)
    - Further evidence of disturbed respiration includes the type of breathing during sleep (open mouth) as well as previous adenoidectomy and/ tonsillectomy
    - Fracture: Condylar fracture leads to facial asymmetry. Trauma to the teeth affect the development of occlusion.

Habits

- Finger/thumb sucking—frequency
- Nail/lip biting—intensity
- Tongue biting/thrusting—duration
- Bruxism
- Mouth breathing.

Physical Growth Evaluation

- This is important to note since rapid growth during the adolescent growth spurt facilitates tooth movement, but significant growth modification may not be possible in a child who is beyond the peak of the growth spurt
- Key point for investigation during the initial orthodontic interview.

Body Type

- Ectomorphic: Tall and thin
- Mesomorphic: Average build
- Endomorphic: Short and fat.

Build

- Aesthetic: They are thin built and usually possess narrow dental arches
- Pletoric: They are obese built and generally have broad dental arches
- Atheletic: Neither thin nor obese and have normal dental arches.

Gait

- It is the act of walking or locomotion
- It is the way person walks
- Abnormalities of gait are usually associated with neuromuscular disorder which may have a dental correlation.

Posture

- This refers to the way a person stands
- Abnormal posture can predispose to malocclusion due to alteration in maxillo-mandibular relationship.

Height and Weight

They give a clue to the physical maturation and growth of the patient, which may have dentofacial correlation relationship.

Clinical Evaluation

- There are two goals of orthodontic clinical examination
- To evaluate and document oral health, jaw function and facial aesthetics
- To decide which diagnostic records are required.

Extra-oral Examination

Cephalic and Facial Examination

- The shape of the head and facial structures are assessed,
- Measurements can be evaluated according to the cephalic index of the head and the morphologic facial index
- Cephalix index (CI): $CI = \frac{\text{Maximum skull width}}{\text{Maximum skull length}}$
  - Maximum cranial breadth is measured wherever it is found between the two most prominent points on either side of the cranium
  - Maximum cranial length is the distance between the glabella and the most prominent point of the occipital bone in the midline.
- Dolicocephalic: Long and narrow head— Narrow (<75.9) dental arch
- Mesocephalic: Average shape of the head— Normal (76.0–80.9) dental arch
- Brachycephalic: Broad and short head— Broad (81.0–85.4) dental arch.

Morphologic Facial Index

- The form of the facial morphology has a certain relationship to the shape of the dental arch
- Morphologic facial index (MFI):

$$MFI = \frac{\text{Morphologic facial height}}{\text{Bizygomatic width}}$$

- Dolicofacial: Long and narrow (88.0–92.9) face.
- Mesofacial: Average (84.0–87.9) face/normal face.
- Brachyfacial: Broad and short (79.0–83.9) face.
- Facial proportion:
  - The proportional relationship of height and width, more than the absolute value of either height or width, establishes the overall facial proportion
  - Prior to the advent of cephalometric radiography dentist and orthodontists often used anthropometric measurements, to help establish facial proportion.
- Facial profile **(Fig. 11.1)**:
  - A careful examination of the profile yields some information
  - The technique of facial profile has sometimes been called the "poor man's cephalometric analysis"

Method to Visualise Facial Profile

Drop two lines :

- One from the bridge of the nose to the base of the upper lip
- Second from that point downwards to the chin.

Depending upon the Angle Formed :

- Divergence of face is defined as an anterior or posterior inclination of the lower face relative to the forehead. It is influenced by the patients' racial and ethnic background
- American, Indians and Orientals have greater anterior divergent face
- Whites of Northern European have posterior divergent face
- A straight profile line, regardless of whether the face is divergent, does not indicate a problem **(Figs. 11.2A to C)**.

Frankfurt Horizontal and Mandibular Plane Angle (FMA)

- The inclination of the mandibular plane to the true horizontal should be noted. The mandibular plane is visualised readily by placing a finger or mirror handle along the lower border
- This is important because a steep mandibular plane angle usually indicates long anterior facial vertical dimensions and a skeletal open-bite tendency, while a flat mandibular plane angle often correlates with short anterior facial height and deep-bite malocclusion.

Nose

- Size, shape and position of the nose determine the aesthetic appearance of the face
- The assessment of the nose in the prognosis of an orthodontic case is therefore of special importance
- Besides the contour of the bridge and the tip of the nose, the size and the shape and width of the nostrils as well as position of the nasal septum should be assessed. These finding can indicate impairment of nasal breathing.

Lips

Configuration of the lips can be assessed by the following criteria:

- Lip length
- Width
- Curvature
- In a balanced situation, the length of the upper lip measures one-third whereas the lower lip and the chin measure two-thirds of the lower face height
- In addition, the length of the upper lip should be assessed in relation to the position of the upper incisal edges
- The observation of the nasolabial angle and in particular the mentolabial fold is indicative of the degree of lip tension
- Apart from ethnic characteristics, lip protrusion is influenced by the thickness of the soft tissues, the tone of orbicularis muscle, position of anterior teeth and the configuration of underlying bony structures
- Morphologically inadequate lips:
  - On rare occasions, the upper lip is morphologically short
  - The significance of the morphologically short upper lip to malocclusion, speech disorders and retention of orthodontically treated cases often is over stated

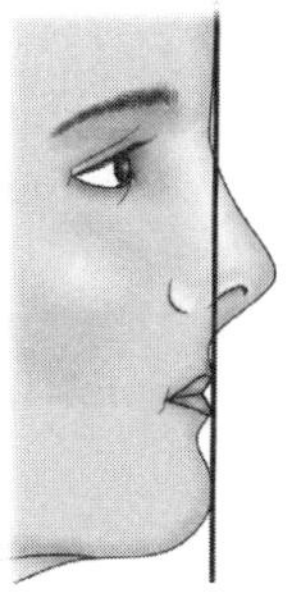

Fig. 11.1: Facial profile

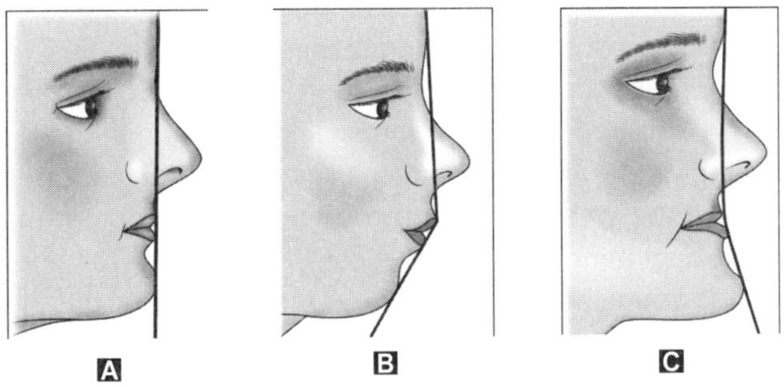

Figs. 11.2A to C: (A) Straight; (B) Convex; and (C) Concave profile

- Lips originally diagnosed as morphologically inadequate may be found satisfactory later because the tooth movements allow normal lip function to return.

- Competent lips:
  - The lips are in contact when the musculature is relaxed.
- Incompetent lips:
  - Anatomically short lips with a wide gap between the upper and lower lip in relaxed position.
- Potentially incompetent lips:
  - The protuding upper incisors prevent the lip closure, otherwise the lips are developed normally.
- Everted lips:
  - These are hypertrophied lips with redundant tissue but weak muscular tonicity.
- Mento labial sulcus:
  - Deep mento labial sulci and hyperactivity of mentalis muscle
  - This habitual pattern of muscle behaviour impedes the forwards development of the anterior alveolar process in the mandible.

Intra-oral Examination

Intra-oral examination should begin by examining the following details:

- Oral hygiene status
- Frenum: In an infant, upper labial frenum extends from the upper lip to the incisive papilla. As the incisors erupt, the frenum usually migrates and gets attached to the labial surface of the alveolar process
  - Occasionally, the frenum will persist and this may be associated with midline diastema. In these cases, the palatine papilla will blanch, the lip is pulled forwards—Blanch test
  - Lower lingual frenum is examined by asking the patient to protrude the tongue. If the patient is not able to protrude the tongue— abnormal lingual frenum also called as tongue tie or ankyloglossia.
- Tongue: Look for the presence or absence of indentations or tooth impression on the sides of the tongue. If present— due to large tongue or macroglossia
  - Changes in the tongue position and mobility are often associated with an abnormal lingual frenum.
- Gingiva: The amount of attached gingiva is the keratinised tissue between the depth of periodontal probing and the beginning of alveolar mucosa
  - In young healthy patients 2–3 mm of attached gingiva is apparent
  - In adults, where recession is apparent, gingival grafting should be taken into consideration
  - Periodontal status may also be checked by tooth movement with the help of mouth mirror and the fingers
  - There should be no pockets above 5 mm for the patients planning to undergo orthodontic treatment.
- Palate: Look for the depth and width of the palate and any other developmental abnormalities like torus palatinus
- Teeth:
  - Teeth present
  - Teeth missing
  - Condition of teeth present: Vitality, carious, fractured, discoloured, hypoplastic, wear facets, malformed teeth, etc.
- Angle's classification: The patient should be made to occlude the teeth in centric occlusion and the relationship of molars, canine and the incisors should be examined to classify it according to Angle's classification
- Arch forms:
  - Tapered
  - Ovoid
  - Square.
- Arch symmetry
- Overjet:
  - Horizontal overlapping of upper and lower teeth is called as overjet
  - It is measured from the labial surface of lower anteriors to incisal edges of upper anteriors. (Most proclined tooth)
  - Normal overjet is 2–3 mm
  - Variations of overjet—decreased, increased, reverse overjet or cross-bite and edge to edge bite.
- Overbite:
  - The vertical overlapping of anterior teeth is called as overbite. Normally, it is 2–3 mm
  - To measure overbite—a mark of the incisal edges of upper anterior teeth are made on the labial aspect of the lower anterior teeth. The distance between the incisal edge of lower incisor to the mark gives overbite in mms
  - Overbite percentage—overbite/clinical length of the tooth x 100. Normal value – 33 1/3%.
- Variations of overbite:
  - Deep-bite—where the overbite is more than 2–3 mm
  - Complete deep-bite where the lower anteriors contact either the upper anteriors or the palatal mucosa
  - Closed bite—where the upper anteriors overlap the lower anteriors completely—class II division 2 malocclusion
  - Open bite—lack of vertical overlapping of teeth.
- Transverse tooth malpositions: Cross-bite or scissors bite
- Individual tooth irregularities: Rotations etc

- Curve of spee:
  - Measured by placing a flat surface touching the incisors and posteriorly up to the second molar
  - Flat curve of spee— all teeth touch the flat surface
  - Deep curve of spee— the occlusal surfaces of posterior teeth form a curve which is more than a mm in depth.
- Midline:
  - Normally the upper and lower midlines coincide
  - Nose tip to mid-sagittal plane
  - Mid-sagittal plane to mid-line of upper arch
  - Upper arch mid-line to lower arch midline
  - Lower arch mid-line to mid-symphyseal plane
  - Mid symphyseal plane to mid-sagittal plane.
- Functional examination:
  - Determination of postural rest position of the mandible and freeway space
  - Examination of temporomandibular joint (TMJ)
  - Assessment of functional status of the lips, cheeks and tongue.
- Determination of postural rest position:
  - The rest position of the mandible depends on head and body posture as they are influenced by gravity
  - The patient is seated upright preferably with back unsupported
  - Several methods are available to determine the postural rest position of the mandible.
    - Phonetic method
    - Command method
    - Non-command method
    - Combined method.

Phonetic Exercises

Patient assumes relaxed upright body posture and is looking straight ahead. The letter m is generally used to start and is repeated 5–10 times.

Repeating or spelling the word "Mississipi" also is a good exercise. After the phonetic exercise, the mandible usually returns to postural rest.

Command Method

The patient is asked to perform selected functions, the mandible returns to the postural rest position after each function.

Patient licks the lips and then swallow which produces the desired relationship, because the mandible returns to postural rest within 2 seconds after the exercise.

Non-command Method

The patient has no idea of the parameter being examined.

Careful observations are made as the patient talks, swallows and turns the head while being questioned on a number of unrelated subjects.

Combined Method

The combined method usually provides the best reproduction of the postural rest position in the mixed dentition. The patient performs a prescribed function (e.g. swallowing) and then relaxes. After instructing the patient not to move, the clinician gently palpates the submental muscles to assess whether they are relaxed.

Normally the lower canine should be 3 mm below the upper in comparison with the occlusal position. An inter-occlusal space of 4 mm may be normal. Registration of postural rest position should be done.

Direct Extra-oral Method

Direct caliper measurements can be made on the patients profile by measuring the distance from soft tissue nasion to menton. This measurement is done in both postural rest and habitual occlusion. The difference between the two measurements constitutes the inter-occlusal clearance.

Direct Intra-oral Method

In addition to visual observation, the clinician can perform a direct intra oral procedure by using a plaster core registration similar to that sometimes used in prosthodontics.

Indirect Extra-oral Method

- Does not come under clinical examination— various adjuncts such as cephalometry, kinesiography, electromyography are all used
- Evaluation of the relationship between rest position and habitual occlusion:
  - The movement of the mandible from rest position to full articulation is analysed three dimensionally in the following planes.
    - Sagittal
    - Vertical
    - Frontal.
  - When closing from rest position, the mandible may undergo both rotational and sliding movements
  - The following movements of the mandible from rest position to habitual occlusion must be differentiated for orthodontic diagnosis
  - Pure rotational movement
  - Rotational movement with anterior sliding component
  - Rotational movement with posterior sliding component.

- Evaluation in the sagittal plane:
  - Class II malocclusion without sliding action
  - Without functional disturbance
  - True class II malocclusion
  - Class II malocclusion with posterior sliding action
  - Excessive overbite
  - Class II malocclusion appears more severe than it actually, is sagittaly
  - Class II malocclusion with anterior sliding action
  - Less frequent
  - Malocclusion is more severe than it appears
  - Class III malocclusion
  - Straight path of closure
  - Successful treatment possible if magnitude is not too much
  - Class III malocclusion with posterior sliding action
  - Prognosis is poorer
  - Class III malocclusion with anterior sliding action
  - Prognosis is much better.
- Evaluation in vertical plane:
  - Pseudo deep-bite
  - Small inter-occlusal space
  - Normal eruption of posterior teeth
  - Associated with horizontal growth pattern the possibilities for correction with functional appliance are limited
  - True deep-bite
  - Large inter-occlusal space
  - Infra-occlusion of the posterior segment
  - Prognosis is good, if the vertical growth pattern is present
  - Functional class II problems with posterior displacement and functional deep overbite problems with large inter-occlusal spaces, functional appliances have good prognosis for successful therapy.
- Evaluation in transverse plane.

Laterognathy

- Cross-bite in which midline shift is present in both occlusal and postural rest position
- True asymmetrical facial skeleton
- Successful functional therapy is not possible.

Latero-occlusion

- Midline shift of the mandible is observed only in occlusal position
- In postural rest position, the midlines are coincident and well centered
- The mandible slides laterally from rest position into a cross-bite, in occlusion
- Caused by tooth guidance
- Treatment by elimination of disturbances in the intercuspation
- Examination of TMJ:
  - The objective of this aspect of functional examination is to assess whether incipient symptoms of TMJ dysfunction are present.
- Early symptoms of TMJ problems include:
  - Clicking and crepitus
  - Sensitivity in the condylar region and masticatory muscles
  - Functional disturbances
  - Radiographic evidence of morphologic and positional abnormalities.
- Crepitus:
  - Observed during opening movement
  - Terminal clicking or crepitation occurs because of hypermobility or too much opening
  - It is usually a sign of peripheral irregularity of the articular disc or unevenness of the condylar surface.
- Clinical functional examination of the TMJ area includes three steps:
  - Palpation:
    - The condyle and fossa are palpated with index finger during opening and closing manoeuvers
    - The posterior surface can be palpated by inserting the little finger in the external auditory meatus
    - The condyles can thus be checked for tenderness, synchrony of action and coordination of relative position in the fossae
    - Palpation of the lateral pterygoid muscle area is done by placing the forefinger behind the maxillary tuberosity right above the occlusal plane, and the palmar surface of the finger directed medially towards the pterygoid hamulus.
  - Auscultation:
    - A stethoscope is used to check for signs of clicking and crepitus
    - A stereostethoscope is better because it allows the operator to determine the magnitude and timing of abnormal sounds for each joint simultaneously
    - The examination is performed by having the patient open and close the jaw into full occlusion
    - If clicking or crepitus is noted, the patient is asked to bite forwards into incision and then repeat it
    - Opening and closing movements
    - Most often sounds disappear in the protruded position.

- Functional analysis:
  - Dislocation of the condyles and discoordination of movements are early symptoms of functional disturbance
  - The extent of maximum opening is measured with a Boley gauge. In over bite cases, this amount should be added to the measurement whereas in open bite cases the distance separating the incisors on full occlusion must be subtracted.
- Several specific measures can be employed to prevent functional temporomandibular disorders (TMDs)
  - Early care of deciduous teeth for caries and interferences
  - Elimination of tooth guidance cross bites and an unwanted translatory condylar movement in the deciduous dentition
  - Elimination of neuromuscular dysfunctions and habits that force the mouth open
  - Assessment of somatognathic dysfunction
    - Swallowing.
  - Observe the tongue during various swallow
    - Unconscious swallow
    - Command swallow of saliva
    - Command swallow of water
    - Unconcious swallow during mastication
    - The tongue tip during normal mature swallow touches the curvature of the palate just behind the maxillary incisors.

Simple Tongue Thrust Swallow

- Typically displays contractions of the lips, mentalis muscle and mandibular elevators
- The teeth are in occlusion as the tongue protrudes into an open bite
- The most primary aetiologic factor for open bite due to tongue thrust is because of thumb sucking.

Complex Tongue Thrust Swallow

- Defined as tongue thrust with teeth apart swallow. Patients with this type of swallow combine contractions of the lips, facial and mentalis muscle, lack of contraction of mandibular elevators, a tongue thrust between the teeth and a teeth apart swallow
- The open bite associated with complex tongue thrust is diffuse and often difficult to define than that seen with a simple tongue thrust
- Patients with complex tongue thrust usually demonstrate occlusal interferences in the retruded contact position.

Retained Infantile Swallow

- Defined as predominant persistence of infantile swallowing pattern after the arrival of permanent teeth
- Patients demonstrate a very strong contraction of the lips and facial musculature
- The tongue thrusts strongly between the teeth in front, and on both sides
- Patients have contact only between one molar in each quadrant
- Retained infantile swallow may be associated with skeletal craniofacial development syndromes or neural deficits
- Usually the treatment of abnormal swallowing pattern can be treated with oral screen type of appliance
- The treatment of simple tongue thrust is usually successful
- In complex tongue thrust, problems treatment leads to improved morphologic relationships, but the atypical functional pattern often persists, requiring prolonged retention
- Lip exercises can improve the oral seal.

Tongue

- Morphologic examination
- Size and shape
- Ask the patient to protrude the tongue and note the symmetry of its position
- Then ask the patient to relax the tongue, allowing it to drape over the lower lip
- Functional asymmetries of tongue change from one position to the other
- Morphologic asymmetries will persist in the draped position
- Observe the posture of the tongue while the mandible is in its postural position
- During mandibular posture, the dorsum touches the palate lightly
- Flat low lying anteriorly postured tongue seen in class III malocclusion
- Drop in mandibular and tongue posture in mouth breathing.

Tongue Function

- The object of the tongue function assessment is to make a differential diagnosis possible and determine the tongue's role in malocclusion
- Functional appliance therapy is indicated, if the role of tongue malfunction is a primary aetiological factor.

Muscles of Mastication

- Morphologic examination: Palpation of each jaw muscle at rest and in function is often useful to reveal asymmetries of muscle size and placement
- Functional examination: Functional analysis of the jaw musculature is best carried out with each particular synchronised function in mind.

Respiration

Methods of Examination

- Study the patients breathing unobserved-Nasal breathers usually show the lips touching lightly during relaxed breathing, whereas mouth breathers must keep the lips parted
- Ask the patient to take a deep breath
- Ask the patients to close the lips and take a deep breath through the nose
- Nasal breathers normally demonstrate good reflex control of the alar muscles, which control the size and shape of the external nares
- Therefore, they dilate the external nares on inspiration
- Mouth breathers, even though they are capable of breathing through the nose, do not change the size or shape of the external nares and occasionally actually contract the nasal orifices while inspiring
- Unilateral nasal function may be diagnosed by placing a small, two surfaced steel mirror on the patients upper lip
- The mirror will cloud with condensed moisture during breathing
- A cotton butterfly may also be used.

CHAPTER 12 Cephalometrics

LONG ESSAYS

Question 1

Describe the landmarks, lines and planes used in Cephalometry?

Answer

Cephalometric Landmarks

Cephalometric Landmarks can be broadly classified into:

Cephalometric Landmarks can be broadly classified into two	
I. Anatomic landmarks	• Represents actual anatomic structures of the skull
II. Derived landmarks	• Landmarks that have been constructed or obtained secondarily from anatomic structures in a cephalogram
Landmarks can also be classified into	
	• Hard tissue landmarks
	• Soft tissue landmarks

Anatomic Landmarks

- **Nasion** – Most anterior point on naso frontal suture
- **Sella** – Midpoint of hypophyseal fossa
- **Si** – Most inferior point of lower contour of sella turcica
- **SP** – Most posterior point on posterior contour of sella turcica
- **Se** – Midpoint of the entrance of sella. At the same level of jugum sphenoidal
- **Point A (subspinale)** – Deepest midline point in the curved bony outline from the base of alveolar process of the maxilla. i.e. between ANS and Prosthion

  According to **Donovan** – Junction of maxillary basal bone and alveolar bone.

  Acoording to **Higley** – Deepest midline point between ANS and Prosthion on the premaxilla.

  According to **Jacobson** – Anterior limit of maxillary denture base
- **Prosthion** – Alveolar rim of maxilla or the lower most anterior point on the alveolar portion of the premaxilla in the median plane between upper central incisors
- **Is (Incisor superious)** – Tip of crown of most anterior maxillary central incisor
- **AP 1 (Apicale 1)** – Root apex of the most anterior mandibular central incisor
- **Ii (Incisor inferius)** – Tip of crown of most anterior mandibular incisor
- **AP 1** – Root apex of most anterior maxillary incisor
- **Point B (Supramentale)** – Most anterior part of mandibular base or it is the most posterior point in the outer contour of the mandibular alveolar process, in the median plane

  According to **Donovan** – It is the Junction of mandibular basal bone and alveolar process.

  According to **Jacobson** – It is the Anterior limit of mandible
- **Pog** – Most anterior point on bony chin in median plane
- **Gn** – According to **Brodie,** this point is located by taking the midpoint between most anterior and inferior points on the bony chin

  According to **Craig** – Point of intersection of facial and mandibular plane.
- **Go** – It is defined as the constructed point at the intersect of lines tangent to posterior margin of ascending ramus and mandibular base
- **Me** – According to **Sassouni** - Most caudal point in the outline of the symphysis or the inferior most point on mandible
- **Ar (Articulare)** - According to **Bjork** – Point of intersection of the posterior margin of ascending ramus and outer margin of cranial base

- **Cd (Condylion)** – Most superior point on the head of the condyle
- **Or (Orbitale)** – Lower most point of the orbit in radiograph
- **ANS** – Tip of bony anterior nasal spine in the median plane
- **PNS** – The intersection of continuation of anterior wall of pterygopalatine fossa and the floor of nose
- **Basion** – Lowest point on the anterior margin of foramen magnum in the median plane
- **Ptm (Pterygomaxillary fissure)** – Anterior wall represents maxillary tuberosity outline, posterior wall represents anterior curve of pterygoid process
- **Po (Porion)** – According to **Tweed** – It is 4.5mm above geometric center of ear rod

  According to **Craig** – It is the Uppermost point on the soft tissues overlying the external auditory meatus
- **BO (Bolton point)** – According to **Broadbent** – Highest point in the upward curvature of the retrocondylar fossa
- **D point** – Center of symphysis given by Steiner
- **Op (Opisthion)** – Most posterior point of the bony margin of the foramen magnum
- **AC (Acanthion)** – Tip of ANS
- **J point** – Located at the junction of the anterior border of ramus and the corpus of mandible
- **DS (Dorsam selae)** – Square bone forms posterior boundary of sella turcica
- **Broadbent registration patient (R)** – Perpendicular from sella on Nasion – Bolton plane.

Lines and Planes of Lateral Cephalometrics

- **Blumenbach's plane (Resting horizontal plane)** - It is the plane formed as the skull, minus the mandible rest on a flat horizontal surface. Entails the skull resting anterior on maxillary teeth and posterior either on occipital condyles or on the mastoid process
- **Broadbent's line (S-N reference line)** – From sella to nasion
- **Broadbent Bolton line** – Line from Bolton patient to nasion
- **Broca's line** – Extends from true anatomic prosthion to the lower most point of the occipital condyle. When skull is resting on horizontal surface
- **Camper's line** – Line extending from tip of ANS to the centre of external auditory meatus. Camper's plane is a triangular plane formed by two lines from tip of ANS to each external auditory meatus
- **Decoster's line** – This is the only line that is not linear connection of two points. It represents an actual anatomical contour of the planoethmoidal line from internal plate of frontal bone down through roof of cribriform plate to the anterior portion of sella turcica
- **Frankfort horizontal plane** – Its origins date back to the international congress on prehistoric anthropology and archaeology, held in **Frankfort in 1882**. The line runs from orbitale to porion. It is supposed to represent the ideal horizontal position of the head when the patient stands erect
- **Palatal plane** – Line running from ANS to PNS
- **His plane** – Runs from acanthion to opisthion
- **Hold way line** – Also referred as harmony line. It was developed by **R.A. Holdaway** and is strictly a soft tissue profile assessment reference line. Runs from soft tissue pogonion to vermilion border of upper lip
- **Huxley's line** – Runs from nasion to basion and referred as **nasion-basion line**. It would be the near perfect base reference line for research purposes on growth and development
- **Mandibular plane** – Four different mandibular planes

  Steiner – Line joining Go and Gn

  Downs – Line joining Go and Me

  Tweed and Ricketts – Straight line tangent to the lower most border of mandible.

  Bimpler's line – Line from menton to antigonial notch.
- **Margolis line** – Line runs from nasion to spheno-occipital-synchondrosis
- **Occlusal plane** – 3 occlusal planes
  - **First plane** – Line joining midpoint of overlap of mesio-buccalcusps of upper and lower first molars with point bisecting overbite of incisors. Used by **Downs and Steiner.**
  - **Second plane** – Used by **Ricketts** and in **Wits** analysis called as functional occlusal plane and is line joining the midpoint of the overlap of mesio- buccal cusp of I[st] molars and buccal cusps of premolars or deciduous molars.
  - **Third plane** – Line joining midsection of molar cusps to the tip of upper incisors.
- **Orbital plane** – Plane perpendicular to Frankfort horizontal plane at orbitale
- **Ramal plane** – Line tangent to posterior border of ramus of mandibular
- **Rickett's esthetic line** –Extends from soft tissue tip of nose to the most anterior portion of soft tissue chin
- **Von Ihering's line** – Orbitale to center of external auditory meatus
- **Y-axis** – Given by **Downs** and extends from sella to gnathion.

Question 2

What is Down's Analysis?

Answer

- Downs analysis was given by W. B. Downs in the year 1948
- This analysis was one of the first to be introduced.

Downs Sample

- The control material studied by downs was derived form 20 white subjects, who ranged in age from 12 to 17 years
- All individuals possessed clinically excellent occlusions.

Various Landmarks Used In This Analysis

- Nasion – is most anterior point on the mid point of fronto nasal suture
- Sella – located at the mid point of sella turcica
- Porion – located on the superior surface of external auditory meatus
- Point A (Subspinale) – Deepest midline point on the concavity of maxilla between ANS and Prosthion
- Point B (Supra mentale) – Deepest midline point of the mandible between Pogonion and Infradentale
- Gnathion – located at the point of inter section of facial mandibular plane

Reference Planes Used in this Analysis

- Most important reference plane (Frankfort horizontal plane) – Extends from Porion to Orbitale
- Other plane (Facial plane) – line from Nasion to Pogonion
- Occlusal plane – line bisecting the occlusion of first molars and incisal over bite
- Mandibular plane – Tangent to the lower border of the mandible and Gonial angle.

Measurements

Downs analysis consist of 10 parameters of which five are used to described the skeletal pattern five described the dental pattern.

Skeletal Pattern

- Facial angle
- Angle of convexity
- A-B plane
- Mandibular plane angle
- Y (Growth) axis.

Dental Pattern

- Cant of occlusal plane
- Inter incisal angle
- Incisor occlusal plane angle
- Incisor mandibular plane angle
- Protrusion of maxillary incisors.

Skeletal Pattern

Defines the underlying facial type:

- Dental pattern establish the lower teeth is placed in position to underlying bony structures
- When observing facial profiles, WB downs noted that generally the position of the mandible could be used in determining whether or not faces were balanced. The 'ideal" profile, which represents the best harmony of features or beauty of form for most people, is one in which the position of the mandible is orthognathic, that is, neither retrusive nor protrusive.

Downs reduced his observations to the following four basic facial types:

- Retrognathic, a recessive lower jaw
- Orthognathic an ideal or average lower jaw
- Prognathic, a protrusive lower jaw
- True prognathism, a pronounced protrusion of the lower face.

Facial Angle

- The facial angle is used to measure the degree of retrusion or protrusion of the lower jaw. This is the inferior inside angle in which the facial line (nasion-pogonion) intersects Frankfort horizontal plane
- The mean reading for this angle is 87.8 degrees (SD, 3.6) with a range of 82 to 95 degrees **(Fig. 12.1)**.

Angle of Convexity

- The angle of convexity is formed by the intersection of line N-point A to point A-pogonion
- This angle measures the degree of the maxillary basal arch at its anterior limit (point A) relative to the total facial profile (nasion-pogonion) **(Fig. 12.2)**.

A-B Plane

- This angle is formed between a line connecting point A and point B and line
  - Joining nasion to pogonion (facial plane)
- The A-B plane is a measure of the relation of the anterior limit of the apical bases to each other relative to the facial plane **(Fig. 12.3)**.

Mandibular Plane Angle

- Mandibular plane according to downs, is tangent to the gonial angle and the lowest point of the symphysis
- The mandibular plane angle is established by relating the MP to the Frank fort horizontal plane
- Increased mandibular plane angle is suggestive of vertical growth with hyper divergent facial pattern
- High mandibular plane angle complicate treatment and prognosis **(Fig. 12.4)**.

Y – (Growth) Axis

- The Y-axis is measured as the acute angle formed by the intersection of a line from the sella turcica to gnathion with the Frankfort horizontal plane
- This angle is larger in class II facial patterns than in class III tendencies
- The y-axis indicates the degree of the downward, rearward, or forward position of the chin in relation to the upper face
- A decrease of the y-axis in serial radiographs may be interpreted as a greater horizontal than vertical growth pattern. An increase in the y-axis is suggestive of vertical growth exceeding horizontal (or forward) growth of the mandible
- The range extends from a minimal of 53 degrees to a maximal of 66 degrees with a mean reading of 59.4 degrees **(Fig. 12.5)**.

Cant of Occlusal Plane

- Downs originally defined the occlusal plane as that line bisecting the overlapping cusps of the first molars and the incisal overbite
- In cases in which the incisors are grossly malpositioned, Downs recommended drawing the occlusal plane through the region of the overlapping cusps of the first premolar and first molars
- It measures the slope of the occlusal plane to the Frankfort horizontal **(Fig. 12.6)**.

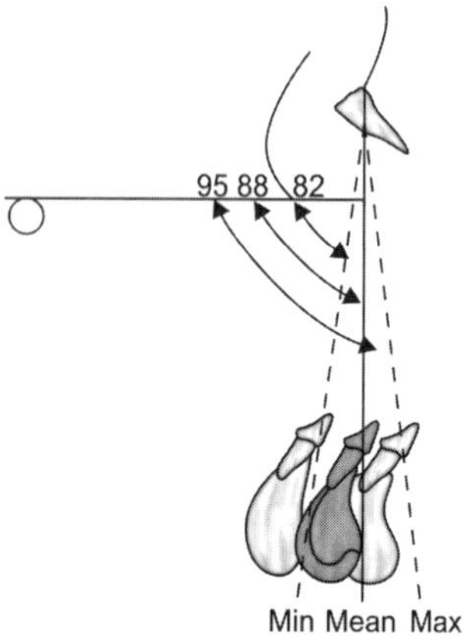

Fig. 12.1: Facial Angle

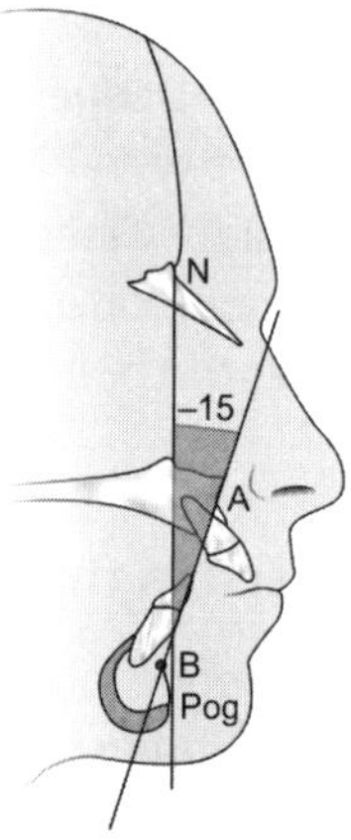

Fig. 12.3: A- B plane

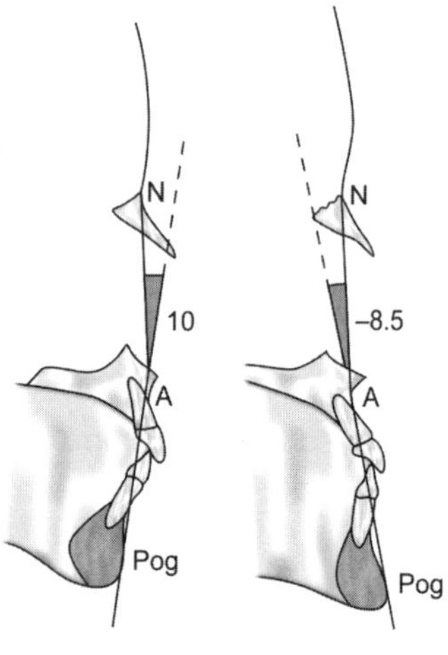

Fig. 12.2: Angle of Convexity

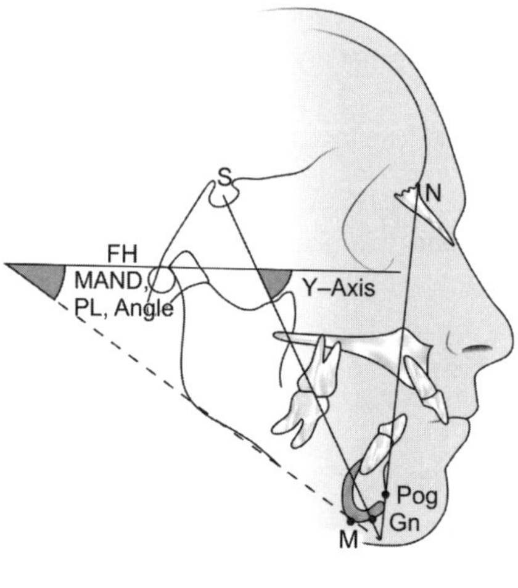

Fig. 12.4: Mandibular Plane Angle

Interincisal Angle

- The interincisal angle is established by passing a line through the incisal edge and the apex of the root of the maxillary and mandibular central incisors
- This angle is decreased in class I bimaxillary protrusion and Class II div1 cases increased in Class II div 2 cases **(Fig. 12.7)**.

Incisor – Occlusal Plane Angle

- The incisor – occlusal plane angle relates the lower incisors to their functioning surface at the occlusal plane and the inferior inside angle is read as a positive or negative deviation from a right angle
- The positive angle increases as the teeth incline forward **(Fig. 12.8)**.

Incisor – Mandibular Plane Angle

The incisor mandibular plane angle is formed by the intersection of the mandibular plane with a line passing through the incisal edge and the apex of the root of the mandibular central incisor **(Fig. 12.9)**.

Protrusion of Maxillary Incisors

- The protrusion of the maxillary incisors is measured as the distance between the incisal edge of the maxillary central incisor to the line from point A-pogonion
- The distance is positive if the incisal edge is ahead of the point A-pogonion line and indicates the amount of maxillary dental protrusion
- The reading is negative if the incisal edge lies behind the point A-pogonion line and suggests a retruded position of maxillary incisors **(Fig. 12.10)**.

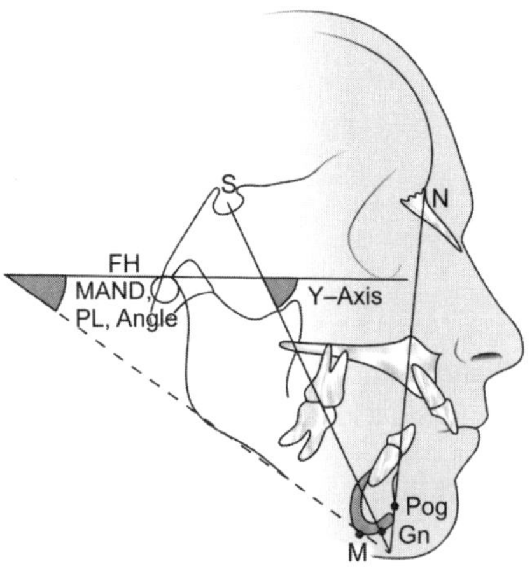

Fig. 12.5: Y Axis

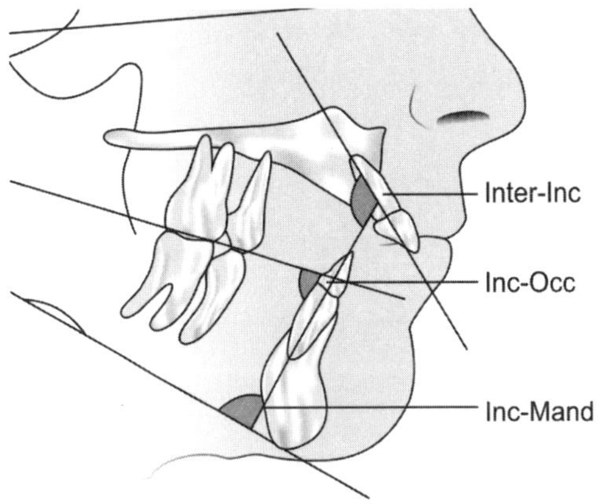

Fig. 12.7: Interincisal Angle

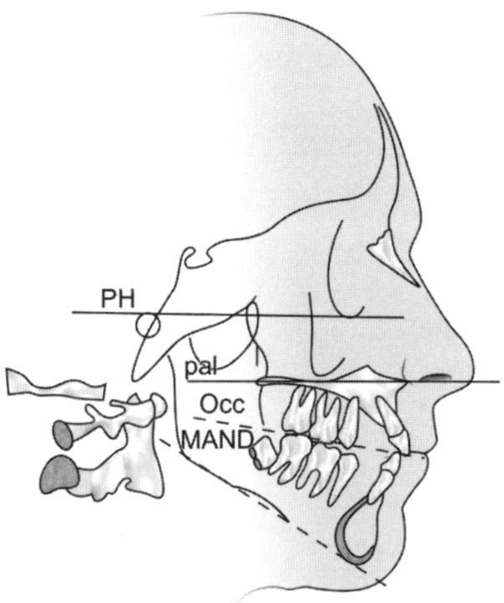

Fig. 12.6: Cant of Occlusal Plane

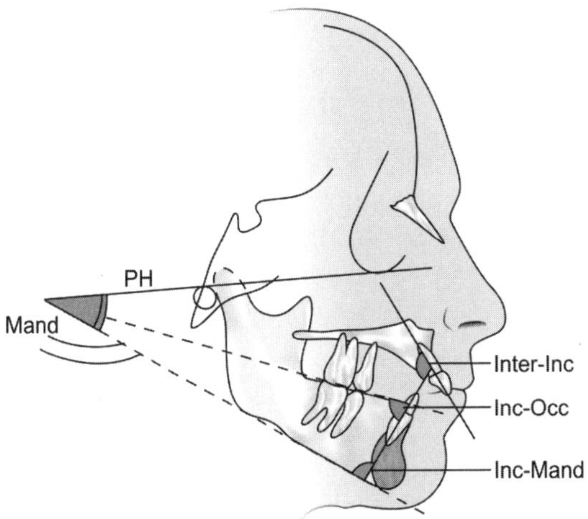

Fig. 12.8: Incisal Occlusal Plane Angle

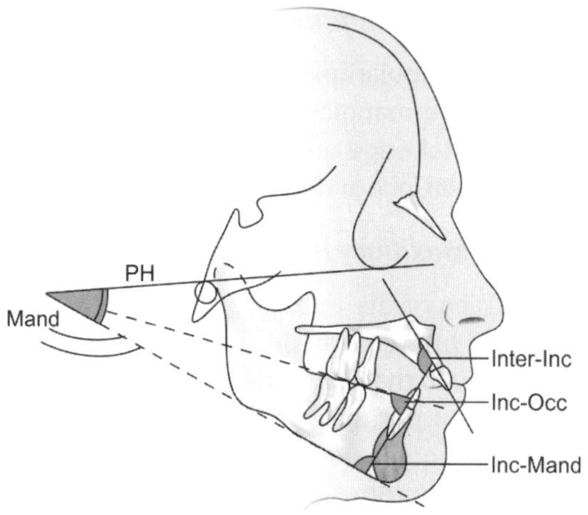

Fig. 12.9: Incisal mandibular plane angle

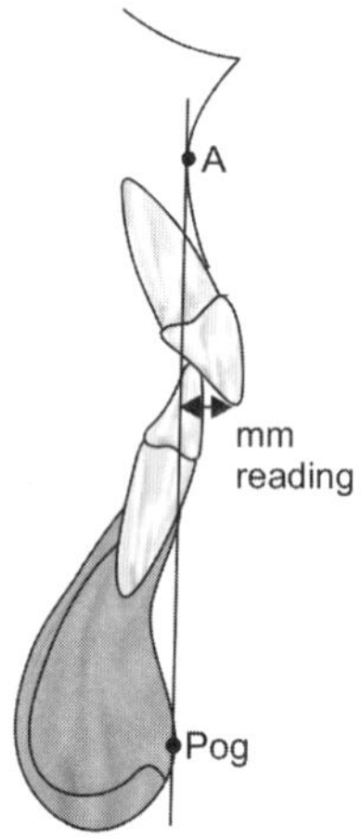

Fig. 12.10: Protrusion of maxillay incisor

Downs' Measurements Used for Cephalometric Polygon

Parameter	Mean (Degrees)	SD
Skeletal Pattern		
Facial angle	87.8	3.6
Angle of convexity	0	5.1
A-B plane angle	-4.6	3.7
Mandibular plane angle	21.9	3.2
Y-axis	59.4	3.8
Dental pattern		
Cant of occlusal plane	+9.3	3.8
U1 to L1	135.4	5.8
U1 to occlusal plane	+14.5	3.5
L1 to mandibular plane	+1.43	3.8
L1 to A-P plane	+2.7 mm	1.8

Question 3

What is Steiner's Analysis?

Answer

This cephalometric analysis was proposed by Cecil C Steiner. He selected what he considered to be the most meaningful parameters and evolved a composite analysis, which he believed would provide maximum clinical information with least number of measurements.

The analysis includes:

- Skeletal Analysis
- Dental Analysis
- Soft Tissue Analysis.

Landmarks used:

- Sella (S)
- Nasion (N)
- Anterior Nasal Spine
- Posterior Nasal Spine
- Pt. A
- Pt. B
- Gonion (Go)
- Gnathion (Gn).

Planes used:

- SN Plane.
- Palatal Plane (ANS- PNS)
- Occlusal Plane
- Mandibular Plane (Go- Gn).

Skeletal Analysis

- SNA angle : 82° ± 2°
- SNB angle : 80° ± 2°
- ANB angle : 2° ± 2°
  - Class- I – ANB : 0-5°
  - Class-II – ANB : ≥ 6°
  - Class-III – ANB : < 0°
- SND angle : 76°
- Mandibular plane to SN : 32°
- Occlusal plane to SN : 14.5°

Dental Analysis

- UI to NA (angle) : 22°
- UI to NA (linear) : 4mm
- LI to NB (angle) : 25°
- LI to NB (linear) : 4mm
- Interincisal angle : 130°

SNA Angle: (Fig. 12.11)

- Orthognathic Maxilla (82° ± 2°)
- Prognathic Maxilla (> 84°)

- Rethrognathic Maxilla (< 80°)

SNB Angle: (Fig. 12.12)

- Orthognathic Mandible (80° ± 2°)
- Retrognathic Mandible (< 78°)
- Prognathic Mandible (> 82°)

ANB Angle: (Fig. 12.13)

- It provides a general idea of the anteroposterior discrepancy of the maxillary to the mandibular apical bases
- The mean reading is 2 degrees
  - >2 degrees indicate class II tendency
  - <2 and below 0 indicate class III tendency.

SN to Occlusal Plane (OP): 14°

It tells us about the rotation of occlusal plane in relation to Anterior Cranial Base **(Fig. 12.14)**.

Go Gn to SN: (Fig. 12.15)

- Indication of vertical proportions of face
- Mean reading: 32°
  - >32° Vertical Growth Pattern
  - < 32° Horizontal Growth Pattern.

Maxillary Incisor Position

- The teeth are related to the NA line **(Fig. 12.16)**
- Two measurements; one in degrees and the other in mm
- Reading in degrees indicates the relative angular relationship of upper incisors to NA
- Reading in mm indicates the a-p positioning of the teeth
- Ideal values are 22 degrees (Angular) and 4mm (Linear)
  - >22°: proclined incisors
  - <22°: retroclined incisors
  - >4mm: protrusive incisors
  - < 4mm: retrusive incisors.

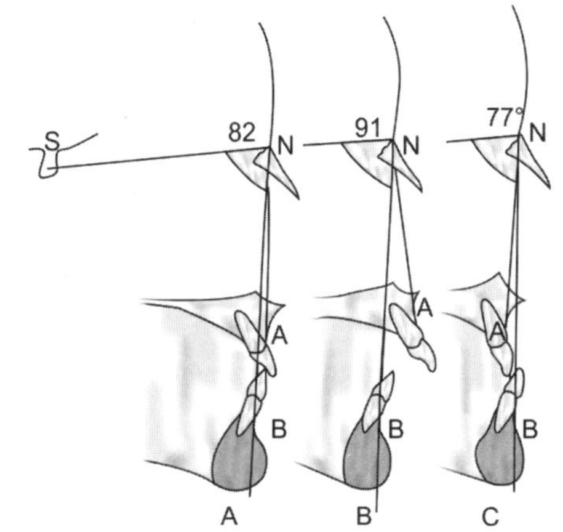

Fig. 12.11: SNA Angle

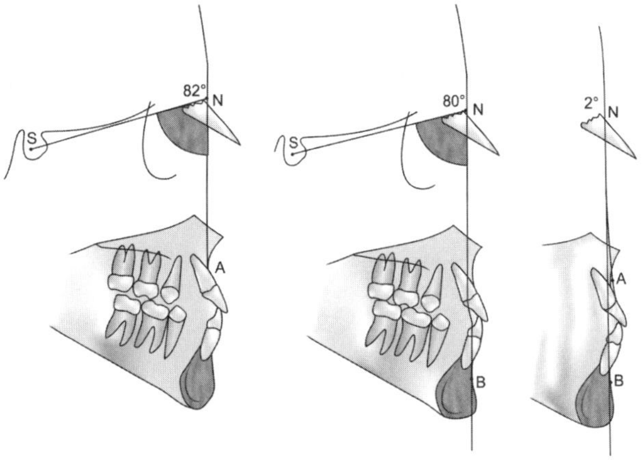

Fig. 12.13: ANB angle

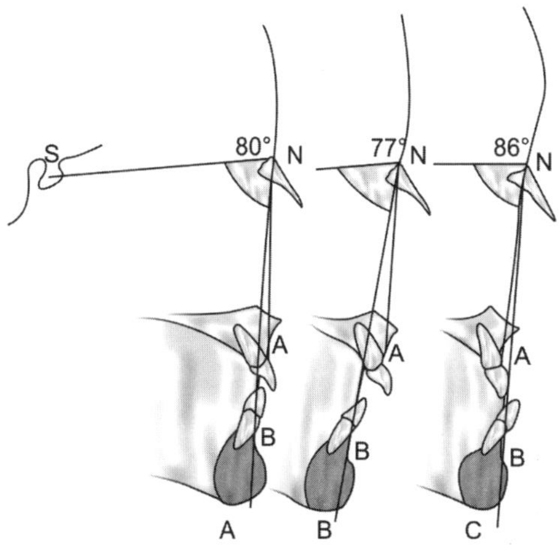

Fig. 12.12: SNB angle

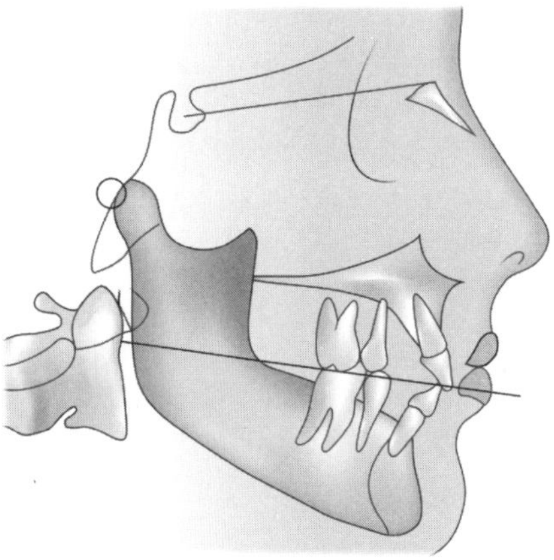

Fig. 12.14: SN to OP

Mandibular Incisor Position

- The teeth are related to the NB line **(Fig. 12.17)**
- Two measurements; one in degrees and the other in mm
- Reading in degrees indicates the relative angular relationship of upper incisors to NB
- Reading in mm indicates the a-p positioning of the teeth
- Ideal values are 25 degrees and 4mm
  - >25°: proclined incisors
  - <25°: retroclined incisors
  - >4mm: protrusive incisors
  - < 4mm: retrusive incisors.

Interincisal Angle

- Relates the upper incisor to the lower incisor **(Fig. 12.18)**
- The mean angle is 130 degrees
- If angle>130, upper and/or lower incisors require advancing anteriorly or correcting of axial inclination
- The offending teeth are determined by maxillary and mandibular tooth positions

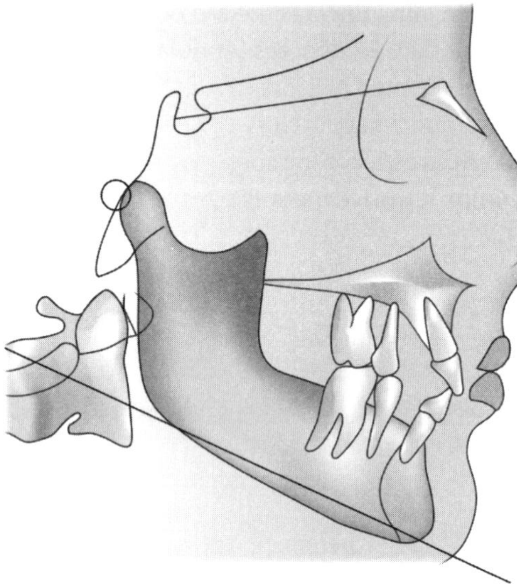

Fig. 12.15: Go Gn to SN

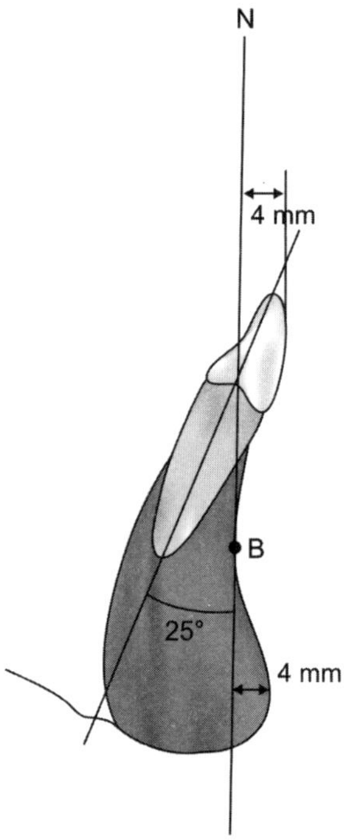

Fig. 12.17: Mandibular incisor position

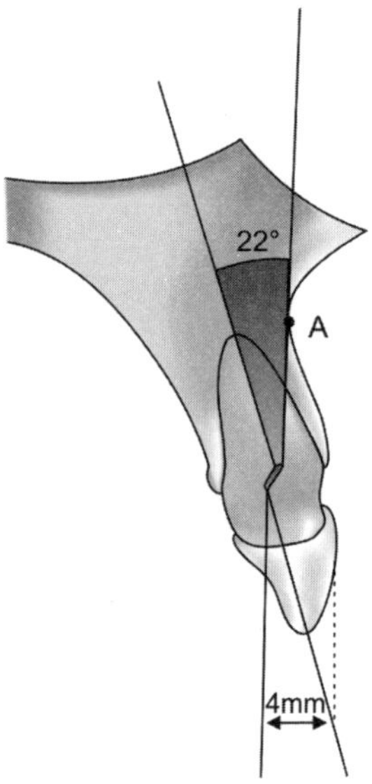

Fig. 12.16: Maxillary incisor position

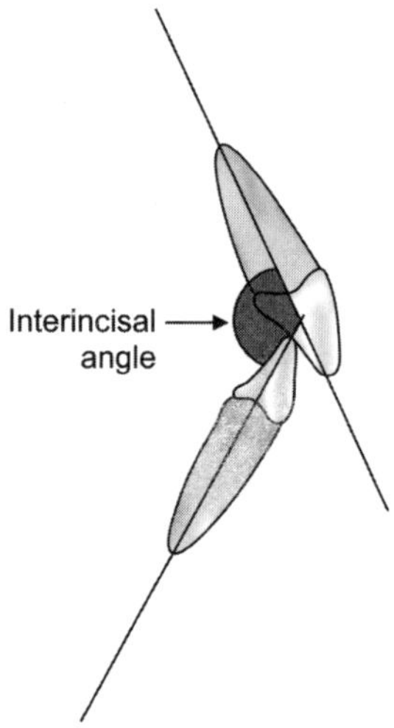

Fig. 12.18: Interincisal angle

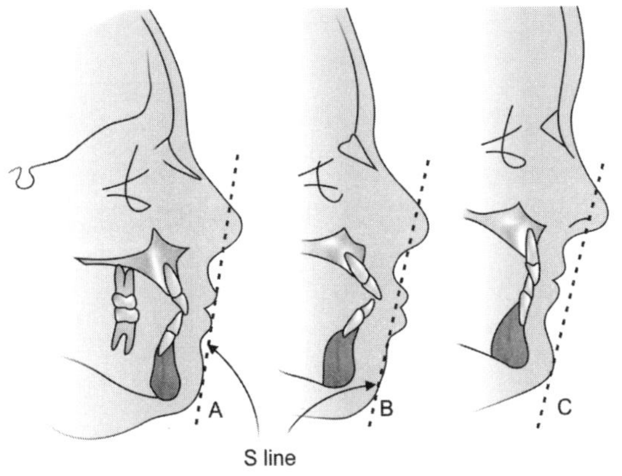

Fig. 12.19: S line

Soft Tissue Analysis

- It is a graphic record of visual observations made in the clinical examination
- It includes an appraisal of the adaptation of soft tissue to the bony profile
- Steiner's "S" line passes through the middle of 's' formed by lower border of nose to the contour of chin **(Fig. 12.19)**
- Lips beyond S-line are procumbent and those within are interpreted as 'concave'
  - Balanced lips
  - Protrusive lips
  - Recessive lips and lower facial profile.

SHORT ESSAYS

Question 1

What is Tweed Analysis?

Answer

Proposed by Dr. Charles Tweed.

- It was developed as an aid to treatment planning, anchorage preparation and determining the prognosis of orthodontic cases
- The analysis is primarily based on the deflection of the mandible as measured by the Frankfort mandibular plane angle (FMA) and the posture of the lower incisor
- Then depending on the space required extractions are planned
- Dr. Tweed established that prognosis could be predicted relatively accurately based on the configuration of the triangle (Tweed's Triangle) **(Fig. 12.20)**.

Tweed's Triangle is Formed by

- Frankfort Horizontal Plane
- The Mandibular plane
- The long axis of lower incisor.

Three Angles thus Formed are

- Frankfort mandibular plane angle (FMA)
- Lower incisor to mandibular plane (IMPA)
- Lower incisor to Frankfort Horizontal (FMIA).
  - FMA = 25 degrees
  - IMPA = 90 degrees
  - FMIA = 65 degrees.

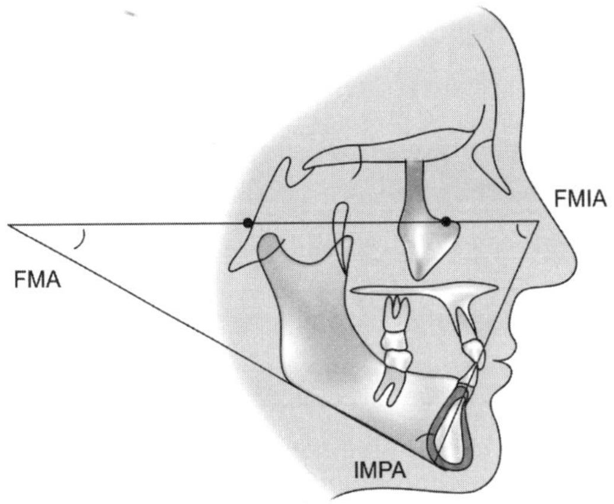

Fig. 12.20: Tweed Triangle

According to Tweed,

- FMA is the basis
- FMA 16-28 degrees ---- good prognosis.

At 16 degrees FMA, the IMPA = 90 + 5 = 95 degrees.
At 22 degrees FMA, the IMPA = 90 degrees.
At 28 degrees FMA, the IMPA = 90 – 5 = 85 degrees.

- Approximately 60% malocclusions have FMA between 16 and 28 degrees
- FMA from 28 to 35 ----fair prognosis. At 35 degrees majority cases require extractions
- FMA above 35 ----Bad prognosis
- FMIA angle to be maintained at 65-70 degrees
- By establishing the position lower incisors should occupy, provisions are made for variations in mandibular position and upper incisors are placed accordingly

- The ideal positioning of the lower incisors helps in the stability of the results achieved thereby indicating good prognosis.

Question 2

What is Wit's Appraisal?

Answer

Jacobson gave the Wits appraisal of jaw disharmony. It is the measure of the extent to which the jaws are related to each other anteroposteriorly.

Construction

Draw perpendicular from point A and B on the maxilla and mandible on to the occlusal plane **(Fig. 12.21)**.

The points of contacts of the perpendicular onto the occlusal plane are labeled AO and BO respectively.

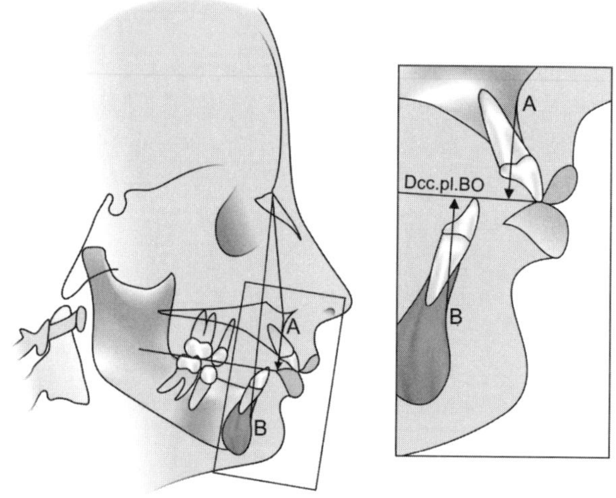

Fig. 12.21: Wits Appraisal

Wits reading

- For males BO ahead of AO by 1 mm
- For females BO coincides with AO
- If AO is ahead of BO it indicates Skeletal class II pattern
- If BO is ahead of AO it indicates Skeletal class III pattern.

SHORT NOTES

Question 1

Define Cephalometrics?

Answer

Cephalometrics includes measurements, description and appraisal of the morphologic configuration and growth changes in the skull by ascertaining the dimensions of lines, angles and planes between anthropometric landmarks established by physical anthropologists and point selected by orthodontists.

CHAPTER 13 Skeletal Maturity Indicators

LONG ESSAYS

Question 1

What are the different skeletal maturity indicators. What is the importance of skeletal maturity indicators?

Answer

- Skeletal maturity indicators are tools used to determine the growth potential of the patient to decide the treatment protocol
- Since chronologic age is a poor indicator of specific stages of maturation, the biologic age is used to determine the dental, morphologic, skeletal age and the onset of puberty
- Since there is a variation in the timing, velocity of growth and the growth remaining of different individuals, skeletal age determination is essential to formulation of a viable orthodontic treatment plan
- Skeletal maturation refers to the degree of ossification in bone
- During the growth period of an individual, all bones goes through a series of morphologic changes that can be visualised radiographically. This sequence of changes is relatively consistent for a given bone in every individual, however the timing varies according to individual.

Different Skeletal Maturity Indicators are:

- Hand and Wrist radiographs
- Radiograph of middle phalanx of third finger
- Cervical vertebrae radiographs.

Hand Wrist Radiographs

The bone in hand and wrist region of an individual undergo specific changes at different growth period and can be visualized easily in a radiograph.

A number of methods have been described to assess the skeletal maturity using hand-wrist radiographs. The following are the most commonly used methods:

- Atlas methods by Greulich and Pyle
- Bjork, Grave and Brown Method
- Fishman's Skeletal Maturity Indicators
- Hagg and Taranger Methods.

Anatomy of Hand – Wrist

The hand-wrist region is made up of the following four groups of bones **(Fig. 13.1)**.

1. Distal ends of long bones of forearm
2. Carpals
3. Metacarpals
4. Phalanges.

Distal Ends of Long Bones of Forearm

The distal ends of radius and ulna, which are long bones of the forearm, form the first group of bones.

The radius and the ulna give rise to a distal projection on their respective sides. These are called the ulna styloid and the radial styloid.

The Carpals

They consist of eight small, irregularly shaped bones arranged in two rows:

1. Proximal row: Scaphoid, lunate, triquetral and pisiform
2. Distal row: Trapezium, trapezoid, capitate, and hamate.

Each of these eight carpal bones ossifies from one primary center, which appears in a predictable pattern.

The Metacarpals

- They are 5 miniature long bones forming the skeletal framework of the palm of the hand
- They are numbered 1-5 from the thumb to the little finger
- Each metacarpal ossifies from one primary center (in its shaft) and a secondary center on the distal end (except for the first metacarpal where it appears at the proximal end).

The phalanges

They are small bones forming the fingers. They are three in number in each finger, except the thumb which has only two phalanges.

The three bones are referred to as the proximal, middle (absent in thumb) and the distal phalanges. The phalanges ossify in 3 stages.

- **Stage 1:** The epiphysis and diaphysis are equal
- **Stage 2:** The epiphysis caps the diaphysis by surrounding it like a cap
- **Stage 3:** Fusion occurs between the epiphysis and diaphysis.

The Sesamoid Bone

The sesamoid bone is a small nodular bone most often present embedded in tendons in the region of the thumb.

Indications for hand-wrist radiographs:

- In patients showing discrepancy in skeletal and chronologic age
- Determination of skeletal growth status prior to Skeletal Class II and III malocclusion treatment
- To predict future skeletal maturation rate and status
- To predict the pubertal growth spurt

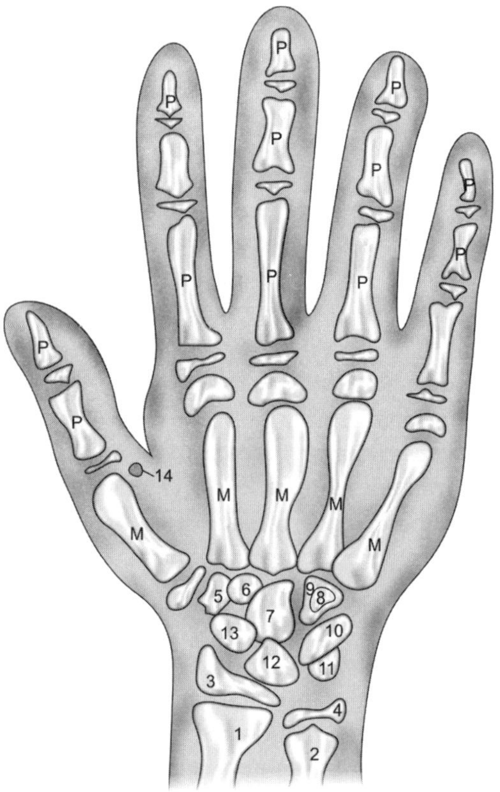

Fig. 13.1: Hand and Wrist Bones

- To study the role of heredity, environment, nutrition etc., on the skeletal maturation pattern
- It is indicated in patients with skeletal malocclusion needing orthognathic surgery, if undertaken between 16-20 years so as to assess the growth status.

Greulich and Pyle Method

- Greulich and Pyle published an atlas showing ideal pictures of the hand wrist of different chronologic ages for both males and females
- Each photograph in the atlas depicts a particular skeletal age. The patient's radiograph is matched with one of the photographs in the atlas.

Bjork, Grave and Brown Method

- They divided skeletal growth in 9 stages
- Each stages represents level of skeletal maturity
- Appropriate chronological age for each of the stages was given by *Schopf* in 1978.
- **Stage One (males 10.6 years, Females 8.1 years) PP2 (=) stage (Fig. 13.2):** The epiphysis and diaphysis of the proximal phalanx of index finger are equal. It occurs approximately three years before the peak of pubertal growth spurt
- **Stage Two (males 12.0 years, Females 8.1 years) MP3(=) stage (Fig. 13.3):** The epiphysis and diaphysis of the middle phalanx of the middle finger are equal
- **Stage Three (Males 12.6 years, Females 9.6 years) Pisi, H1-, and R = stage (Fig. 13.4):** This stage is characterized by presence of 3 areas of ossification:
  1. The hamular process of the hamate exhibits ossification **(Fig. 13.4A)**
  2. Ossification of pisiform **(Fig. 13.4B)**
  3. The epiphysis and diaphysis of radius are equal **(Fig. 13.4C).**
- **Stage Four (Males 13.0 years, Females 10.6 years) S- and H2 stage:** This stage marks the beginning of the pubertal growth spurt. It is characterized by:
  1. Initial mineralization of the ulnar sesamoid of the thumb **(Fig. 13.5A)**
  2. Increased ossification of the hamular process of the hamate bone **(Fig. 13.5B).**
- **Stage Five (Males 14.0 years, Female 11.0 years) MP3 cap, PP1 cap and R cap stage (Fig. 13.6):** This stage signifies the peak of the pubertal growth spurt. It is characterized by union between epiphysis and diaphysis of the distal phalanx of the middle finger
- **Stage six:** Union of epiphysis and diaphysis of middle phalanx of third finger

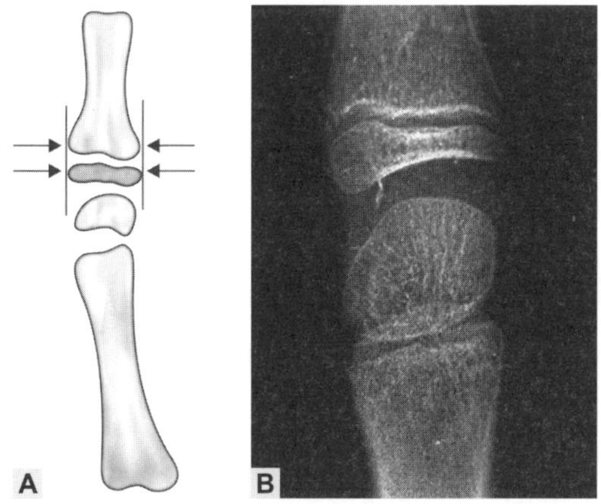

Figs. 13.2A and B: The epiphysis and diaphysis of the proximal phalanx of index finger are equal

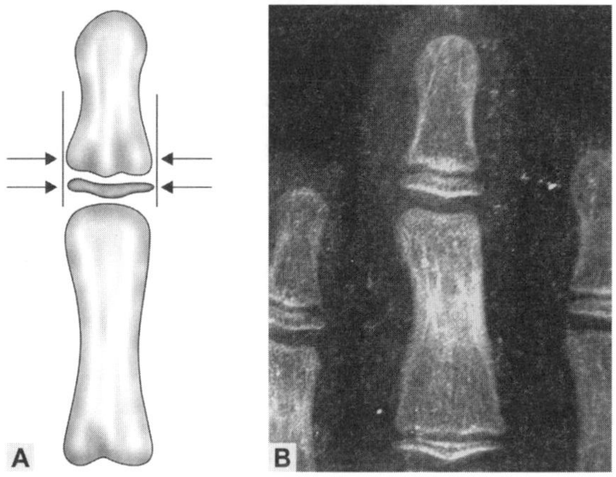

Figs. 13.3A and B: The epiphysis and diaphysis of the proximal phalanx of index finger are equal

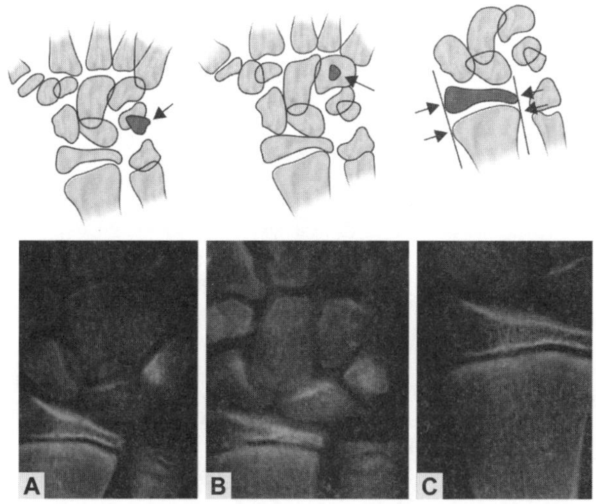

Figs. 13.4A to C: Areas of ossification. (A) The hamular process of the hamate exhibits ossification; (B) Ossification of pisiform; (C) The epiphysis and diaphysis of radius are equal

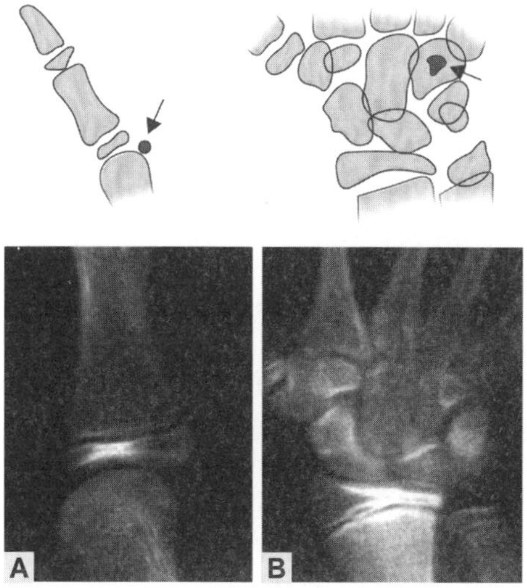

Figs. 13.5A and B: Beginning of the pubertal growth spurt. (A) Initial mineralisation of the ulnar sesamoid of the thumb; (B) Increased ossification of the hamular process of the hamate bone

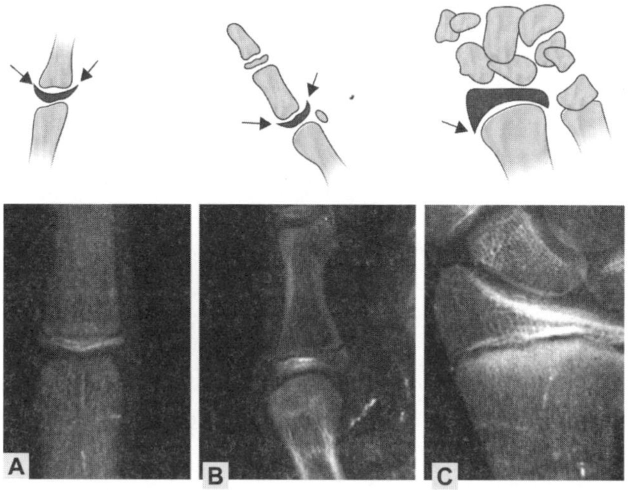

Figs. 13.6A to C: Union between epiphysis and diaphysis of the distal phalanx of the middle finger

- **Stage Seven (Males 15.9 years, Females 13.3 years) DP3 U stage (Fig. 13.7)**: Union of epiphysis and diaphysis of the proximal phalanx of the little finger occurs. This stage marks the end of pubertal growth spurt
- **Stage Eight (Males 15.9 years, Females 13.9 years) PP3 U stage (Fig. 13.8)**: This stage shows fusion between the epiphysis and diaphysis of the middle phalanx of the middle finger
- **Stage Nine (Males 18.5 years, Females 16.0 years) (Fig. 13.9)**: This is the last stage and it signifies the end of skeletal growth. It is characterized by fusion of epiphysis and diaphysis of the radius.

Fishman's Skeletal Maturity Indicator

- A system for evaluation of skeletal maturation was proposed by **Leonord S. Fishman in 1982**
- In his system Fishman uses only four stages of bone maturation **(Fig. 13.10)**
- The sequence of the four ossification stages progresses through **(Fig. 13.11)**.
  1. Widening of epiphyses on selected phalanges
  2. Ossification of the adductor sesamoid of thumb
  3. The capping of particular epiphyses over the diaphysis
  4. Fusion of selected epiphyses and diaphysis.

Width of epiphysis as wide as diaphysis

- Third finger – Proximal phalanx
- Third finger – Middle phalanx
- Fifth finger – Middle phalanx.

Ossification

Adductor sesamoid of thumb.

Capping of epiphysis

- Third finger – Distal phalanx
- Third finger – Middle phalanx
- Fifth finger – Middle phalanx.

Fusion of epiphysis and diaphysis

- Third finger – Distal phalanx
- Third finger – Proximal phalanx
- Third finger – Middle phalanx
- Radius.

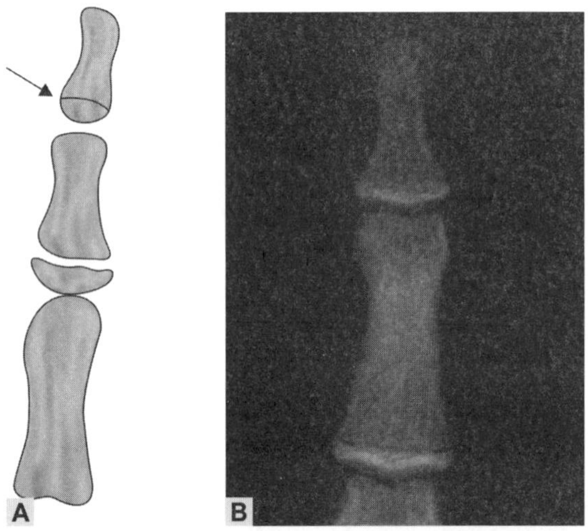

Figs. 13. 7A and B: Union of epiphysis and diaphysis of the proximal phalanx of the little finger occurs

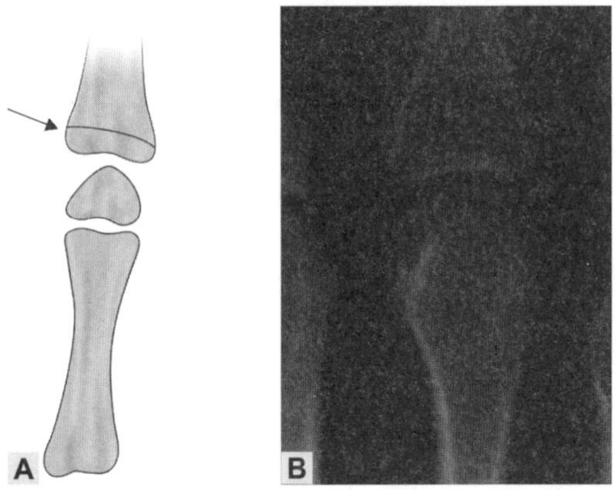

Figs. 13.8A and B: Fusion between the epiphysis and diaphysis of the middle phalanx of the middle finger

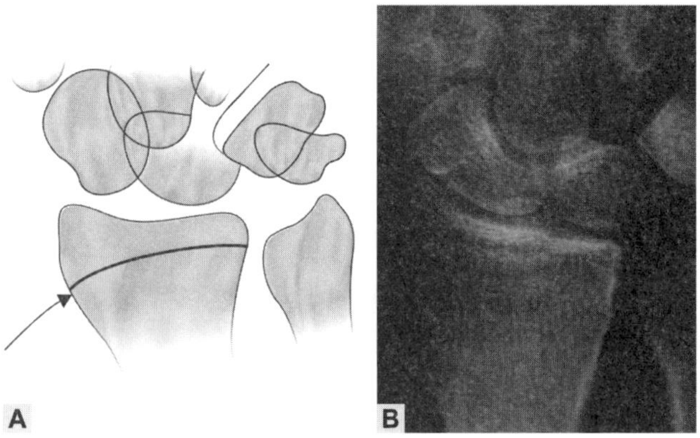

Figs. 13.9A and B: Last stage and it signifies the end of skeletal growth and characterised by fusion of epiphysis and diaphysis of the radius

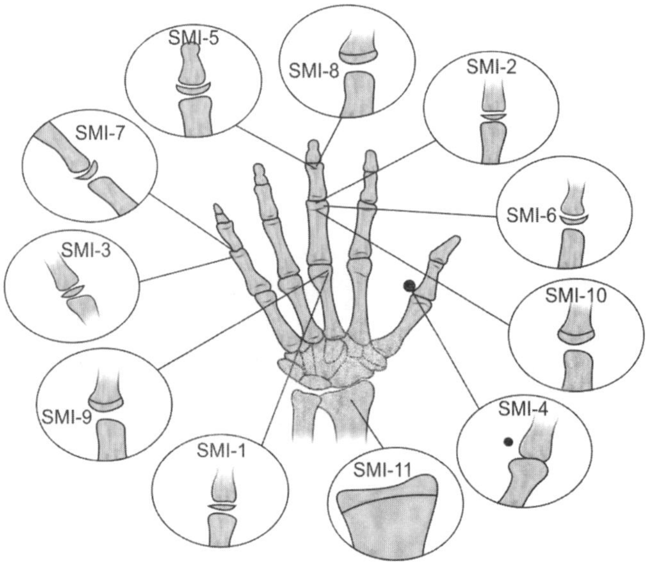

Fig. 13.10: Fishman's skeletal maturity indicators

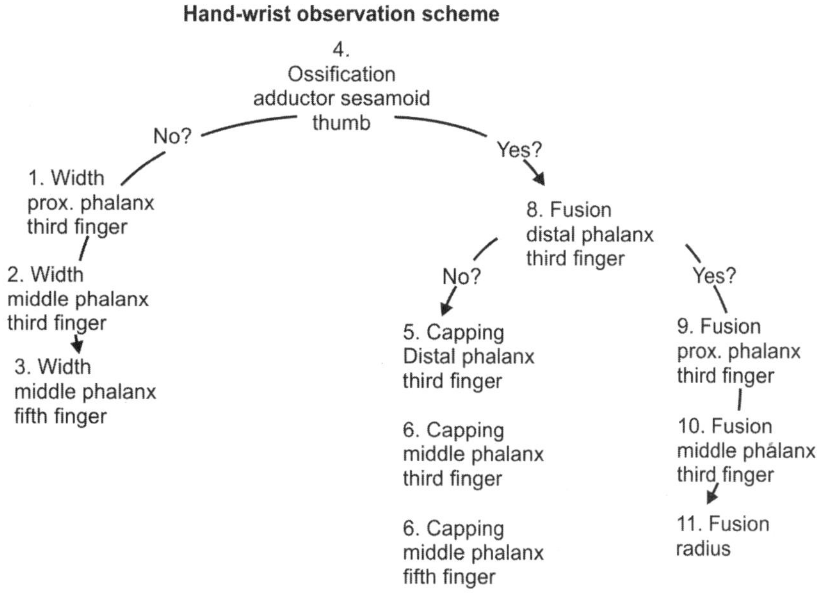

Fig. 13.11: Hand-wrist observation scheme

Maturation Assessment by Hagg and Taranger (1982)

Skeletal development in the hand and wrist in analyzed by assessment of the ossification of the ulnar sesamoid of the metacarpophalangeal joint of the first finger (S) and certain specified stages of three epiphyseal bones: the middle and distal phalanges of the third finger (MP3 and DP3) and the distal epiphysis of the radius (R).

Sesamoid

Fusion of Sesamoid is usually attained during the acceleration period of the pubertal growth spurt (onset of P.H.V.: Peak Height Velocity).

Third Finger Middle Phalanx

- **MP3-F**: The epiphysis is as wide as the metaphysis. This stage is attained before onset of P.H.V.
- **MP3-FG**: The epiphysis is as wide as the metaphysis and there is distinct medial and/or lateral border of the epiphysis forming a line of demarcation at right angles to the distal border. This stage is attained 1 year before or at P.H.V.
- **MP3-G**: The sides of the epiphysis have thickened and also cap its metaphysis, forming a sharp edge distally at one or both sides. This stage is attained at or 1 year after P.H.V.
- **MP3-H**: Fusion of the epiphysis and metaphysis has begun and is attained after PHV but before end of growth spurt
- **MP3-I**: Is attained before or at end of growth spurt

Third Finger Distal Phalanx

DP3-I: Fusion of the epiphysis and metaphysis is completed. This stage signifies the fusion of the epiphysis and metaphysis and is attained during the acceleration period of the pubertal growth spurt (i.e. end of P.H.V.).

Radius

- **R-I**: Fusion of the epiphysis and metaphysis has begun. This stage is attained 1 year before or at the end of growth spurt.
- **R-IJ**: Fusion is almost completed but there is still a small gap at one or both margins.
- **R-J**: Is characterized by fusion of the epiphysis and metaphysis.

Maturational Assessment with Middle Phalanx of Third Finger

The radiographs of middle phalanx of third finger were taken using dental x-ray unit with dental x-ray film by the method described by Hassam M., Abdul Kader.

- **MP3-F stage (onset or start of the curve of pubertal growth spurt);** Epiphysis is as wide as metaphysis **(Fig. 13.12A)**
- **MP3-FG stage (acceleration part of the curve of pubertal growth spurt);** Epiphysisis as wide as the metaphysis and there is a distinct medial and/or lateral border of the epiphysis forming a line of demarcation at right angle to the distal border **(Fig. 13.12B)**

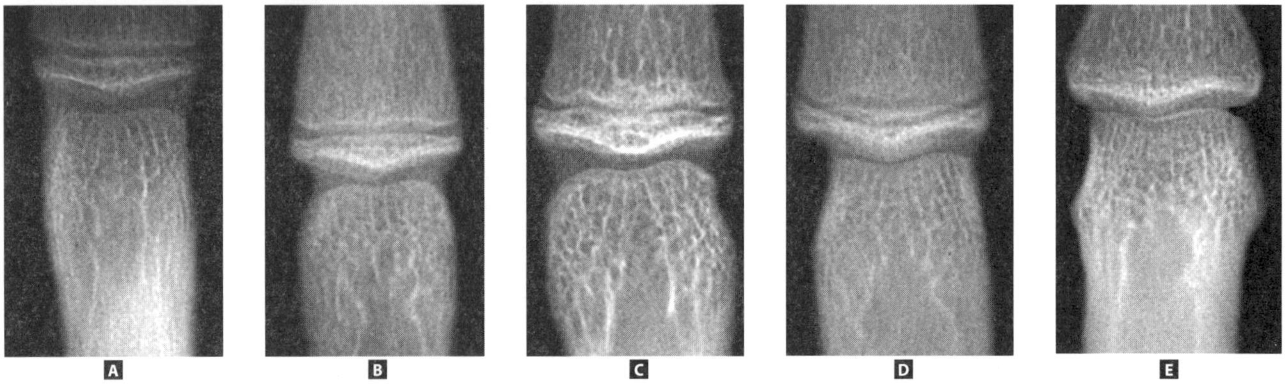

Figs. 13.12: (A) MP3 F, (B) MP3 FG, (C) MP3G, (D) MP3 H (E) MP3 I

- **MP3-G stage (peak-PTV, the point of maximum pubertal growth spurt);** Sides of the epiphysis have thickened and cap its metaphysis forming a sharp edge distally at one or both sides **(Fig. 13.12C)**
- **MP3-H stage (deceleration part of the curve of pubertal growth spurt);** Fusion of epiphysis and metaphysis has begun **(Fig. 13.12D)**
- **MP3-I stage (end of pubertal growth spurt);** Fusion of epiphysis and metaphysis is completed **(Fig. 13.12E)**.

Skeletal Maturation using Cervical Verterbrae (CVMI)

This method utilizes the skeletal changes in the cervical vertebra during the growth of an individual to determine the growth status **(Fig. 13.13)**.

Hassel and Farman have put forward the following six stages in vertebral development:

- **Stage 1**: This stage is called as **Initiation**. It refers to the beginning of adolescent growth with 80% to 100% of adolescent growth remaining
  - Inferior borders of C2, C3 and C4 are flat at this stage
  - The vertebrae are wedge shaped, and the superior vertebral borders tapers from posterior to anterior direction.
- **Stage 2**: The second stage is termed **Acceleration**
  - Growth spurt initiates in this stage, with 65% to 85% of adolescent growth remaining
  - Concavities start developing on the inferior borders of C2 and C3, while the C4 remains flat
  - The bodies of C3 and C4 are nearly rectangular in shape.
- **Stage 3**: The third stage called **Transition**, and it corresponds to acceleration of growth towards peak height velocity with 25% to 65% of adolescent growth remaining
  - Distinct concavities can be appreciated in the inferior borders of C2 and C3, while concavity begins to emerge in the inferior border of C4

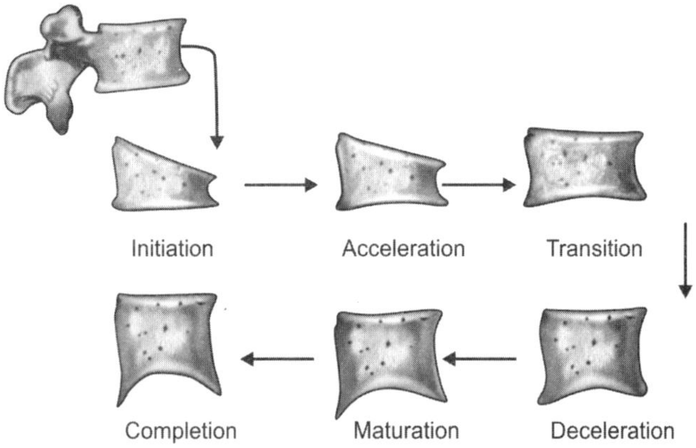

Fig. 13.13: Assessment of skeletal maturation using the vertebral column

  - The bodies of C3 and C4 were rectangular in shape.
- **Stage 4**: This stage called **Deceleration** corresponding to deceleration of adolescent growth spurt with only 10% to 25% of adolescent growth left
  - Distinct concavities can be seen in the inferior borders of C2, C3 and C4
  - The vertebral bodies of C3 and C4 start appearing more square in shape.
- **Stage 5**: The fifth stage is called **Maturation**. Final maturation of the vertebrae took place during this stage, with 5% to 10% of adolescent growth left
  - More accentuated concavities are seen in the inferior borders of C2, C3 and C4
  - The bodies of C3 and C4 were almost square in shape.
- **Stage 6**: This stage called **Completion** and it corresponds to completion of growth. Growth ceases in this stage
  - Deep concavities are seen in the inferior borders of C2, C3 and C4
  - The bodies of C3 and C4 are square or greater in vertical dimension than in horizontal dimension.

CHAPTER 14

Model Analysis

LONG ESSAYS

Question 1

What is model analysis? Describe different model analyses for permanent dentition.

Answer

Model analysis is one of the essential diagnostic aids. Study models help us to visualise the patient's occlusion from all aspects and also help us in making the necessary measurements of the arch teeth, the dental arches and the basal bone to carry out the various types of model analyses. Model analysis provides valuable information and when it is correlated with the other diagnostic aids, will help in diagnosing and treatment planning of a case.

Advantages of Model Analysis

- Better understanding the case for treatment planning
- Visual aid for the dentist to monitor tooth movement
- Serve as pre- and post-treatment comparison motivating tool
- Prediction values from different analysis
- Help judge between extraction and non-extraction cases
- Lingual occlusion can be visualised.

Model Analyses for Permanent Dentition

- Pont's index
- Linder Harth index
- Korkhaus analysis
- Arch perimeter analysis
- Carey's analysis
- Bolton tooth size ratio
- Ashley Howe's analysis
- Peck and Peck index.

Pont's Index

In 1909, Pont devised a method of pre-determining an ideal arch width based on the mesio-distal width of the crown of the maxillary incisors. Pont suggested that the ratio of combined incisors to transverse arch width was ideally 0.8% in bicuspid area and 0.64% in first molar area. He also suggested that the maxillary arch be expanded 1–2 mm more during treatment than is ideal to allow for relapse.

Procedure

- Measure the mesio-distal width of maxillary central and lateral incisors on either side **(Fig. 14.1)**
- Sum up the mesio-distal width of left upper central incisor, right upper lateral incisor let the value be "X"
- Measure the arch width in premolar region from the distal pits of upper first premolars
- Measure the arch width in molar region from the mesial pits of upper first permanent molar **(Fig. 14.2)**
- Calculate the ideal arch width in premolar region using the formula $\frac{X}{8} \times 100$
- Calculate the ideal arch width in molar region using the formula $\frac{X}{64} \times 100$.

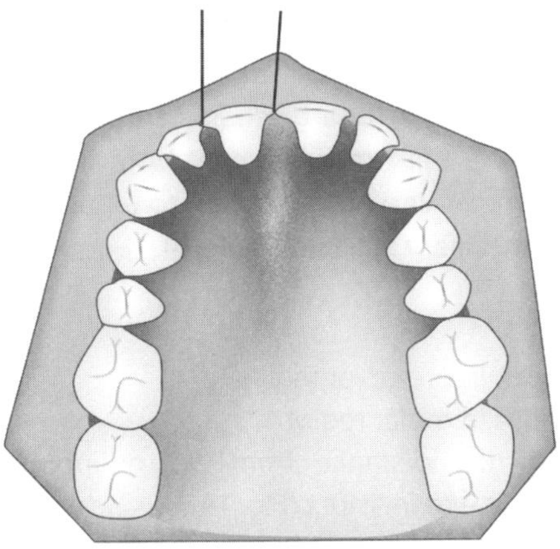

Fig. 14.1: Determination of the mesio-distal width of maxillary central incisor

Inference

- If the calculated value is greater than the measured value, then the arch is narrow for the sum of incisors width and the arch needs expansion
- If the measured value is greater than the calculated value, then the arch is wider for the sum of incisors width and there is no scope for expansion.

Drawbacks

- This analysis is based on the study of French population and hence, its universal validity is questionable
- This analysis does not take into consideration the alignment of teeth
- This analysis does not consider the malformation of the teeth for example, peg laterals.

Linder Harth Index

It is similar to Pont's index and is used to determine dental arch width in the premolar and molar regions.

As the study is carried out over German population, a different set of standards have been proposed, while the basic procedure is same.

$$\text{Anterior arch width} = \frac{\text{S.I.} \times 100}{85}$$

$$\text{Posterior arch width} = \frac{\text{S.I.} \times 100}{65},$$

where S.I. is the sum of incisors.

Korkhaus Analysis

- This analysis is similar to Pont's analysis
- Korkhaus used Linder Harth's measurements
- An orthometer was devised by Korkhaus and from that ideal arch width in premolar region and molar region can be determined
- The perpendicular distance from the inter-premolar line to the incisor for a given S.I can be determined.He introduced a third measurement from the midpoint of inter-premolar line of upper arch to a point in between the two maxillary incisors **(Table 14.1)**.

Measurements

- Arch width in premolar region
- Arch width in molar region
- Perpendicular distance from the midpoint of inter-premolar line to incisiors **(Fig. 14.3)**
- For a particular width of incisors there is a specific value of distance from the incision to the inter-premolar line according to Korkhaus **(Fig. 14.4)**.

Inference

- This analysis tells about the arch width. If the perpendicular distance is more than ideal, then anterior teeth are proclined
- If the perpendicular distance is less than the ideal, then the anterior teeth are retroclined
- For the values noted the mandibular value (Ll) should be equal to the maxillary value (Lu) in millimeters minus 2 mm **(Fig. 14.5)**.

Arch Perimeter Analysis

This analysis helps to find out the difference between the basal bone and the tooth material in maxilla.

Upper Arch Procedure

- Measure the mesio-distal width of all the teeth from the second premolar on one side to the second premolar on the other side and sum it up. This gives us the tooth material or the space required
- Measure the arch perimeter using brass wire from the mesio-buccal line angle of maxillary first permanent molar and pass the wire along the contact of premolar, and

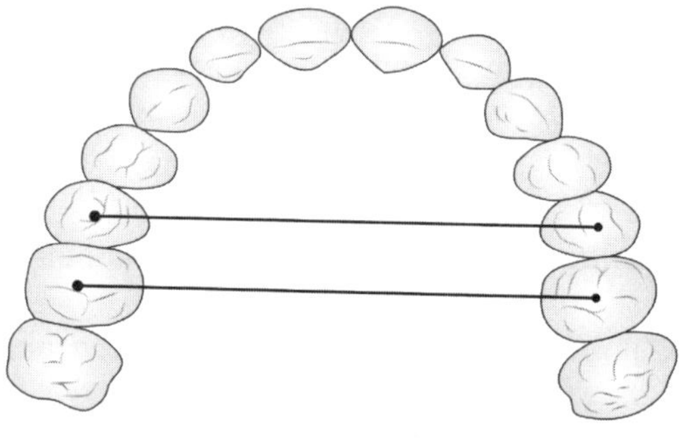

Fig. 14.2: Determination of arch width in molar region

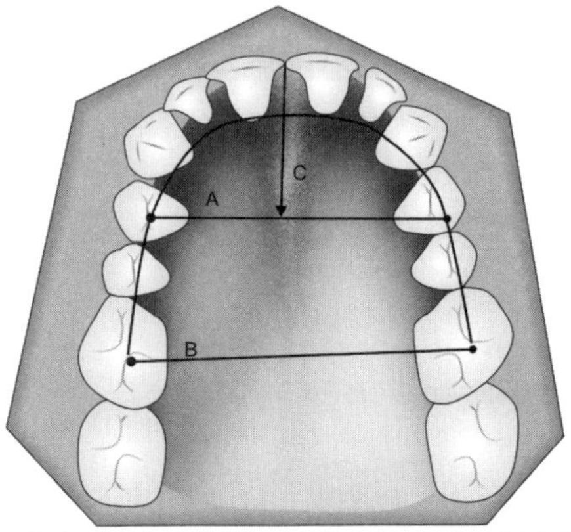

Fig. 14.3: A: Arch width in premolars, B: Arch width in molars, C: Perpendicular distance from midpoint of inter-premolar line to incisiors

Table 14.1: Korkhaus measurements

S. No.	Sum of incisors (in mm)	Arch width in premolar region (in mm)	Arch width in molar region (in mm)	Perpendicular distance form incision to inter-premolar line (in mm)
1.	27	32	41.5	16
2.	27.5	32.5	42.3	16.3
3.	28	33	43	16.5
4.	28.5	33.5	43.8	16.8
5.	29	34	44.5	17
6.	29.5	34.7	45.3	17.3
7.	30	35.5	46	17.5
8.	30.5	36	46.8	17.8
9.	31	36.5	47.5	18
10.	31.5	37	48.5	18.3
11.	32	37.5	49	18.5
12.	32.5	38.2	50	18.8
13.	33	39	51	19
14.	33.5	39.5	51.5	19.3
15.	34	40	52.5	19.5
16.	34.5	40.5	53	19.8
17.	35	41.2	54	20
18.	35.5	42	54.5	20.5
19.	36	42.5	55.5	21

through the incisive papilla on an imaginary repositioned arch from, and through premolar of the opposite side up to mesio-buccal line angle of maxillary first permanent molar. **(Fig. 14.6)**

- In case of proclined anteriors, the wire is passed along the cingulum of anterior teeth
- If the anterior teeth are retroclined, the brass wire in the anterior segment passes labial to the teeth
- If the anterior teeth are well aligned the wire passes over the incisal edge of anteriors
- By comparing the tooth material and arch length required, we can obtain the extent of arch length discrepancy
- If the tooth material is more than the space available there can be crowding/space shortage
- If the tooth material is less than the space available, then there can be spacing/space excess.

Inference

- It is between 0 mm and 2.5 mm—non-extraction case
- If it is between 2.5 mm and 5 mm—extraction of second premolar is recommended
- If it is more than 5 mm—extraction of first premolar is recommended.

Carey's Analysis (Mandible)

- Measure the mesio-distal width of all the teeth from the second premolar on one side to the second premolar of the other side and sum it up. This gives us the tooth material or space required
- Take a brass wire, place it on the mesio-buccal line angle of lower first permanent molar and pass it along the buccal cusp tips of premolars and the cingula of aligned anterior teeth and pass it along the buccal cusp tips of premolars up to the mesio-buccal line angle of the opposite side lower first permanent molar. This gives us the space available.

Inference

Depending upon the space shortage, line of suggested treatment planning is as follows:

- If it is between 0 mm and 2.5 mm—non-extraction case
- If it is between 2.5 mm and 5 mm—extraction of second premolar is recommended
- If it is more than 5 mm—extraction of first premolar is recommended.

Bolton Tooth Size Ratio

According to Bolton, there exists a ratio between the mesio-distal widths of maxillary and mandibular teeth. The Bolton's analysis helps in determining disproportion in size between maxillary and mandibular teeth.

He devised a procedure for determining the ratio of total mandibular versus maxillary tooth size and anterior mandibular versus anterior maxillary tooth size.

Study of these ratios helps in examining:

- The overjet and overbite relationship that will likely be obtained after treatment is finished
- The effects of contemplated extraction of posterior occlusion and incisor relationship
- And the identification of occlusal misfit produced by interarch tooth size incompatibilities.

Procedure

Measure the mesio-distal width of:

654321	123456
654321	123456

Determination of Overall Ratio

According to Bolton, the sum of mesio-distal widths of the mandibular teeth anterior to the second permanent molar is 91.3% the mesio-distal widths of the maxillary teeth mesial to the second molars.

$$\text{Overall ratio} = \frac{\text{Sum of mandibular 12}}{\text{Sum of maxillary 12}} \times 100$$

- Ratio is less than 91.3% shows maxillary tooth material excess
- Ratio more than 91.3% shows mandibular tooth material excess.

Determination of Anterior Ratio

The sum of mesio-distal width of the mandibular anteriors to the mesio-distal width of the maxillary anteriors should be 77.2%.

$$\text{Anterior ratio} = \frac{\text{Sum of mandibular 12}}{\text{Sum of maxillary 12}} \times 100$$

- Ratio less than 77.2%, shows maxillary anterior excess
- Ratio more than 77.2%, shows mandibular anterior excess.

If the anterior ratio exceeds 77.2%, the discrepancy is in excessive mandibular anterior. From the standard chart given by Bolton; locate the patient's maxillary 6 measurement and check for the mandibular value for the same. It is the correct mandibular measurement.

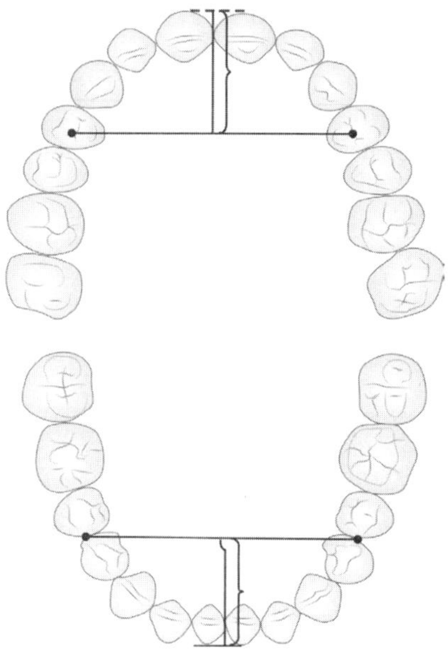

Fig. 14.4: Korkhaus Analysis

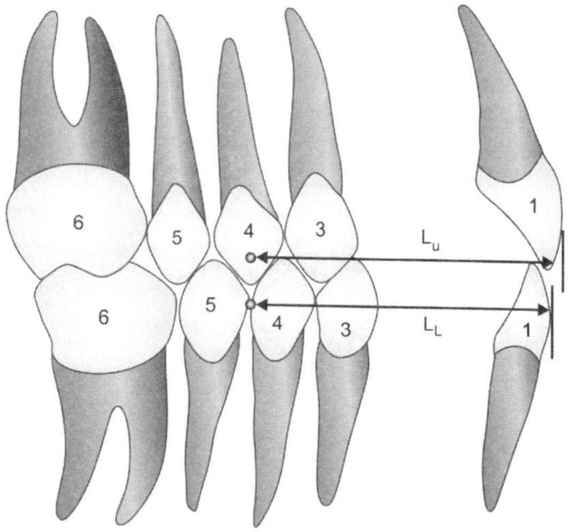

Fig. 14.5: Maxillary (Lu) and Mandibular Values (Ll)

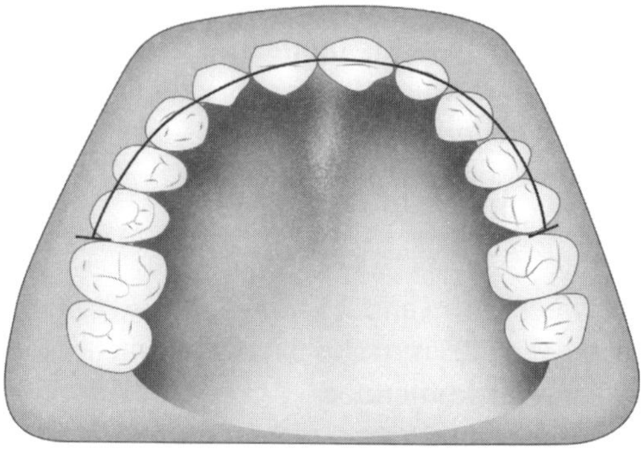

Fig. 14.6: Arch Perimeter

Table 14.2: Bolton values for maxillary and mandibular 6 anterior teeth

Sum mandibular 6 ______ mm = Anterior Ratio × 100 = ______ % Anterior Ratio				Mean	77.2 = 0.22
Sum maxillary 6 ______ mm.				S.D.	(s) 1.65
				Range	74.5 – 80.4

Maxillary 6	Mandibular 6	Maxillary 6	Mandibular 6	Maxillary 6	Mandibular 6
40.0	30.9	45.5	35.1	50.5	39.0
40.5	31.3	46.0	35.5	51.0	39.4
41.0	31.7	46.5	35.9	51.5	39.8
41.5	32.0	47.0	36.3	52.0	40.1
42.0	32.4	47.5	36.7	52.5	40.5
42.5	32.8	48.0	37.1	53.0	40.9
43.0	33.2	48.5	37.4	53.5	41.3
43.5	33.6	49.0	37.8	54.0	41.7
44.0	34.0	49.5	38.2	54.5	42.1
44.5	34.4	50.0	38.6	55.0	42.5
45.0	34.7				

Table 14.3: Bolton values for maxillary and mandibular 12 teeth.

Sum mandibular 12 ______ mm = Anterior Ratio × 100 = ______ % Ove-all Ratio				Mean	91.3 = 0.26
Sum maxillary 12 ______ mm.				S.D.	(s) 1.91
				Range	87.5 – 94.8

Maxillary 12	Mandibular 12	Maxillary 12	Mandibular 12	Maxillary 12	Mandibular 12
66	77.6	94	85.8	103	94.0
86	78.5	95	86.7	104	95.0
87	79.4	96	87.6	105	95.9
88	80.3	97	88.6	106	96.8
89	81.3	98	89.5	107	97.8
90	82.1	99	90.4	108	98.6
91	83.1	100	91.3	109	99.5
92	84.0	101	92.2	110	100.4
93	84.9	102	93.1		

The difference between the actual and correct mandibular measurement is the amount of excessive arch length (**Table 14.2**).

If the overall ratio is more than 77.2%, Actual mandibular 6 (mm)—ideal mandibular 6 (mm) = excess.

If the overall ratio is less than 77.2%, Actual maxillary 6 (mm)—ideal maxillary 6 = excess.

If the overall ratio exceeds 91.3%, the discrepancy is in excessive mandibular overall teeth size. From the standard chart given by Bolton (**Table 14.3**); locate the patient's maxillary 12 measurement and opposite; it is the correct mandibular measurement. The difference between the actual and correct mandibular measurement is the amount of excessive arch length.

If the overall ratio is more than 91.3%, Actual mandibular 12 (mm)—ideal mandibular 12 (mm) = difference.

If the overall ratio is less than 91.3%, Actual maxillary 12—ideal maxillary 12 = difference.

Table 14.4: Values of the index ($\frac{MD}{FL} \times 100$) for the mandibular incisors

Group (famale)	N	Mean	SD	Range	d	t
Central incisors						
Prrfect alignment	90	88.4	4.3	78.2 – 97.7		
					6.0	9.30*
Control populatiom	130	94.4	4.9	80.0 – 105.3		
Lateral incisors						
Prrfect alignmen	90	90.4	4.8	78.0 – 101.9		
					6.4	9.27*
Control populatiom	130	96.8	5.2	85.7 – 112.7		

N = Number of teeth.
d = Difference between the means.
*Very highly significant difference, $p < 0.001$.
SD = Standard deviaion.
t = test value.

Peck and Peck Analysis or Index

Harvey Peck and Sheldon Peck present a new method of detecting and evaluating tooth shape deviations of the mandibular incisors **(Table 14.4)**.

It is based on the observation that the persons with ideal incisal arrangement have smaller mesio-distal width and comparatively larger labio-lingual width than in person's with incisal crowding.

Procedure

- Measure the mesio-distal width of lower incisor individuals
- Measure the labio-lingual width of lower incisors individually
- Then the ratio of mesio-distal width and labio-lingual width is to be calculated separately for lower centrals and laterals.

$$\text{Index} = \frac{\text{Mesio-distal}}{\text{Facio-lingual (FL)/Labio-lingual (LL)}} \times 100$$

- MD/FL index as a numerical expression of crown shape as viewed incisally is confined to the mandibular incisors
- And this can be compared with ideal mean values.

Ideal mean values:

- For lower centrals—88–92%
- Lower laterals—90–95%.

Inference

- Lower incisors within or below these ranges are considered favourably shaped
- Lower incisors with MD/FL index above these ranges considered to have crown shape deviations contributing to crowding phenomenon
- If the calculated value is greater than mean value it is suggestive of the fact that mesio-distal width is more than labio-lingual width
- Hence, proximal stripping can be indicated, to relieve the crowding and thereby to alter the ratio so that it is in favourable range for long-term post-retention stability.

Ashley Howe's Analysis

- Ashley Howe considered tooth crowding to be due to deficiency in arch width rather than arch length
- He found a relationship between total width of 12 teeth anterior to the second molars and the width of the dental arch in the first premolar region
- Howe's (1944, 1954) devised a formula for determining whether the apical bases (or basal arches) could accommodate the patient's teeth.

Procedure

Measure the mesio-distal width of:

123456	123456
123456	123456

- Sum up the mesio-distal width separately for upper and lower teeth—tooth material(TM)
- Premolar diameter (PMD) is measured from the buccal cusp tips of the first premolars on one side to the buccal cusp tip on the other side.

Premolar Diameter Basal Arch Length

- Premolar basal arch width (PMBAW) or canine width is measured from the root apices of the first premolar on one side to the first premolar on the other side

Table 14.5: Ashley Howe's Analysis

	Upper	Lower
Tooth material	85-98	78.5-89
Premolar Diameter PMD TM	39-45 43.5-48.5	31-37.5 39.5-43
Premolar basal Arch width PMBAW/TM %	40.5-48 45.5-51.5	37.543.5 45.5-51.5
Basal arch length BAL % TM	29.5-36.5 32.5-39.5	29-34.5 35.5-39

- Basal arch length is the perpendicular distance from the tangent drawn on the distal aspect of the first permanent molar to the anterior limit of the arch

  Calculate: $\frac{\text{PMBAW}}{\text{TM}} \times 100$
- Compare the values with the standard values given by Howe (**Table 14.5**).

Inference

- If PMD is greater than PMBAW, expansion is contraindicated
- If PMBAW is greater than PMD, expansion is indicated
- If $\frac{\text{PMBAW}}{\text{TM}} \times 100$
- Is less than 37% Howe considered it as a basal arch deficiency case requiring.

Extraction of teeth to manage the case:

- If it is 44%, it is an ideal case and extraction is not required
- If it is between 37 and 44% it is a borderline case, which may/may not require extraction
- If it is less then 37%, extraction is required.

Question 2

What are the different mixed dentition analyses?

Answer

Mixed Dentition Analyses

- Huckaba's analysis
- Hixon and Oldfathers method
- Tanaka and Johnston analysis
- Nance and Carey's analysis
- Moyer's mixed dentition analysis
- Total space analysis.

Huckaba's Analysis (Radiographic Method)

- He uses both study casts and radiograph for determining the width of unerupted tooth
- With any type of radiograph, it is necessary to compensate for enlargement of the radiographic image. This can be done by measuring an object that can be seen both in radiograph and on the cast, such as primary tooth. A simple proportional relationship can then be established as follows:

$$\frac{\text{Actual width of primary molar (X1)}}{\text{Apparent width of primary molar (X2)}}$$

$$\frac{\text{Apparent width of primary molar (X2)}}{\frac{\text{Actual width of un erupted premolar (Y1)}}{\text{Apparent width of unerupted premolar (Y2)}}}$$

$$\text{Or } Y1 = \frac{X1 \times Y2}{X2}$$

- Accuracy of this method of determining the width of the unerupted tooth is fair to good, depending upon the quality of the radiographs and this position in the arch
- This technique can be used in maxillary and mandibular arches for all entire groups.

Hixon and Oldfather's Method

- The mesio-distal width of the mandibular central and lateral incisor is obtained from the casts
- The width of the premolars is determined from the intra-oral periapical radiographs made using long cone technique
- Sum up the width of the central and lateral incisor along with the width of unerupted premolars of that particular side
- The estimated sum total width of the cuspids and bicuspids of that particular side can be obtained from the following. Every measured sum width of incisors and bicuspids has a corresponding sum width of the cuspids and bicuspids in the following Table.

Measured values in mm		Estimated tooth size
46	→	18.4
47	→	18.7
48	→	19.0
49	→	19.4
50	→	19.7
51	→	20.0
52	→	20.3
53	→	20.7
54	→	21.0
55	→	21.3

56 ⟶ 21.6
57 ⟶ 22.0
58 ⟶ 22.3
59 ⟶ 22.6
⟶

Moyer's Mixed Dentition Analysis

Basis for Moyer's Mixed Dentition Analysis

There is high correlation among the sizes of different groups of teeth in a particular individual. Thus, by measuring one group of teeth, it is possible to make a prediction of the size of other groups of teeth with a fair degree of accuracy.

Procedure

- The sum mesio-distal width of the mandibular incisors is measured
- Align the mandibular incisor well on the cast and then measure the space left for the cuspids and bicuspids on either side separately from the distal aspect of the aligned lateral incisor to the distal aspect of the first permanent molars
- Similarly align the maxillary incisors on the cast and then measure the space left in the arch for the cuspids and bicuspids
- Using the Moyer's probability chart, the sum total of mesio-distal width of upper and lower cuspids and bicuspids from upper and lower charts is found out respectively, for the given sum width of the lower central and lateral incisors at 75% probability **(Table 14.6).**
  - The space available and space required in all the four quadrants are compared to determine the arch length discrepancy.

Reason for Choosing the Mandibular Incisors

- They erupt first and offer the earliest opportunity of measurement
- They are less variable and more reliable than maxillary incisor.

Advantage

- It has minimal error and the range of possible error is precisely known
- It can be done with equal reliability either by a beginner or by an expert
- It is not time—consuming
- It requires no special equipment
- It can be done in the mouth as well on the cast
- It may be used for both the arches.

Tanaka and Johnston Analysis

This method is used for quick chair side prediction of the size of unerupted canines and premolars.

Method

- Calculate ½ of M-D width of lower incisors
- Add 10.5 mm to predict combined width of mandibular cuspid and bicuspid
- Add 11 mm to predict combined width of maxillary cuspid and bicuspid
- Compute the amount of space left in the arch for molar adjustment by subtracting the space required from space available.

Predicted width of maxillary canine and premolar =

$$\frac{\text{Sum of mandibular incisors} + 11}{2}$$

Predicted width of mandibular canine and premolar =

$$\frac{\text{Sum of mandibular incisors} + 10.5}{2}$$

Procedure in the Maxillary Arch

The procedure is similar to that for lower arch width except:

- A different predictability chart is used for predicting the sum of upper cuspid and bicuspid
- Allowance must be made for overjet correction when measuring the space to be occupied by the aligned incisors.

Table 14.6: Moyer's prediction values at 75% level

Total mandibular Incisor width	19.5 20.0 20.5 21.0 21.5 22.0 22.5 23.0 23.5 24.0 24.5
Width of 3 4 5 (male)	20.6 20.9 21.2 21.3 21.8 22.0 22.3 22.6 22.9 23.1 23.4
Width of 3 4 5 (female)	20.1 20.4 20.7 21.0 21.3 21.6 21.9 22.2 22.5 22.8 23.1
Total maxillary incisor width	25.0 25.5 26.0 26.5 27.0 27.5 28.0 25.5 29.0
Width of 3 4 5 (male)	23.7 24.0 24.2 24.5 24.8 25.0 25.3 25.6 25.9
Width of 3 4 5 (female)	23.4 23.7 24.0 24.3 24.6 24.8 25.1 25.4 25.7

Nance Carey's Analysis

This analysis is similar to arch perimeter analysis of the permanent dentition.

Procedure

- Measure the mesio-distal width of the erupted permanent teeth
- The width of each unerupted tooth, cuspids and bicuspids is measured from the intra—oral periapical radiographs
  - The total mesio-distal width of all the teeth in each quadrant will indicate space required to accommodate the permanent teeth
  - Using brass wire, measure the arch perimeter
  - Compare the space required and space available to arrive at the arch length discrepancy.

Total Space Analysis

Total space analysis was developed by Levern Merrified of the Tweed foundation in order to overcome certain disadvantages of conventional dental oriented mixed dentition analysis.

- This method divided the lower dental arch into three areas, i.e., anterior, middle and posterior—to analyse the space requirement in the lower arch, measurements form the study casts and cephalograms are used in this analysis
- This discrepancy for each area has to be calculated and the resultant value is added together to yield the discrepancy of the arch.

Anterior Area

- Space required
  - Measure the width of the mandibular incisors on the casts and the width of the cuspids from the radiographs
  - Cephalometric correction for the incisor positioning is calculated according to the Tweed's method. Frankfort mandibular incisor angle (FMIA) is taken into consideration instead of incisor mandibular plane angle (IMPA) of Tweed. The incisors are repositioned and the difference in the actual and proposed FMIA is determined. The difference is angulation is multiplied by 0.8 to get the difference in millimeteres
  - Soft tissue modification: Upper lip thickness was measured from the vermilion border of the upper lip to the greatest curvature of the labial surface of the central incisors. The total chin thickness was measured from the soft tissue chin to the N-B line
  - If the lip thickness was greater than chin thickness, the difference was determined and multiplied by 2 and added to the space required. If it was less than or equal to chin thickness, no soft tissue modification was necessary
  - Measure the 'Z' angle of Merrifield and add the cephalometric correction to it. If the corrected 'Z' angle was greater than 80° the mandibular incisor angulation was modified as necessary (up to an IMPA of approximately, 92° degrees). If the corrected angle was less than 75° degrees, additional uprighting of the mandibular incisor was necessary.

Space available: Measure the space available by using a brass wire from the mesio-buccal line angle of first primary molar of one side to the other.

Middle Area

- Measure the mesio-distal width of the first permanent molars on the cast and measure the width of the unerupted premolar from the radiographs
- Curve of occlusion : A flat object is placed on the occlusal surface of mandibular teeth contacting the incisors and the first permanent molars. The deepest point between this flat surface and the occlusal surface of primary molars was measured on both the sides
- The following formula was applied to known the space required for flattening the curve of occlusion.

$$\frac{\text{Depth on right side + depth of left side + 5 mm}}{2}$$

Space available: Space available is measured using a brass wire from the mesio-buccal line angle of first primary molar to the disto-buccal line angle of first permanent molar on either side.

Posterior Area

Space required: Mesio-distal width of second and the third molars is obtained from the radiographs as they might be unerupted. If the molars are not visible on the radiographs, Wheeler's method issued for calculation, i.e.,

$$X = \frac{Y - X^1}{Y^1}$$

Where

X = Estimated value of the third molar in the individual patient
Y = Actual size of permanent mandibular
X1 = Wheeler's value of third molars
Y1 = Wheeler's value for first molars.

Space available: The amount of space available consisted of space presently available on the casts and the estimated increase.

Space presently available: This was obtained by measuring the distance on the occlusal plane tangent to distal surface of first permanent molars to the anterior border of ramus on a lateral cephalogram.

Estimated increase or Prediction: The estimated increase in 3 mms per year, i.e., 1.5 mms on either side until 14 years of age in girls and 16 years in boys. The age of the patient is subtracted from 14 or 16 according to the sex of the patient and is multiplied by 3 to obtain the estimated increase.

Total space deficit/discrepancy: The total deficit or the discrepancy is derived by comparing the space required and space available in anterior, middle and posterior areas. Thus this analysis tells us precisely where the discrepancy is present, i.e., in the anterior, middle or the posterior areas.

CHAPTER 15

Biology of Tooth Movement

LONG ESSAYS

Question 1

Describe the theories of tooth movement?

Answer

There are three main theories of tooth movement:

1. The bioelectric theory.
2. Pressure tension theory.
3. Fluid dynamic theory.

Bioelectric Theory

It is proposed by Farrar in 1876.

It has been shown that distortion of cells and extracellular matrix is associated with alteration in tissue and cellular electric potentials.

Bones generally have a remarkable ability to remodel their structure in such a way that the stress is optimally resisted.

It has been hypothesised that mechanical deformation of the crystalline structure of the hydroxyapatite and the crystalline structure of collagen induce migration of electrons that generate local electric fields. This phenomenon is called "piezoelectricity".

- Such signals die away quickly even though the force is maintained
- But when the force is released and the crystal lattice returns to the original shape, a reverse flow of electrons occurs. Rhythmic activity would cause a rhythmic flow of electrons in both directions
- Cells are sensitive to this piezoelectric effect. It has been assumed that bending of bone may create negative fields occurring in the concave aspect of the bone surface leading to deposition.

Areas of convexity are associated with positive charges and evoke bone resorption. Further, ions in the fluids surrounding the living bone interact with these electrical fields. These currents of small voltages are called "streaming potentials" **(Fig. 15.1)**.

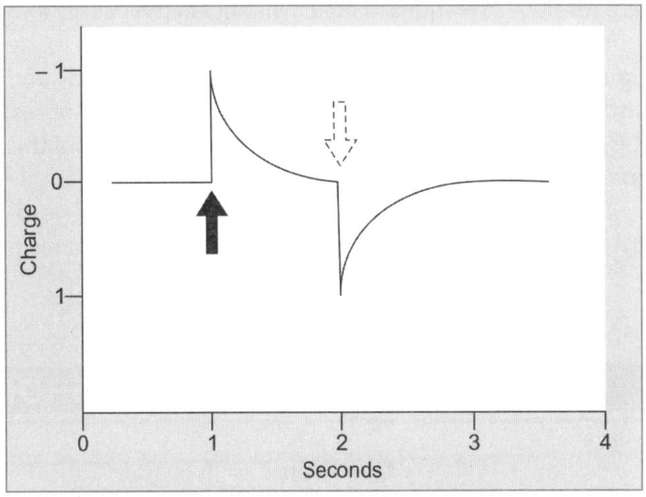

Fig. 15.1: Areas of convexity with positive charges and evoke bone resorption

Recent in vivo experiments conducted by Roberts et al. have revealed that a negative electrical field is created in the areas where the periodontal ligament (PDL) is widened.

Pressure Tension Theory

This classic hypothesis on the mechanism of tooth movement, based on the work of Oppenheim (1911), Sandstedt (1905), and Schwarz (1932), postulate the movement of the tooth within the periodontal space, generating a "pressure" side and a "tension" side.

Schwarz hypothesized that the PDL space is a continuous hydrostatic system, and forces applied to this environment by means of mastication or orthodontic appliances create a hydrostatic pressure that would be, in accordance with Pascal's law, transmitted equally to all regions of the PDL.

On the "pressure" side, cell replication is said to decrease as a result of vascular constriction, causing bone resorption.

On the "tension" side, cell replication is said to increase because of the stimulation offered by the stretching of the fibre bundles of the PDL, thus causing bone deposition.

In terms of fibre content, the PDL on the "pressure" side is said to display disorganisation and diminution of fibre production, while on the "tension" side, fibre production is said to be stimulated.

Fluid Dynamic Theory (Bien 1966)

This theory is also called the blood flow theory as proposed by Bien. According to this theory, tooth movement occurs as a result of alterations in fluid dynamics in the PDL.

The periodontal space contains a fluid system made up of interstitial fluid, cellular elements, blood vessels and viscous ground substance in addition to periodontal fibres. It is a confined space and passage of fluid, in and out of this space is limited.

The contents of the PDL thus create a unique hydrodynamic condition resembling a hydraulic mechanism and a shock absorber. When the force is removed, the fluid is replenished by diffusion from capillary walls and recirculation of interstitial fluid.

But when a force of greater magnitude and duration is applied during orthodontic tooth movement, the interstitial fluid in the periodontal space gets squeezed out and moves towards the apex and cervical margins which results in decreased tooth movement. This is called the "squeeze film effect" as proposed by Bien.

When an orthodontic force is applied, it results in compression of the PDL. Blood vessels of the PDL gets trapped between the principal fibres and this results in their stenosis.

Bien suggested that there is an alteration in the chemical environment at the site of vascular stenosis due to a decreased oxygen level in the compressed areas as compared to the tension side.

The formation of these aneurysms and vascular stenosis causes blood gases to escape into the interstitial fluid thereby creating a favourable local environment for resorption.

SHORT ESSAY

Question 1

What are the histologic changes seen during orthodontic tooth movement?

Answer

When orthodontic force is applied upon the tooth to carry out orthodontic tooth movement, areas of pressure and areas of tension are generated around the tooth depending to direction of force.

Areas of pressure are generated in the direction of tooth movement whereas areas of tension are formed in the opposite direction.

Bone resorbs in the areas of pressure while bone gets deposited in the areas of tension.

Histologic changes seen during orthodontic tooth movement can be broadly classified in two headings:

1. Changes seen upon application of mild forces.
2. Changes seen upon application of heavy forces.

Changes upon Application of Mild Forces

As described earlier areas of pressure and areas of tension are seen after application of any kind of force.

Changes on Pressure Side

- The periodontal ligament (PDL) gets compressed to one-third of original thickness in the direction of tooth movement
- Vascularity increases due to increase in capillary blood supply
- Increased vascularity leads to increased mobilisation of fibroblasts and osteoclasts
- Bone resorbing cells/osteoclasts are lined along the socket wall on the pressure side in shallow depression called Howship's lacunae
- Orientation of bony trabeculae changes from being parallel to long axis of tooth to being parallel to direction of application of orthodontic force, i.e., horizontal to long axis of tooth
- This change revert backs to being parallel during the retention phase post-orthodontic therapy
- When the forces applied are within physiologic limits, the resorption is seen in the alveolar bone immediately adjacent to the ligament
- This is known as frontal resorption.

Changes on Tension Side

- This is the side opposite to the direction of force
- In the area upon application of force, the PDL membrane gets stretched leading to increase in the distance between alveolar process and the tooth
- There is an increase in the vascularity which causes mobilisation of cells like fibroblasts and osteoblasts
- The traction force leads to the formation of osteoid by the osteoblasts adjacent to the lamina dura. This osteoid is lightly calcified and in due course of time it matures into woven bone.

Secondary Remodelling Changes

In addition to the osteoclastic and osteoblastic activity on the pressure side and tension side respectively, bony changes are seen elsewhere to maintain the width or thickness of the alveolar bone. These changes are referred to as secondary remodelling changes.

Changes upon Application of Heavy/ Extreme Forces

When extreme forces are applied on tooth/teeth, it causes crushing or complete compression of the PDL leading to necrosis.

On the Pressure Side

- The root of the teeth closely approximates the lamina dura thus, compressing the PDL leading to occlusion of blood vessels. Due to reduced blood supply because of occlusion of blood vessels, the PDL is deprived of the nutritional supply leading to hyalinisation
- In such cases, the bone does not resorb in the frontal portion adjacent to the teeth, rather resorption is seen in the adjacent marrow spaces and in the alveolar bone below, i.e., behind and above hyalinised zone. This kind of resorption is termed as undermining or rearward resorption.

On the Tension Side

- The PDL gets over stretched leading to tearing of blood vessels and ischemia
- Thus, on application of extreme forces there is net increase in osteoclastic activity as compared to osteoblastic activity, leading to loosening of tooth within the socket
- In addition, pain and hyperaemia of gingiva may also occur due to application of extreme forces during the orthodontic treatment.

Question 2

What is hyalinisation?

Answer

During the crucial stage of the initial application of force, compression in limited areas of the membrane frequently impedes vascular circulation and cell differentiation, causing degradation of the cells and vascular stimulus rather than proliferation and differentiation. The tissue reveals a glass-like appearance in light microscopy—Hyalinisation.

Hyalinisation is caused partly by anatomic and partly by mechanical factors, and is almost unavoidable in the initial period of tooth movement in clinical orthodontics. It represents a sterile necrotic area, generally limited to 1 or 2 mm in diameter.

The process displays three main stages:

1. Degeneration.
2. Elimination of the destroyed tissue.
3. Establishment of a new tooth attachment.

Degeneration starts where the pressure is highest and the narrowing of the membrane is most pronounced, i.e., around bony spicules. It may be limited to parts of the membrane or extend from the root surface to the alveolar bone. Electron microscopy has shown that advanced cellular and vascular changes may occur within a few hours of the application of the force. Retardation of the blood flow is followed by disintegration of the vessel walls and degradation of blood elements, all occurring by mechanisms different from those seen during physiologic breakdown.

In hyalinised zones the cells cannot differentiate into osteoclasts and no bone resorption can take place from the PDL membrane. Tooth movement stops until the adjacent alveolar bone has been resorbed, the hyalinised structures removed and the area repopulated by cells. A limited hyalinised area occurring during the application of light forces may be expected to persist from 2–4 weeks in a young patient. When high density is present, the duration is longer.

The peripheral areas of the hyalinised compressed tissues are eliminated by an invasion of cells and blood vessels from the adjacent undamaged PDL. The hyalinised materials are ingested by the phagocytic activity of macrophages and are completely removed.

The adjacent alveolar bone is removed by indirect resorption of cells that have differentiated into osteoclasts on the surface of adjacent marrow spaces.

When the orthodontic force applied to human teeth are kept within the optimal range used in orthodontic practice, the osteocytes of the alveolar bone adjacent to the hyalinised PDL reveal no signs of degeneration or cell death with necrosis of the bone.

Re-establishment of the tooth attachment in the hyalinised areas starts by synthesising new tissue elements as soon as the adjacent bone and degenerated membrane tissue have been removed. The ligament space is now wider than before treatment started, and the membranous tissue under repair is rich in cells.

SHORT NOTES

Question 1

Describe optimum orthodontic force?

Answer

Optimum orthodontic force refers to the force which carries out desired orthodontic tooth movement efficiently, i.e., rapidly with minimum tissue damage and clinical discomfort.

According to Oppenheim and Schwarz, optimum orthodontic force should be equivalent to capillary pressure or 20–26 g/cm of root surface area.

Forces which are below optimum orthodontic force does not carry out orthodontic tooth movement while forces above, lead to tissue necrosis which causes hyalinisation.

Characteristics of optimum orthodontic force clinically:

- Produces rapid orthodontic tooth movement
- Patient discomfort is minimum
- Lag phase of tooth movement is minimum
- Lack of marked mobility of tooth/teeth being moved.

Characteristics of optimum orthodontic force histologically:

- Tooth vitality and integrity of periodontal ligament is maintained
- Initiates maximum cellular response
- Produces frontal resorption.

Optimum force for various orthodontic tooth movements:

- Tipping: 35–60 g
- Rotation: 35–60 g
- Extrusion: 35–60 g
- Intrusion: 10–20 g
- Root uprighting: 50–100 g
- Bodily movement: 70–120 g.

Question 2

What are the phases of tooth movement?

Answer

The phases of tooth movement are as follows **(Fig. 15.2)**:

Initial Phase

- Rapid tooth movement over a short distance which then ceases

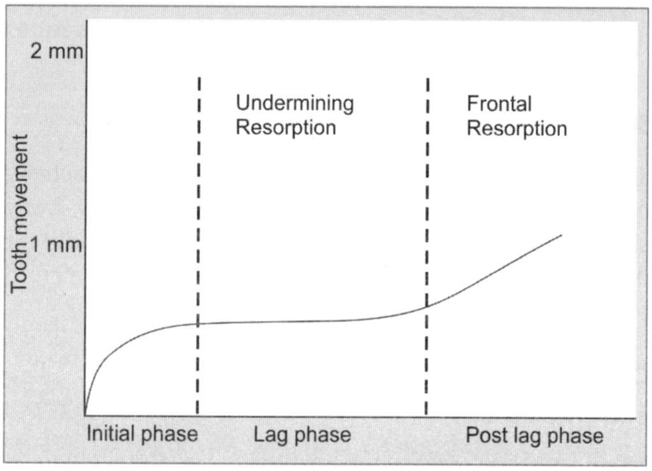

Fig. 15.2: Phases of tooth movement

- Displacement of tooth in PDL and bending of alveolar bone takes place
- In this phase, both light and heavy forces have same effect, i.e., the tooth displaces the same distance with both heavy and light forces
- During this phase, the tooth moves by approximately, 0.4–0.9 mm in a week.

Lag Phase

- Little or no tooth movement
- Formation of hyalinised tissue
- This hyalinised tissue has to be resorbed before further tooth movement takes place
- Duration of this phase depends on the amount of the force used to move the tooth
- On application of light forces, this phase is small as the amount of hyalinise tissue formed is less which as on application of heavy forces, this phase is longer because of the formation of more amount of hyalinised tissue formed
- This phase generally lasts for 2–3 weeks but may extend up to 10 weeks, depending on the amount of forces used
- Lag phase also depends on the density of alveolar bone and the age of the patient besides the amount of hyalinised tissue formed.

Post-lag Phase

- Rapid tooth movement as hyalinised tissue is removed
- Osteoclasts are found over a larger surface area which results in the resorption of bony surface facing the PDL.

Interrupted Lag Phase

Reitan initially observed that little or no movement occurs during the hyalinisation period or lag phase. But movement can occur following reactivation of spring force before undermining resorption has eliminated the hyalinised areas resulting from the previous activation. This might be termed an "interrupted lag phase".

Question 3

Illustrate biochemical reactions to orthodontic tooth movement with the help of a flowchart?

Answer

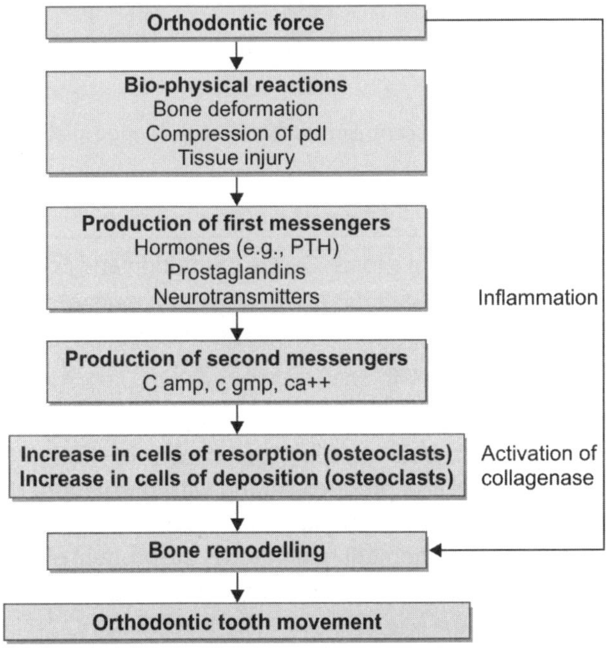

Abbreviations: PDL: Periodontal ligament; PTH: Parathyroid hormone; cAMP: Cyclic adenosine monophosphate; cGMP: Cyclic guanosine monophosphate

Question 4

Describe the different types of orthodontic forces.

Answer

"Orthodontic forces" comprises of those forces whcih affect periodontal ligament and alveolar process, whereas "orthopaedic forces" are more powerful and act on the basal parts of the jaws.

The decisive variables regarding these forces at the cellular level are application, magnitude, duration, and direction of force.

Types of Forces

Two different types of force exist:

1. Continuous (fixed appliances).
2. Intermittent (removable appliances).

Continuous Forces

- Modern fixed appliance systems are based on light continuous forces from the arch wire
- However, a continuous force may be interrupted after a limited period (interrupted continuous force), e.g. the movement that occurs when a tooth is ligated to a labial arch, the tooth being held in position after the force is no longer acting; torquing movement performed by an edgewise arch wire
- Although the typical continuous force acts for longer periods, the interrupted force is of comparatively short duration (3–4 weeks on average).

Intermittent Forces

- Such a force act during a short period and is induced primarily by removable appliances, especially functional appliances
- This also applies to springs resting on the tooth surface that produces impulses and stimuli of short duration as the appliance moves during speech and swallowing
- The intermittent action may then to a varying extent result in less compression on the pressure side and shorter hyalinisation periods, unlike elicited by continuous forces
- Experiments have shown that movement effected by an intermittent force depends on the length of time of application and on the magnitude of force
- The disadvantage of intermittent tooth movement is the mode of displacement, which always occurs in the form of tipping.

CHAPTER 16 Biomechanics

LONG ESSAYS

Question 1

Describe centre of resistance (Cres)?

Answer

- Every free body or an object can be balanced at a single point, which is known as center of gravity. At this point whole of the weight of the body is supposed to be concentrated
- The relationship of a line of action to the centre of gravity of a free body determines the movement upon application of force
- However, a tooth cannot move freely upon application of force as it is partly embedded into the socket with root being surrounded by periodontal fibres which are unevenly distributed
- In a restrained body like a tooth, a point called as center of resistance (analogous to center of gravity of a free body) is used. When a force is applied at center of resistance of a restrained body, translation occurs

The center of resistance for:

- Single-rooted tooth : along the long axis of the tooth, between one third and half of the root length apical to the alveolar crest. The level of the alveolar crest determines the center of resistance
- For a multirooted tooth : the center of resistance lies between the roots, 1 or 2 mm apical to the furcation area.

Factors influencing center of resistance are:

- Root length & morphology : teeth with longer roots will have centre of resistance away from crown as compared to teeth with shorter roots
- Number of roots
- Level of alveolar bone support : with decreased or less bone support, the centre of resistance shifts apically **(Fig. 16.1)**.

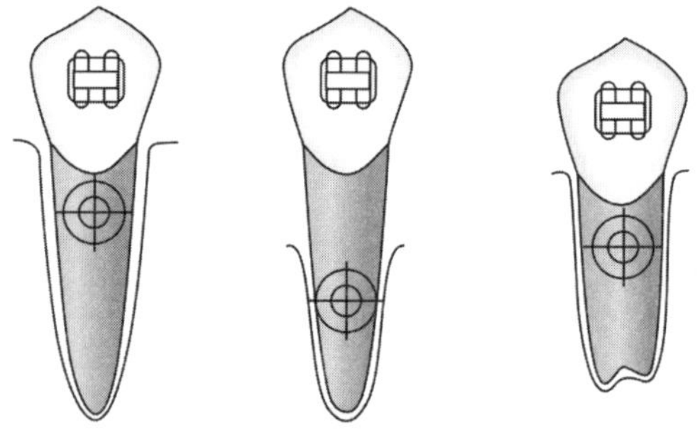

Fig. 16.1: Change in centre of resistance with change in alveolar bone level

Question 2

Describe Moment of a force, Centre of rotation and Couple?

Answer

Moment of a Force

When the line of action of force applied in a restrained body does not pass through the center of resistance, some rotation is also produced along with translation. This rotation is termed as moment.

The amount of moment generated is the product of force applied with the perpendicular distance between center of resistance and the line of action of force applied.

- Moments is depicted by curved arrows
- In two-dimensional diagrams, clockwise moment is depicted as positive while counterclockwise moment as negative
- Values can then be added together to determine the net moment on a tooth relative to a particular point, such as the center of resistance.

Centre of Rotation (Crot)

Center of rotation of a body is a point in the body on which it rotates, as determined from initial and final positions.

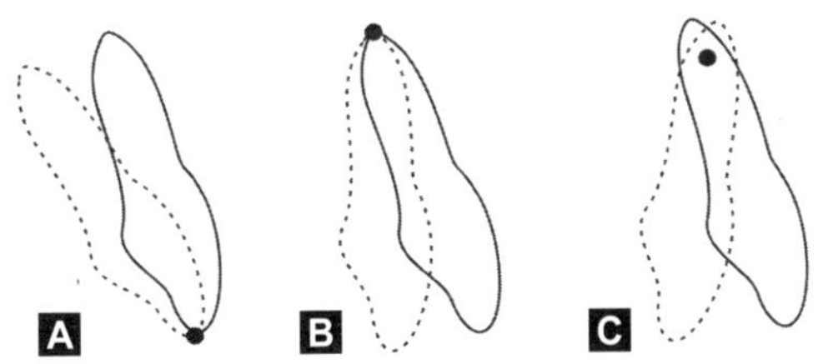

Fig. 16.2: Centre of rotation

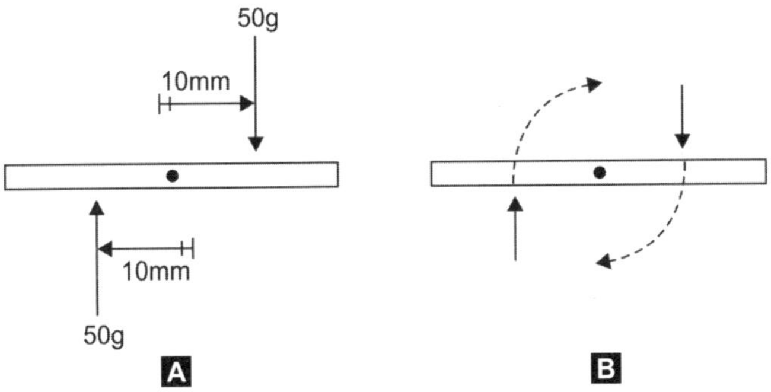

Fig. 16.3A & B: Couple and its movement

For Example

- In **Fig. 16.2A** the incisal edge is fixed, while force is applied at the apex of the tooth causing movement of only the portion apical to the incisal edge, thus, the incisal edge becomes centre of rotation.
- In **Fig. 16.2B** the root apex is fixed, and the other portion of the tooth rotates, thus making the apex as centre of rotation.
- In **Fig. 16.2C** both the apex and incisal edge are rotation opposite to each other, making the point slightly incisal to apex as centre of rotation.

Couple

- A couple consists of two equal forces in opposite direction which are parallel but non-collinear **(Fig. 16.3A)**
- The magnitude of a couple is the product of the magnitude of forces by the distance between them **(Fig. 16.3B)**.

Moment of a Couple

- It is the tendency of a couple force to produce rotation around the Cres (center of resistance)
- Direction of rotation can be determined by following the direction of either force around the Cres to the origin of opposite force.

Question 3

Discuss Tipping, Bodily movement, Intrusion and Extrusion?

Answer

Tipping

- In this tooth movement, movement of crown occurs in one direction while the root tends to move in the opposite direction
- Tipping occurs when the application of force occurs on the crown of the tooth on a single point
- Tipping tends to concentrate compression on a small periodontal area **(Fig. 16.4)**.

Uncontrolled Tipping: This takes place when the center of rotation is close or apical to the center of resistance. In this the crown and root move in opposite direction **(Fig. 16.5A)**.

Controlled Tipping: In this, the center of rotation is at the apex, thus only the crown moves in one direction while the root does not move **(Fig. 16.5B)**.

Bodily Movement

- Translatory movement of a tooth/teeth in mesio- distal or labio-lingual direction is called as bodily movement. It occurs when the applied force has two point contact on the tooth surface
- In this the tooth moves parallel to the long axis, thus the applied force is distributed over large areas of the alveolar bone

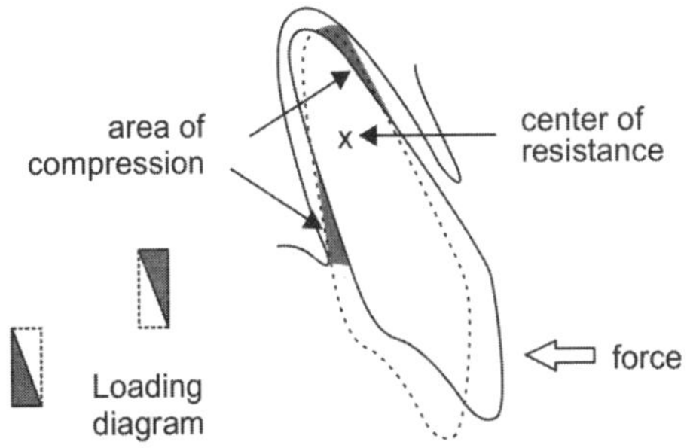

Fig. 16.4: Tipping

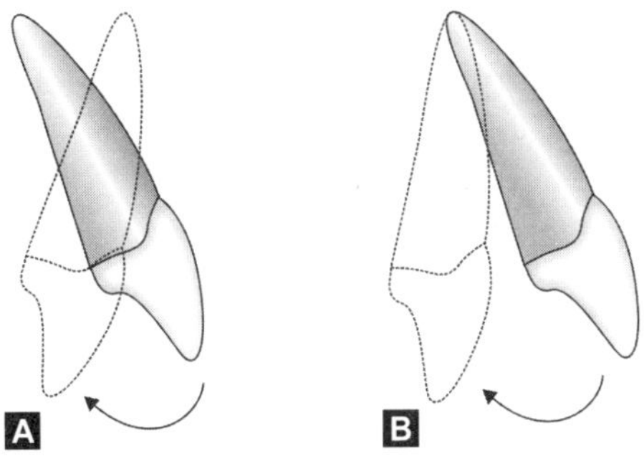

Fig. 16.5: Controlled and uncontrolled tipping

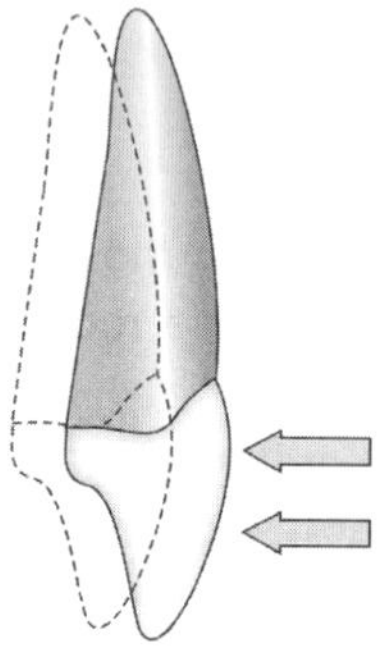

Fig. 16.6: Bodily movement in arrows depicting 2 point contact

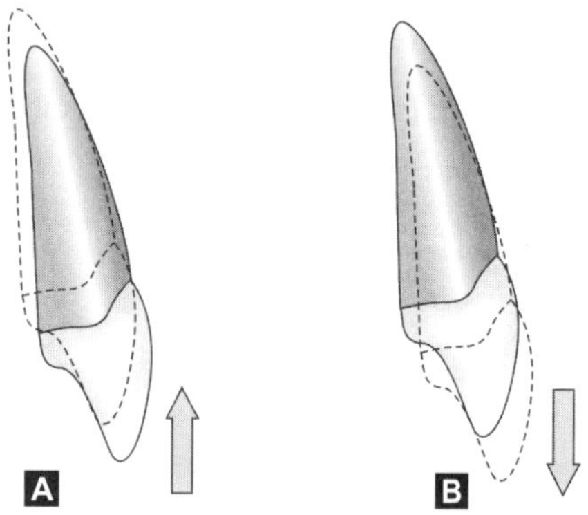

Fig. 16.7A and B: (A) Intrusion (B) Extrusion

- The hyalinesed zones produced are smaller as the force applied on single point on the bone is small as the force is distributed over a large surface area, thus allowing the resorption of the alveolar bone to occur **(Fig. 16.6)**
- The tooth movement following such applied force is quite favorable since there is steady bone resorption as well as steady periodontal fibers on the tension side.

Intrusion

- The movement in which the translation of tooth/teeth occurs along its long axis in an apical direction is termed as intrusion **(Fig. 16.7A)**
- In this, there is a high concentration of force occurring at the root apex
- Since the area of application of force is small, light force are used to carry out intrusion to prevent root resorption
- Intrusion— 10-20 gm.

Extrusion

- The movement in which the translation of tooth/teeth occurs along its long axis in an occlusal direction is termed as extrusion **(Fig. 16.7B)**
- Ideally it produces only tension and no compression. But as we extrude if the tooth tips, areas of compression are created
- Even if compressed areas could be avoided heavy forces in pure tension would be undesirable. So the force should be in the same magnitude as those for tipping
- Extrusion – 35-60 gms.

Question 4

Discuss type of Forces?

Answer

Forces can be divided as:

Continuous

Force is maintained at same appreciable fraction of the original from one patient visit to the next.

Interrupted

Force levels which decline to zero between activations. Fixed appliances that are constantly present can produce both continuous and interrupted forces.

Intermittent

Force levels decline abruptly to zero intermittently and return to original level some time later. When tooth movement occurs force levels will decrease as they would with a fixed appliance (Intermittent force could become interrupted between the adjustments of the appliance).

Intermittent forces are produced by all patient activated appliances such as:

- Removable plates
- Headgear
- Elastics

Forces generated during normal function like chewing, swallowing and speaking are also intermittent applied forces, which are not maintained for enough hours per day to have significant effect on the position of the teeth.

CHAPTER 17 Anchorage

LONG ESSAYS

Question 1

Define and classify anchorage and write in brief about each of them?

Answer

Anchorage is Defined As

- According to "Graber", Anchorage in orthodontics is defined as "the nature and degree of resistance offered by an anatomic unit for the purpose of affecting tooth movement"
- According to "White and Gardiner", it is defined as "the site of delivery from which force is exerted"
- According to "Proffit", it is defined as "resistance to unwanted tooth movement"
- According to "Moyers", it is defined as "resistance to displacement".

Classification

Moyer's Classification

I. According to the Manner of Force Application

- **Simple anchorage**: Force application tends to change axial inclination of anchor teeth
  - Resistance of anchor unit to tipping forces is utilised to move other teeth.
- **Stationary anchorage**: Force application tends to displace the anchorage unit bodily in space
  - Anchorage value is greater than simple anchorage.
- **Reciprocal anchorage**: Two or more teeth moving in opposite directions and pitted against each other by the appliance
  - Usually the resistance to each other is equal and opposite
  - For example: Cross bite elastics, dental expansion.

II. According to the Jaws Involved

- **Intra-maxillary**: Anchorage units are located in the same jaw
- **Inter-maxillary (Baker's anchorage)**: Anchorage distributed to both the jaws, e.g., class II (elastic traction), and class III (elastic traction).

III. According to Site of Anchorage

- **Intra-oral**: Anchorage established within the mouth, that is utilizing the teeth, mucosa or other intra-oral structures
- **Extra-oral**: Anchorage obtained outside the oral cavity
  - Cervical—utilizing neck for anchorage, e.g., neck strap
  - Occipital—utilizing occipital region for anchorage, e.g., headgears
  - Cranial—utilizing cranium for anchorage, e.g., high headgears
  - Facial—involving aspects of forehead and chin as a source of anchorage, e.g., face masks.
- **Muscular**: Anchorage derived from action of muscles, e.g., vestibular shields.

IV. According to Number of Anchorage Units

- Single or primary anchorage: Anchorage involving only one tooth
- Compound anchorage: Anchorage involving two or more teeth
- Reinforced anchorage: The addition of non-dental anchor units, e.g., mucosa, muscle, head, upper anterior inclined plane, transpalatal arch, and lingual stabilizing arch.

According to Anchorage Loss Permissible (Marcotte's)

- **Minimum anchorage**: In cases with low anchorage demand, more than half of extraction space can be lost by anchor teeth moving mesially.

- **Moderate anchorage**: In these cases, anchor teeth can move forward into one-fourth to one-half of extraction space
- **Maximum anchorage**: In these cases, anchor teeth can move forward into less than one-fourth of extraction space. Anchorage in these patients should be augmented to avoid unwanted movement of anchor teeth.

Nanda's Classification

- **Group A anchorage (critical/severe)**: Seventy-five per cent of the extraction space is required for the retraction of anterior teeth
- **Group B anchorage (moderate)**: Fifty per cent of the extraction space is utilized for the retraction of anterior teeth
- **Group C anchorage (mild/non-critical)**: Twenty-five per cent of the extraction space is used for the retraction of the anterior teeth.

Burstone Classification

- **Group A arches**: Are those in which 75% of the extraction space is utilized for retraction of the anterior teeth
- **Group B arches**: Are those where only 50% of the extraction space is utilized for anterior retraction
- **Group C arches**: Involve minimal anterior retraction (only about 25%)

Simple Anchorage

- In this type of anchorage, the force applied changes the axial inclination of the tooth/teeth that form the anchorage unit in the plane of space in which force is being applied
- Here application of force tends to change the axial inclination of the tooth or teeth that form the anchorage unit. Thus, the resistance of the anchorage unit to tipping is utilized to move another tooth or teeth.

Stationary Anchorage

- In this upon application of force, the body tends to gets displaced bodily in the plane of space in which the force has been applied
- In this the body translates, and the amount of force required to carry out the movement is greater than the force required for axial movement
- It refers to the advantage that can be obtained by pitting bodily movement of one group of teeth against tipping of another. Since the resistance offered by the teeth to bodily movement is considerably more than tipping, it brings about efficient movement of teeth by tipping.
- For example: Retraction of maxillary incisors using first molars as anchorage in a Begg's appliance **(Fig. 17.1)**. Since, in this case the molars are not free to tip due to the presence of a two-point contact in the molar but the incisors are free to tip on the unipoint contact, it is an example of stationary anchorage.

Reciprocal Anchorage

- Anchorage in which the resistance of one or more dental units is utilized to move one or more opposing dental units
- The term generally refers to the resistance offered by two malposed units when the dissipation of equal and opposite forces tends to move each unit towards a more normal occlusion **(Fig. 17.2)**.

Examples of reciprocal anchorage include closure of a midline diastema, correction of posterior cross bite through cross elastics, etc.

Intra-maxillary Anchorage

When all the resistance units are situated within the same jaw **(Fig. 17.3)**.

Inter-maxillary Anchorage (Baker's Anchorage)

The resistance units are situated in one jaw and are used to effect tooth movement in the other jaw **(Fig. 17.4)**.

For example: Class II and Class III elastics.

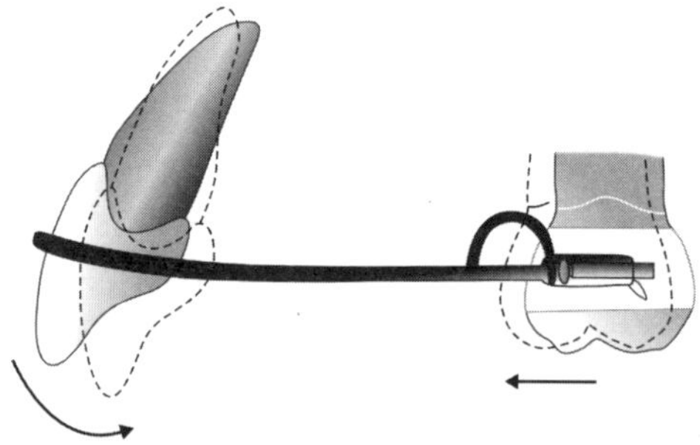

Fig. 17.1: Anchorage in a Begg's appliance

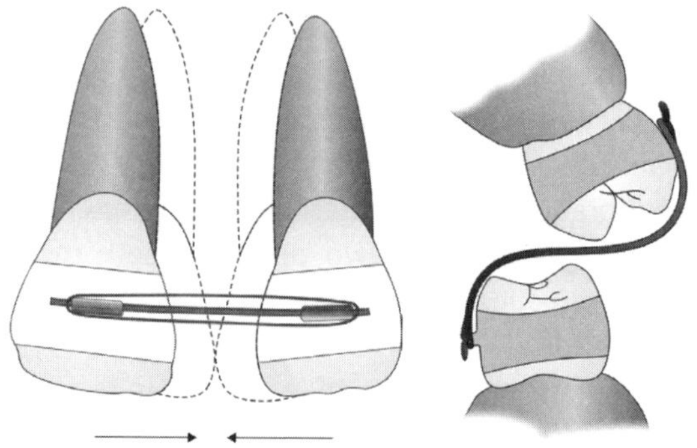

Fig. 17.2: Reciprocal anchorage

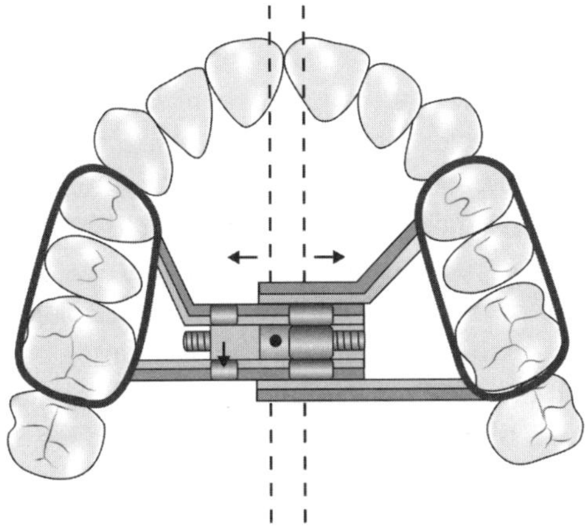

Fig. 17.3: Intramaxillary anchorage

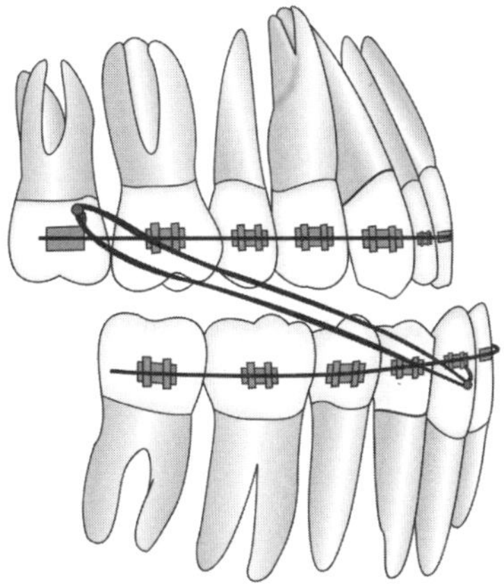

Fig. 17.4: Intermaxillary anchorage

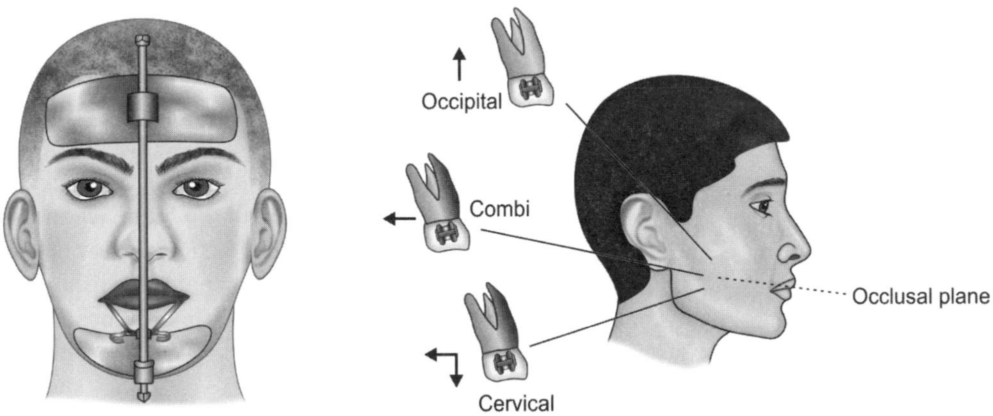

Fig. 17.5: Extraoral anchorage

Intra-oral Anchorage

In this all the resistance units are situated within the oral cavity. The intraoral anatomic units that are used for providing anchorage are teeth, palate and alveolar bone.

Extra-oral Anchorage

Anchorage in which one of the anchorage units is situated outside the oral cavity is termed extra-oral anchorage **(Fig. 17.5)**

For example, headgear and face mask which utilize resistance provided with different parts of head and neck like occipital bone, back of neck, cranium, chin and forehead.

- Cervical—utilizing neck for anchorage, e.g., neck strap
- Occipital—utilizing occipital region for anchorage, e.g., cervical pull headgears
- Cranial—utilizing cranium for anchorage, e.g., high pull headgears
- Facial—involving aspects of face as a source of anchorage, e.g., face masks.

Single or Primary Anchorage

In this the single tooth with greater alveolar support is used to move another tooth with lesser alveolar support.

Compound Anchorage

In this, the anchorage is augmented by adding multiple dental units.

Reinforcing the anchorage by adding multiple dental units is effective because with more teeth (or extra-oral structures) in the anchorage, the reaction force is distributed over a larger periodontal ligament (PDL) area. This reduces the pressure on the anchor units, moving them down the slope of the pressure-response curve.

Multiple or Reinforced Anchorage

In this, anchorage is augmented by adding multiple units by different means like extra-oral appliances, upper anterior inclined planes, Nance palatal buttons, transpalatal arch, lingual stabilizing arch.

Question 2

Write in detail about sources of anchorage?

Answer

These are anatomical units and/or regions which are used for the purpose of providing the resistance to movement, i.e., anchorage. These are further divided into two groups depending upon their location as:

- Intra-oral sources
- Extra-oral sources.

Intraoral Sources

Alveolar Bone

Within limits the alveolar bone resists deformation. This can be seen from the arrangement of trabecular pattern within the alveolar bone. Once the forces generated exceed those that can be resisted by the alveolar bone, it permits tooth movement by bone remodelling.

Less dense alveolar bone offers less anchorage. More mature bone increases anchorage. This takes place because of two factors; one the bone becomes more calcified and dissolution takes time, and two, the regenerative capacity of the bone increases. Forces that are dissipated over a larger bone surface area offer increased anchorage.

Teeth

Teeth by themselves resist movement. Forces can be exerted from one set of teeth can move certain other teeth. The anchorage potential of teeth depends upon a number of factors including the root form, size of the roots, the position of the teeth, the axial inclination of the teeth, their intercuspation, etc.

- **Root form**: The root form to a large extent is responsible for the degree of anchorage provided by a tooth. The root in cross section can be either round, flat (mesio-distally) or triangular. The distribution of the periodontal fibres on the root surface aids in anchorage. The more the fibres, the better is the anchorage potential. The direction of attachments of fibres also effects anchorage offered by a tooth. Round roots have only half of their periodontal fibres stressed in any given direction. Hence, offers least anchorage. Mesio-distally flat roots are able to resist mesio-distal tooth movement better as compared to the relatively narrow labial and lingual surfaces. Triangular roots, like those of the canines are able to provide greater anchorage. Their flatness adds to the resistance
  - The tripod arrangement of roots, like that seen on maxillary molars also aids in increasing the anchorage
  - The round palatal root resists extrusion and the two flat buccal roots resist intrusion and the mesio-distal stresses
  - Under clinical situations where the buccal tube is bonded/welded on the buccal aspect of these teeth they show a tendency to roll mesially, the crown rotating mesio-palatally under mesially directed forces.
- **Size of the roots**: The larger or longer the roots, there is more anchorage potential. The maxillary canines because of their longer roots can be at times, be the most difficult teeth to move in certain clinical situations
- **Number of roots**: The greater the surface area, the greater the periodontal support and hence, greater the anchorage potential. Multirooted teeth provide greater anchorage as compared to single rooted teeth with similar root length
- **Position of tooth**: Sometimes the position of the teeth in the individual arches also helps in increasing their anchorage potential. As in the case of mandibular second premolars, which are placed between two ridges—the mylohyoid and the external oblique, they provide an increased resistance to mesial movement
- **Axial inclination of the teeth**: When the tooth is inclined in the opposite direction to that of the force applied, it provides greater anchorage resistance or anchorage
- **Root formation**: Teeth with incomplete root formation are easier to move and are able to provide lesser anchorage
- **Contact points**: Teeth with intact contacts and/or broad contact provide greater anchorage
- **Intercuspation**: Good intercuspation leads to greater anchorage potential. This is mainly because the teeth in one jaw are prevented from moving because of the contact with those of opposing jaw, this is especially true for teeth, in the posterior segment which also show the presence of attrition facets.

Basal Bone

Certain areas of the basal bones like the hard palate and the lingual surfaces of the mandible in the anterior regions can be used to augment the anchorage. The Nance palatal button is one such appliance that makes use of hard palate to provide resistance to the mesial movement of the maxillary molars.

Cortical Bone

Ricketts floated the idea of using cortical bone for anchorage. The intention being that the cortical bone is denser with decreased blood supply and the bone turn over. Hence, if certain tooth are torqued to come in contact with the cortical bone they would have a greater anchorage potential. The idea as such remains controversial as tooth roots also show resorption in such conditions and the risk of non-vitality of such teeth is also more.

Musculature

Under normal circumstances the perioral musculature plays an important part in the growth and development of the dental arches. Hypertonicity of the perioral musculature enhances the anchorage potential of the mandibular molars, preventing their mesial movement.

Methods of Obtaining Anchorage

Reinforcement of Anchorage

- Depends on the type of the teeth movement desired. Anchorage can be reinforced by including as many teeth as possible in the anchorage unit.
- The ratio of PDL area of anchorage unit to PDL area of tooth movement unit should be 2:1 without friction and 4:1 with friction.
- By addition of teeth from the opposite dental arch to anchor unit.
- By patient wearing extraoral appliance (headgear) placing backward force against the upper arch.
- Use of skeletal anchorage systems.

Subdivision of Desired Tooth Movement

A common way to improve anchorage control is to pit the resistance of a group of teeth against the movement of a single tooth rather than dividing the arch into or less equal segments, e.g., to reduce strain on posterior anchorage—retraction of canine individually.

Tipping/Uprighting

Another possible strategy for anchorage control is to tip the teeth and then upright them rather than moving them bodily.

Friction and Anchorage Control Strategies

In a typical extraction case, it is desired to close the extraction space 60% by retraction of anterior teeth and 40% by forward movement of posterior segments. This can be obtained by three approaches:

1. One step space closure with a frictionless appliance
2. Two step procedure by sliding the canine, then retracting the incisors (tweed technique)
3. Two step closure by tipping the anterior segment with some friction and then uprighting the tipped teeth.

Cortical Anchorage

Cortical bone is more resistant to resorption; tooth movement is slowed when root contacts it. By torquing the roots of posterior teeth outward against the cortical plate it inhibits the mesial movement when extraction spaces are to be closed.

Nance Holding Arch, Transpalatal Arch and Lower Lingual Holding Arch

The Nance holding arch can be used to maintain maxillary arch length. The arch consists of a wire embedded in an acrylic button on the anterior palate and soldered to bands on the maxillary first permanent molars **(Fig. 17.6)**.

A transpalatal arch consists of a wire passing over the palatal vault and soldered to the first permanent molars. The purpose of these arches is to maintain arch width and molar position after buccal expansion of the maxillary arch and to keep molars from tipping buccally in response to forces from an occipital pull face bow headgear.

Fixed or removable transpalatal arches are used to maintain, expand or constrict intermolar width to rotate, upright mesially tipped molars and to torque maxillary molars **(Fig. 17.7)**.

Lower lingual holding arches comes in fixed and fixed-removable versions. The fixed holding arch is most commonly used to maintain arch width and arch length. A

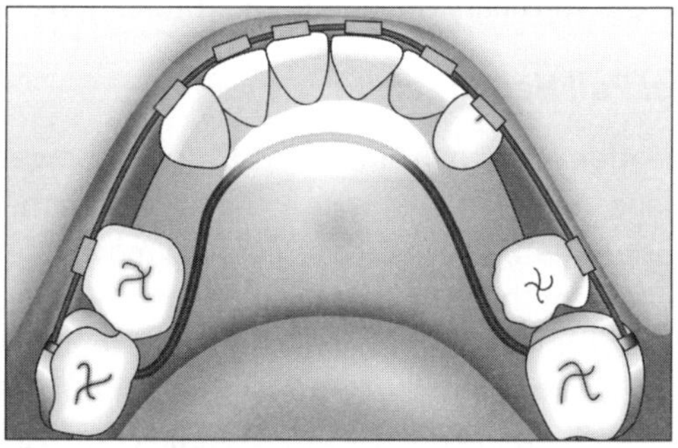

Fig. 17.6: Nance holding arch

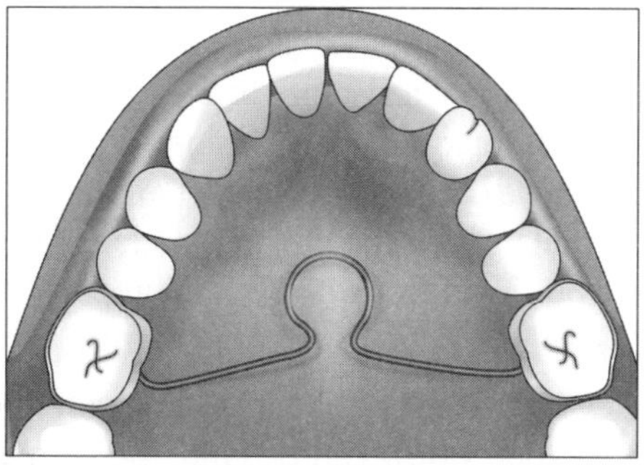

Fig. 17.7: Transpalatal arch

wire with adjustment loop is soldered to bands cemented on the first permanent molars. The wire should rest on the cingula of the mandibular incisors. Adjustment loops allow clinicians to shorten, lengthen raise or lower the wire into passive contact with the incisor cingula **(Fig. 17.8)**.

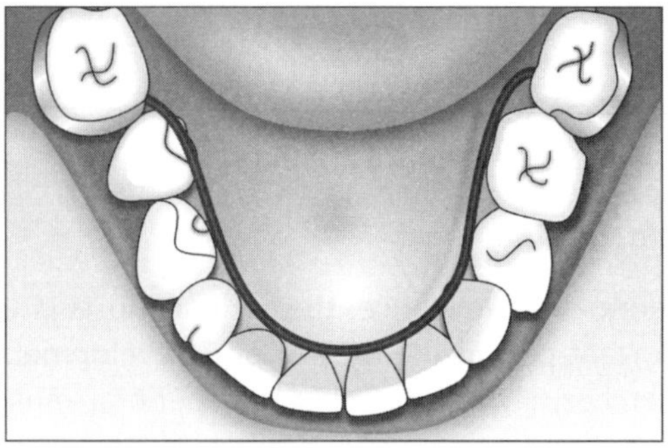

Fig. 17.8: Lower lingual holding arch

Class II Elastics

Inter-maxillary elastics put the upper teeth to the lower teeth and are common means of gaining differential tooth movement. The direction of the elastic defines its force vector and the terminology used to describe it. Class II elastics attach to the anterior maxillary teeth and the posterior mandibular teeth. Thus, a Class II elastics acts to correct a Class II relationship by proving a retraction force to the upper anterior teeth and a simultaneous protraction force to the lower molars **(Fig. 17.9)**.

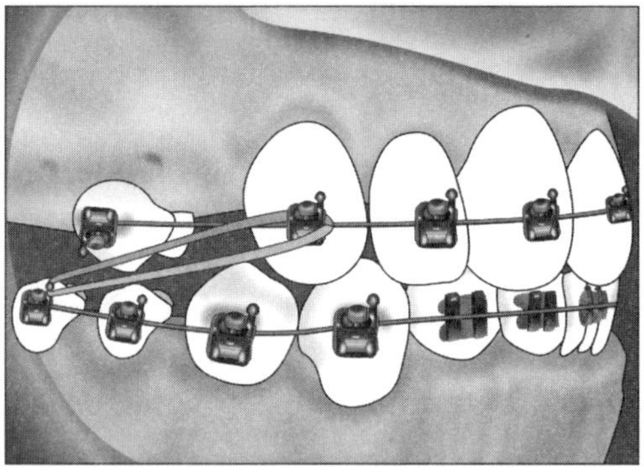

Fig. 17.9: Class II elastics

Alternatively, a Class III elastic hooks from the lower anterior teeth to the upper posterior teeth, creating a force for lower anterior retraction and upper protraction for the resolution of a Class III occlusion.

The major limitation of elastics as an anchorage technique is their dependence on patient compliance. Without patient cooperation these methods are incapable of influencing the treatment results. Many approaches have been devised to eliminate patient compliance as a crucial factor in anchorage control. Ultimately, these techniques attempt to establish anchorage with intra-arch appliance designs.

Extra-oral Method of Anchorage

Head gears are again classified according to the point of origin of force as follows:

- Cervical-anchorage derived from the nape of neck
- Occipital-anchorage obtained from the back of the head
- Parietal-anchorage obtained from the upper part of the head.

Another classification is as follows:

- **High pull headgear**: Anchorage obtained from the upper part of the head and direction of the pull is always above the centre of resistance of the dentition
- **Straight pull headgear**: Anchorage obtained from the back of the line of traction is parallel to the occlusal place
- **Cervical pull headgear**: The combination of cervical pull and high pull headgear with varying proportions of force to each, depending on case requirements.

Another variable in the headgear is the outer bow of the face bow. The outer bow can be long, medium and short. The site of the point of origin of force is the relatively fixed by the position of the headgear strap, and the centre of resistance of the molar remain constant till the tooth has moved.

Therefore, inclination of the line of action may be altered only by variations in the position of the bow. They can be achieved by varying the length of the outer bow, the angulation between the inner and outer bow or a combination of both. The centre of resistance of the maxilla is in the area of postero-superior aspect of zygomatico-maxillary suture.

The centre of resistance of the maxillary dentition is situated between the roots of the premolars. The centre of resistance of maxillary molar is in the trifurcation area.

Cervical Pull Headgear

In this headgear when the inner and the outer bow are in the same plane, there is a clockwise rotation of both the maxilla and the dentition. The incisor region will move inferiorly to a greater extent than the molar region.

The outer bow is bend upwards so that the direction of the traction between the centre resistance of the maxilla and the dentition in an anti-clockwise direction. Hence, the molars will experience a more downward pull than incisors.

Parietal Pull/High Pull Headgear

When the direction of traction is placed behind the centre of resistance of the maxilla and the dentition, a clockwise rotational effect on maxilla and the dentition is observed.

Hence, the molars intrude, incisors extrude. Least vertical dimension and rotational changes are observed when the applied force vector passes through the centre of resistance of the maxilla and the dentition. This is therefore, the preferred setup for the vertical control. But so far it has not been possible to construct a stable head strap for anchoring such a steep force vector.

Combee Type Headgear

This allows a distal force through the centre of resistance of the dentition having equal parietal and cervical components. When the outer bow is angled upward to pass through the centre of resistance. Hence, the centre of rotation is at infinity. This allows for more distalization of the molar with minimum rotational effect.

Question 3

Write in detail about absolute anchorage/skeletal anchorage/mini implants?

Answer

Skeletal anchorage is applied to orthodontic tooth movement when "absolute anchorage" is necessary. With various skeletal fixtures forces might be applied to produce tooth movement in any direction without detrimental reciprocal forces.

Methods of Obtaining Skeletal Anchorage

- Conventional dental implants
- Palatal endosseous implants
- Onplant
- Mini-implant
- Spider Screw
- Micro-implant
- C-orthodontic micro-implant
- Impacted titanium post
- Transitional implants
- Mini plate
- Zygoma anchorage system
- Zygomatic ligatures.

Implants in Orthodontics

- According to Boucher, Implants are alloplastic materials which are surgically inserted into our jaw bone
- According to TM Graber, Implant is a mechanical device made from one or more biomaterials that is intentionally placed within our body either totally or partially buried beneath an epithelial surface
- Implants solve one of the orthodontists' dilemmas, anchorage control. The innate ability of an osseointegrated implant can provide this advantage
- The reliance on patient cooperation would be minimized because the use of headgear and elastics would be eliminated.

Parts of an Implant

The commonly used implant screw has two parts **(Fig. 17.10)**:

- **Implant head**: It serves as the abutment and in the case of an orthodontic implant, it is the source of attachment of elastics or coil springs
- **Implant body**: It is the part embedded inside bone. This may be a screw type or a plate type.

Sites for Implant Placement

The various sites for implant placement reported are:

- Maxillary zone
  - Infrazygomatic crest area
  - Maxillary tuberosity area
  - Anterior nasal spine
  - Midpalatal area
  - Alveolar ridge
  - Extraction site.
- Mandibular zone
  - Retromolar area
  - Symphysis area
  - Lingual plate
  - Interdental region.
- Extra-orally
  - Temporal buttress
  - Zygomatic buttress.

Selecting the Site for Insertion of an Implant

It involves considering several factors:

- The primary purpose of the implant
- The patient's skeletal age
- The quality and quantity of bone available
- Pathologies in operation site
- Anatomical structures
- Biomechanical requirements and the specific therapeutic indication.

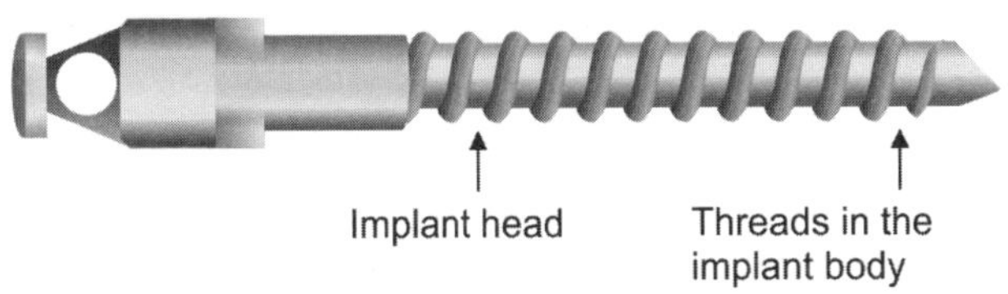

Fig. 17.10: Parts of an implant

Applications of Implants in Orthodontics

The anchorage derived from implants is categorized into:

- Direct anchorage in which an endosseous implant is used as an anchorage site
- Indirect anchorage in which implants are used for preserving anchorage.

The various applications of implants in orthodontic perspective includes:

- Orthopaedic anchorage
- Maxillary expansion
- Maxillary protraction
- Headgear like effects
- Dental anchorage
- Space closure
- Intrusion of anterior teeth
- Intrusion of posterior teeth
- Distalisation
- In conjunction with prosthetic rehabilitation (direct anchorage).

Types

According to exposure of head:

- **Open method**: Head is exposed to the oral cavity
- **Closed method**: Head is embedded in the soft tissue

According the method of placement:

- **Self-tapping method**: First a tunnel is drilled into bone and then the implant is tapped in.
- **Self-drilling method**: Implant itself drills into the bone.

According to path of insertion:

- **Oblique direction**: The micro-implant is inserted at an angle of 30–60° to the long axis of the tooth.
- **Perpendicular**: The micro-implant is inserted perpendicular to the bony surface.

The biomechanics of type of tooth movement required determines the vertical placement of micro implant **(Fig. 17.12)**

Maxillary sites for placement of implant and the functions:

- Infra-zygomatic crest **(Fig. 17.11A)**:
  - **Purpose**: To retract entire maxillary dentition to correct Class II canine and molar relationship, intrusion of maxillary molars.
  - **Size**: Diameter of 1.3 mm and length of 5–6 mm.
- Maxillary tuberosity **(Fig. 17.11B)**:
  - **Purpose**: For retracting the maxillary posterior teeth.
  - Used when the third molars are missing or extracted and the healing is completed.
  - **Size**: 1.3–1.5 mm diameter and 7–8 mm length.
- Between the first and second molar buccally **(Fig. 17.11C)**:
  - **Purpose**: Second choice to retract the anterior teeth when the placement of implant fails between first molar and second premolar
  - Used to apply intrusive force on molars
  - **Size**: 1.2–1.3 mm diameter and length of 7–8 mm.
- Between the first molar and second premolar buccally **(Fig. 17.13A)**:
  - **Purpose**: Site of choice for retraction of anterior teeth and molar intrusion
  - **Size**: 1.2–1.3 mm diameter and 7–8 mm in length.

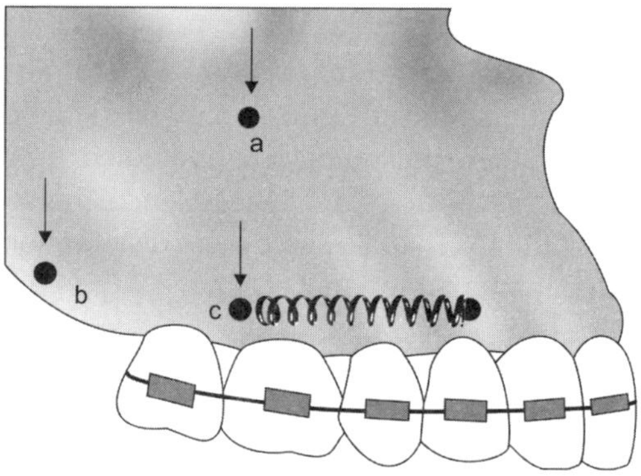

Fig. 17.11A to C: (A) Infrazygomatic crest (B) Maxillary tuberosity and (C) Between the first and second molar buccally

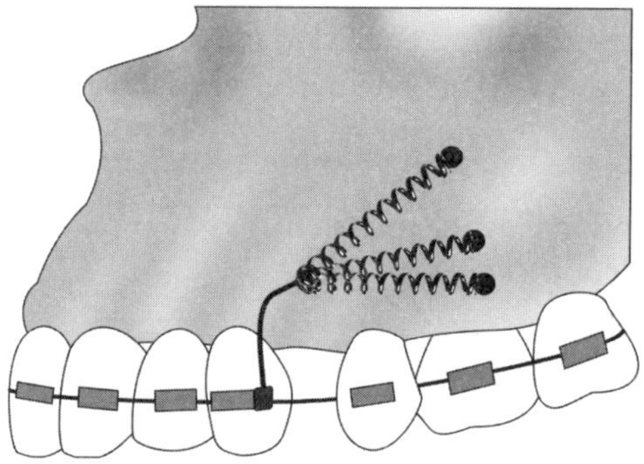

Fig. 17.12: The vertical placement of a micro-implant is determined by biomechanical considerations

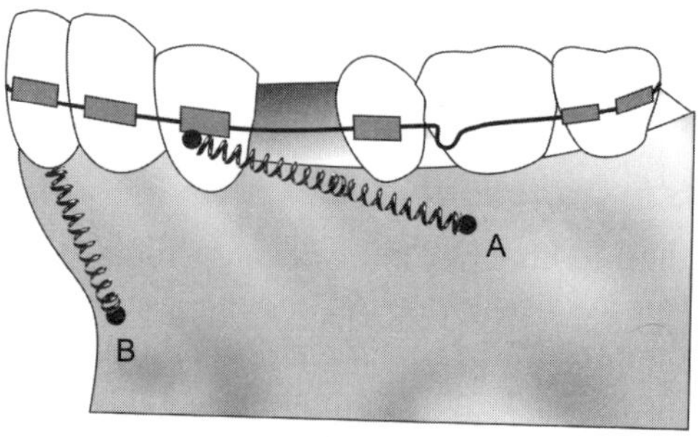

Fig. 17.13: A: Between the first molar and second premolar bucally; B: Between the maxillary incisors facially

- Between the canine and premolar buccally:
  - **Purpose**: Useful for moving the maxillary molars distally or mesially and for intrusion of buccal segments
  - **Size**: 1.2–1.3 mm diameter and 7-8 mm length.
- Between the maxillary incisors facially **(Fig. 17.13B)**:
  - **Purpose**: For intrusion and torque control of the maxillary incisors
    - Implant is placed between the roots
    - Ligature wire should be attached to the head, as the soft tissue tends to grow around it
    - Microimplants placed between the central and lateral incisors bilaterally can be used to correct the cant in occlusal plane.
  - **Size**: 1.3–1.6 mm in diameter and 7–8 mm length.
- Between second premolar and first molar buccally and between first and second molar palatally:
  - **Purpose**: For anchorage in lingual orthodontics and intrusion of molars to correct open bite
  - **Size**: 1.3–1.6 mm diameter and 10–12 mm length.
- Midpalatal area:
  - **Purpose**: For any kind of movement of the posterior teeth
    - Unilateral constriction of arch
    - Attached to transpalatal appliance for augmenting anchorage and distalizing molars.
  - **Size:** 1.5–1.8 mm and 5–6 mm length.

Mandibular sites for placement of implant and the functions:

- Retromolar area:
  - **Purpose**: Uprighting of tilted mandibular molars, retraction of teeth, buccal uprighting of second molar and distalization
  - **Size**: 1.4–1.6 mm diameter and 5–10 mm length.
- Between the first and second molars buccally:
  - **Purpose**: For retraction of anteriors, intrusion and distal movement of mandibular molars and correction of scissor bite
  - **Size**: 1.3–1.6 mm diameter and 5–7 mm length.
- Between first molar and second premolar buccally:
  - **Purpose**: Retraction of anterior teeth, intrusion of posterior teeth, moving molars buccally and distally
  - **Size**: 1.3–1.6 mm diameter and 5–7 mm length.
- Between canine and premolar:
  - **Purpose**: For protraction of mandibular molars
  - **Size**: 1.3–1.6 mm diameter and 5–7 mm length.
- Mandibular symphysis facially:
  - **Purpose**: Intrusion of mandibular incisors
  - **Size**: 1.3–1.5 mm diameter and 5–6 mm length.

CHAPTER 18 Age Factors in Orthodontics

SHORT NOTES

Question 1

What are the differences between young and an adult patient in case of orthodontics?

Answer

The difference between a young and an adult patient are as follows:

- **Growth to work with**: In a young patient, orthodontist has growth potential to work with whereas an adult patient lacks growth thus an orthodontist merely depends on orthodontic tooth movement or surgery in an adult patient
- **Diagnosis**: Most of the diagnostic aids can be used in both young as well as adult patients
  - An adult patient has more possibility of dormant pathosis, periodontal problems, impaction, faulty restoration, tooth decay, attrition of dentition, etc
  - Some of these factors might interfere with orthodontic therapy
- **Appliance selection**: Younger patient who are in growth phase respond effectively to the orthopaedic and myofunctional appliances whereas in an adult patient the options are less and are restricted to only orthodontic tooth movement and surgery.
  - Also, the young patients can tolerate most of the appliances and are not much concerned by the appearance of the appliance whereas adult patients are concerned about the appearance of the appliance.
- **Periodontal problems**: In an adult patient, the periodontal problems are more common as compared to the young patient
- **Patient motivation and cooperation**: Adult patients are more motivated as compared to the young patients
- **Tissue vitality**: In a young patient, tissue vitality and patient response to orthodontic/orthopaedic force is much more when compared to an adult patient because of decreased vascularity and cellularity in an adult patient
- **Treatment objectives**: There are three treatment objectives, i.e., function, aesthetics and stability, which may not be achieved in an adult patient
- **Treatment appreciation**: Adult patient can appreciate the treatment result more as compared to young patients.

Question 2

What are the age factors in orthodontics?

Answer

Age factors in orthodontics are as follows:

- Utilization of growth potential to work with
- Various diagnostic methods used
- Periodontal problems
- Selection of appliance
- Patient motivation and cooperation
- Tissue vitality
- Treatment objectives
- Treatment appreciation.

Question 3

What is the ideal age for various orthodontic treatments?

Answer

The age of the patient influence orthodontic therapeutic interventions and prognosis:

- The effectiveness of functional appliances like twin block, bionator, Frankel appliance and orthopaedic appliances like headgears to correct skeletal malocclusions are effective during growing stage of the patient

- Maxillary expansion procedures are carried out before the fusion of palatal sutures during early age
- After growth cessation in adult patient, orthognathic surgeries are undertaken to correct skeletal problems.

Question 4

Write a short note on adult orthodontics?

Answer

Orthodontic treatment in adult patient is referred to as adult orthodontics. In adult patients, orthodontic treatment can be classified into two types:

1. Adjunctive orthodontic treatment
2. Comprehensive orthodontic treatment.

Adjunctive Orthodontic Treatment

Adjunctive orthodontic treatment procedures are carried out to facilitate other dental procedures to control diseases and restore function, e.g., uprighting of molars, crossbite correction, forced eruption, diastema closure, etc.

Comprehensive Orthodontic Treatment

Comprehensive orthodontic treatment is the essential treatment procedure carried out for correction of malocclusion.

Response to orthodontic force is slightly slower in adult as compared to children.

CHAPTER 19

Preventive Orthodontics

LONG ESSAYS

Question 1

Define Preventive Orthodontics. Describe in brief the various procedure of preventive orthodontics.

Answer

Graber (1966) defined preventive orthodontics as "the action taken to preserve the integrity of what appears to be normal occlusion at a specific time".

Profit and Ackerman (1980) defined as "prevention of potential interference with occlusal development".

Various procedure in Preventive orthodontics are:

- Parent counseling
  - Prenatal
  - Postnatal.
- Control of caries
- Maintainance of space in case of premature extraction of deciduous teeth
- Extraction of over retained or carious deciduous teeth
- Treatment of abnormal frenal attachments
- Treatment of locked permanent first molars
- Abnormal oral habits.

Parent Counselling

Parents should be educated regarding

- Increase in food intake to meet the special physiological changes in the body to support the growth of the foetus and facilitate normal labour
- Dental development of their child
- Dental disease process
- Oral hygiene measures appropriate for infants
- Expecting mothers should be educated on proper nursing and care of the child
- In case the child is being bottle-fed, the mother is advised to use physiologic nipple and not the conventional nipple.
- As the child grows, parents should be educated regarding the need for maintaining good oral hygiene
- In infants small gauze is used over the ridge of top and bottom jaws for cleaning
- Proper brushing techniques and brushing habits to be explained and evaluated periodically
- Fone's method of brushing is preferred in children
- Fluoride application and dental checkup every 6 months.

Caries Control Procedures

- Diet and oral hygiene Maintenance
- Regular Checkup
- Fluoride applications
- Prophylactic odontomy
- Pit and fissure sealants
- Restorative procedures like silver amalgam, glass ionomers, cermets, stainless steel crown
- Immunization.

Diet and Oral Hygiene Maintenance

- Balanced diet which contains varieties of food, in such quantity and proportion that the need for energy, amino acids, vitamins, fats, carbohydrates and other nutrients is adequately met for maintaining health
- The cariogenic potential of food depends on many variables such as presence of fermentable sugar like sucrose. The parents should be advised to avoid such foods
- The solid foods containing sucrose are more cariogenic than liquid foods
- The frequency in time of ingestion of foods are also important. The sucrose containing food becomes more dangerous if it is eaten more frequent
- The patient should be aided in identification of those foods which are likely to cause oral diseases

- The 3 to 6 yrs olds require parental assistance to achieve effective plaque removal
- Parents should be instructed to brush for the child at least once a day
- Bedtime is the ideal time to establish this routine because the salivary flow rate slows during sleep
- Additional brushings may be performed by the child
- Parents need to remain active in supervising the home care practices of 6-12 yrs old.

Regular Check-up

- The parents should be advised to bring their child for his/ her first dental visit early at least by the time the baby is 6 months of age
- Frequency of recall visits have to be decided according to the individual needs. Usually a 3 monthly recall checkup is advised to monitor oral hygiene status
- Half yearly visit to the dentist should be routine.

Care of Deciduous Dentition

- Deciduous teeth act as natural space maintainers until the developing permanent teeth are ready to replace them into the oral cavity
- All efforts should be taken to prevent early loss of deciduous teeth
- Preventive procedures such as proper and timely application of fluoride topically/ pit and fissure sealant application should be done to prevent caries
- More complex treatment procedures to prevent the natural space maintainer includes pulp therapy (pulpotomy, pulpectomy) and stainless steel crown
- Bite wing radiographs should be taken in order to detect caries
- Once caries is detected proper restoration of affected teeth should be undertaken immediately to prevent loss of arch length
- Restoration should restore the mesio-distal dimension of tooth, but should not be over/under extended allowing drift of contiguous teeth or promote food impaction
- Re- establishment of proper inclined plane relationship with proper anatomic carving will be esthetic and results in normal function and stability of occlusion.

Pit and Fissure Sealants

Indications

- Newly erupted both primary molars and permanent bicuspids and molars with open and/or sticky grooves and fissures
- Stained pits and fissures with minimum decalcification
- The tooth should have erupted less than 4 years ago.

Contraindications

- Child with no previous caries experience
- Proximal caries should not be sealed
- Wide and self-cleansable pit and fissures
- Pit and fissures that have remained carious free for 4 years or longer.

Prophylactic Odontomy

As a preventive procedure the pit and fissure may be minimally prepared and restored before visible attack by caries.

Maintenance of Shedding / Eruption Timetable

- As a rule of Thumb, the shedding of the deciduous dentition should be kept on schedule by extracting the tooth or teeth on one side of the arch, when they have been lost through natural process on the other side to prevent supra eruption
- Should not wait longer than 3 months for nature to do the job, particularly when there is radiographic evidence of abnormal resorption which would otherwise lead to malocclusion
- According to Moyers, normal sequence of eruption provides the highest percentage of normal occlusion
- Eruption in Maxillary arch - 6124537
- Mandibular arch - 6124357
- Abnormal order of arrival may permit shifting of the teeth, with resultant space loss
- Change in the sequence of eruption is a much more reliable sign of a disturbance in normal development than generalized decay or acceleration
- The more a tooth deviates from its expected position in the sequence, the greater the likelihood of some problem.

Space Maintainance

Maintenance of arch length during the primary, mixed and early permanent dentition is of great significance for the normal development of future occlusion.

Causes of space loss:

- Trauma
- Interproximal caries in primary molars
- Ectopic eruption of first perm molars
- Delayed eruption
- Congenital absence of permanent teeth
- Microdontia can cause arch length deficiency

Space maintainers are appliances used to maintain the space created by the loss of deciduous teeth prior to eruption of its successor to prevent drifiting of adjacent teeth into that space.

Classifications

According to Hitchcock

- Removable or fixed or semi fixed
- With bands or without bands
- Functional or non functional
- Active or passive
- Certain combinations of above.

According to Raymond C. Thurow

- Removable
- Complete arch
  - Lingual arch
  - Extra oral anchorage.
- Individual tooth.

According to Hinrichsen

Fixed space maintainers:

- Class I
  - Non functional types
    - Bar type
    - Loop type.
  - Functional type.
    - Pontic type
    - Lingual arch type.
- Class II.
  - Cantilever type
  - Distal shoe
  - B and E loop.

Removable and fixed:

- Removable
  - Non functional—acrylic plate
  - Functional—acrylic plate with teeth
  - Active—acrylic plate with clasps, spring
  - Passive—acrylic plate with clasps.
- Fixed
  - Band and loop
  - Crown and loop
  - Band and bar
  - Distal shoe/eruption guidance
  - Lingual arch
  - Nance palatal arch
  - Transpalatal arch.
- Semi fixed
  - Removable archwire with molar bands.

Pre-requisites

- Should maintain the Mesio distal dimension of the space created by lost tooth
- Should be as simple and strong as possible
- Should be functional, if possible, atleast to the extent of preventing the overeruption of the opposing tooth
- Should not interfere with normal occlusal adjustments
- Must not endanger the remaining teeth by imposing excessive stresses on them
- Should not interfere with the erupting teeth
- Should not interfere with normal vertical eruption of the adjacent teeth
- Should have a simple design permitting easy construction and placement
- Should be easily adjustable
- Space maintainer should be constructed in a manner so that they do not restrict normal growth and developmental processes
- Should not interfere with oral functions such as mastication, speech or deglutition
- Must be easily cleansable and not serve as traps for food debris
- Reasonable in cost.

Indications

- If space after premature loss of deciduous teeth shows signs of closing
- If use of space maintainer will aid in or make the future orthodontic treatment less involved
- If the need for treatment of malocclusion at a later date is not indicated.

Contraindications

- 1/3rd of the root of succedaneous tooth is already calcified
- Space left is less than the space needed for the permanent successor
- Space shows no signs of closing
- Would further complicate existing malocclusion
- Succidaneous tooth is absent
- Well developed occlusion and cuspal interdigitation or over eruption of opposing tooth prevent space closing.

Removable Space Maintainers

Indications

- If abutment teeth cannot support the fixed appliance
- Cleft palate has to be closed with the denture
- Bands cannot be adopted, it is advised to use a removable space maintainer can be give
- Multiple loss of deciduous teeth.

Contraindications

- Lack of patients cooperation
- Patients allergic to acrylic materials
- Epileptic patients who have uncontrolled seizures.

Advantages

- Easy to clean and permit maintenance of proper oral hygiene
- Maintains and restores the vertical dimension
- It can be worn part time allowing circulation of the blood to soft tissues
- Functions like aesthetic/mastication/phonetics
- Dental checkup for carries detection can be done easily
- Stimulate eruption of permanent teeth
- Room can be made for permanent teeth to erupt without changing the appliance
- They prevent development of tongue Thrust habit into the extraction space
- More than one tooth can be replaced
- Being tissue-borne, they impose less stress on remaining teeth
- Easier to fabricate, less chair time.

Disadvantages

- Patient may not wear it, patient compliance in 3-6 year age group and uncooperative children is poor
- It may be lost or broken by the patient
- It may restrict lateral growth of the jaws if clasps are incorporated
- May cause irritation of the underlying soft tissues.

Fixed Space Maintainers

Advantages

- Do not interrupt with passive eruption of teeth
- Do not interfere with Normal Jaw growth
- Permanent successor teeth can erupt freely
- No patient co-operation required.

Disadvantages

- Elaborate instrumentation with expert skill is needed
- Tooth structure under the bands may decalcify
- Supra eruption of opposing teeth can take place.

Band and Loop

Consist of a band and loop. The tooth distal to the extraction space is banded and a loop made up of 0.036" wire is soldered to the band with the mesial end in contact with the distal surface of tooth mesial to the extraction space.

Indications

- Unilateral loss of primary first molar before or after the eruption of permanent first molars
- Bilateral loss of single primary molar before eruption of permanent incisors
- When second primary molar is lost after the eruption of first permanent molar
- Sometimes its given in cases of premature loss of primary canines.

Advantages

- Effective for unilateral loss of single tooth in buccal segments
- Economical
- Construction-simple
- Takes little chairside time.
- Adjusts easily to accommodate the changing dentition.

Disadvantages

- Requires constant supervision
- Can cause decalcification
- Does not prevent the continued eruption of the opposing teeth
- Limited to maintainance of single tooth space.

Lingual Arch

- The lingual arch is the most effective appliance for space maintenance in posterior region and minor tooth movement in the lower arch **(Fig. 19.1)**
- The lingual arch space maintainer consists of two bands cemented to the 1st permanent molars or sometimes 2nd deciduous molars, which are joined by a SS wire butting against four incisors
- Usually indicated to preserve the spaces created by multiple loss of primary molars when there is no loss of space in the arch
- The use of lingual arch is a good preventive measure, since it helps in maintaining the arch perimeter by preventing both mesial drifting of the molar teeth and also lingual collapse of the anterior teeth
- Spurs that is Projections of wire, may be used as stoppers distal to anterior teeth to prevent their migration distally in the arch
- These help in maintaining symmetry of centre lines, especially in cases of unilateral tooth loss.

Advantages

- Causes little inconvenience to patient
- Less bulky them removable acrylic space maintainers
- Less conspicuous than other space maintainers
- Serves as a space maintenance for more than one succedaneous tooth in the arch
- Prevents arch collapse
- Prevents mesial migration of banded tooth.

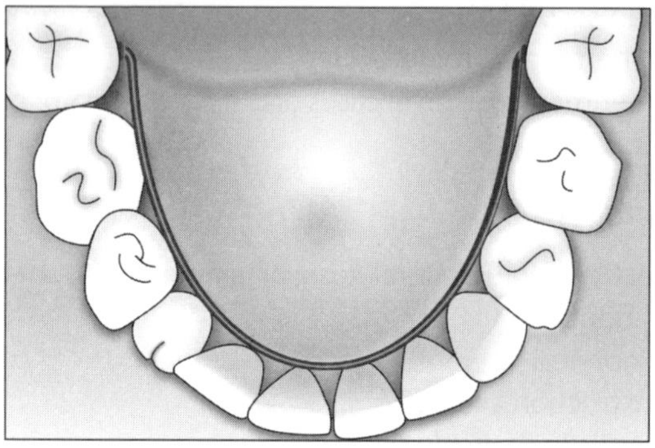

Fig. 19.1: Lingual arch space maintainer

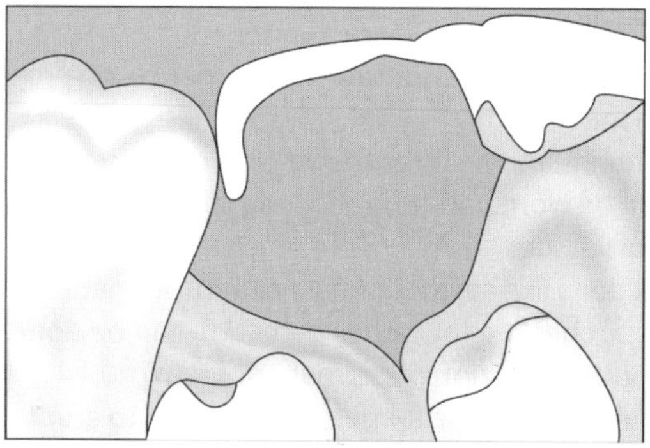

Fig. 19.2: Distal shoe space maintainer

Disadvantages

- Prolonged use of orthodontic bands—decalcification of the tooth
- Arch wire may become embedded into the soft tissue. This seems to occur more often in patients with poor oral hygiene
- Wire may become distorted by masticatory forces and move teeth into undesirable positions
- Appliance should be removed every year and inspected for damage and further usefulness, recemented after topical fluoride treatment.

Transpalatal Arch

- Recommended for stabilizing the maxillary first permanent molars
- Best Indication for transpalatal arch is when one side of the arch is intact, and several primary teeth on the other side are missing
- Also indicated when primary molars are lost bilaterally
- Appliance is designed to prevent the molars from rotating around the palatal roots, which is the first movement resulting in loss of space in the arch perimeter
- The transpalatal arch runs directly across the palatal vault connecting the permanent first molars, avoiding contact with the soft tissue.

Advantages

- No food lodgment
- Simple design
- No inflammatory changes in palate.

Disadvantages

- If given in case of bilateral missing deciduous molar, it cannot prevent drifting of abutment teeth
- If not passive, unexpected vertical and transverse movement of the permanent molars can occur.

Distal Shoe Appliance/Intra-alveolar appliance

- The distal shoe appliance is used to maintain the space created by loss of premature loss of primary second molar **(Fig. 19.2)**
- Also called as erupting guidance appliance as it helps in guiding the eruption of unerupted tooth
- Normally, the distal surface of the 2nd primary molar provides a guide for the unerupted 1st permanent molars
- When the 2nd deciduous molar is extracted prior to the eruption of the first permanent molar, the Distal Shoe appliance provides a path of eruption for the unerupted tooth and prevents undesirable mesial migration.

Indications

When 2nd primary molar is extracted or lost before the eruption of first permanent molar.

Contraindications

- Poor oral hygiene
- Medically compromised patients like patients with congenital heart disease, juvenile diabetics, Rheumatic fever, immunosupression
- If several teeth are missing in same quadrant as there lack of abutment
- Lack of patient cooperation.

Nance Palatal Holding Arch

Consist of an acrylic button resting against the rugae area attached to the bands on molar distal to the extraction space with helps of a wire framework. Indicated in premature loss of first deciduous molar.

- Advantages:
  - Economical
  - Allows growth transversely in the inter-canine areas.
- Disadvantages:
  - Requires more clinical skill
  - Palatal button may cause food accumulation.

CHAPTER 20 Interceptive Orthodontics

LONG ESSAYS

Question 1

Define interceptive orthodontics. Explain in brief the various procedures undertaken in interceptive orthodontics.?

Answer

American Association of Orthodontists defines interceptive orthodontics as "that phase of the science and art of orthodontics, employed to recognize and eliminate potential irregularities and appositions in the developing dentofacial complex".

"Interceptive orthodontics" basically refers to measures undertaken to prevent a potential malocclusion from progressing into a more severe one and is thus undertaken at a time when the malocclusion has already developed or procedures, which are aimed at elimination of factors that may lead to malocclusion.

Indications of Interceptive Treatment

Indications for early interceptive treatment are:

- Dental and/or skeletal class II
- Dental and/or skeletal class III
- Posterior or anterior cross bites
- Greater than 6 mm of overjet, especially in females
- Maxillary midface deficiency
- Moderate incisor crowding
- Ectopic eruptions.

Interceptive Procedures

- Serial extraction
- Correction of developing crossbite
- Space regaining
- Muscle exercises
- Interception of skeletal malrelations
- Removal of bony or soft tissue barrier to enable eruption of teeth.

Serial Extraction

It is defined as timed, planned extraction regimen involving deciduous teeth, followed by extraction of the permanent teeth in order to alleviate crowding as well as the duration of fixed mechanotherapy. Kjellgren coined the term "serial extraction".

Indications

Class I malocclusion with:

- Arch length deficiency
- Absence of physiologic spacing
- Premature loss of primary canine
- Crowded upper and lower anteriors
- Mal positioned lateral
- Localized gingival recession
- Ectopic eruption of teeth
- Mesial migration of buccal segment
- Abnormal eruption pattern and sequence
- Ankylosis
- Growth not enough.

Contraindications

- Congenital absence of teeth
- Mild-moderate crowding
- Deep bite
- Severe Class II, III of dental/skeletal origin
- Cleft lip and palate
- Spaced dentition.

Disadvantages

- Requires clinical judgement
- Prolonged treatment time
- Patient compliance
- Developing tongue thrust
- Arch length reduction
- Ditching between canine and second premolar
- Axial inclination.

Methods

- Dewel's method
- Nance method
- Tweed method

Dewel's method: Extraction of deciduous canines, followed by deciduous first molars and finally first premolars (CD4).

Nance method: Extraction of deciduous first molars, followed by first premolars and then deciduous canines (D4C).

Tweed method: similar to the Nance method except that extraction sequence may involve the deciduous laterals also.

Serial Extraction in Class I Treatment

Group A: Anterior Discrepancy (Crowding)

- Step 1: Extraction of deciduous canines

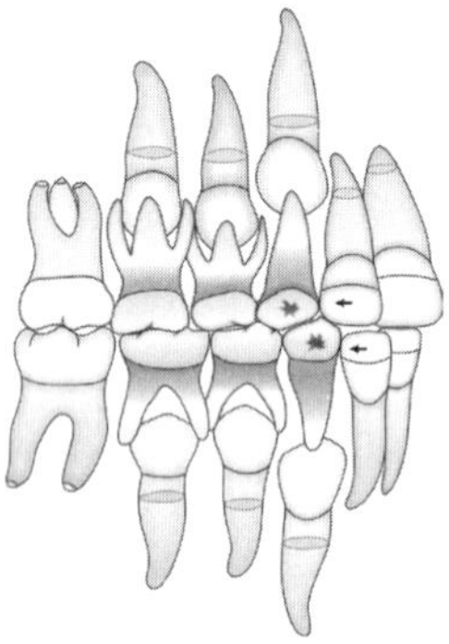

- Step 2: Extraction of deciduous first molar

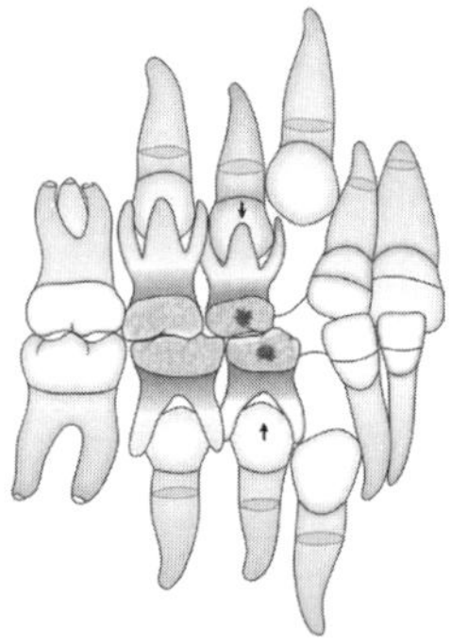

- Step 3: Extraction of first premolar

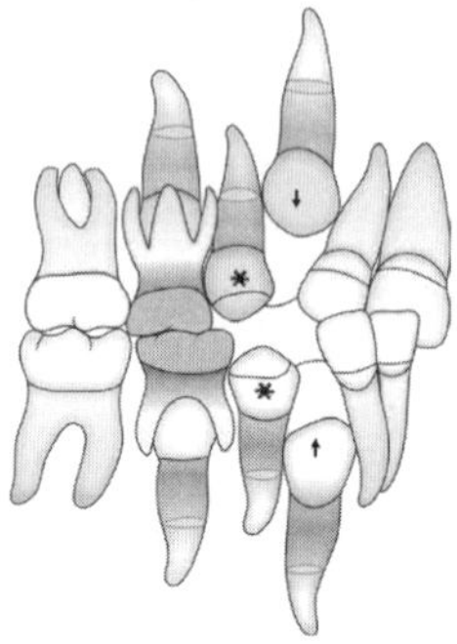

- Step 4: Fixed orthodontic therapy

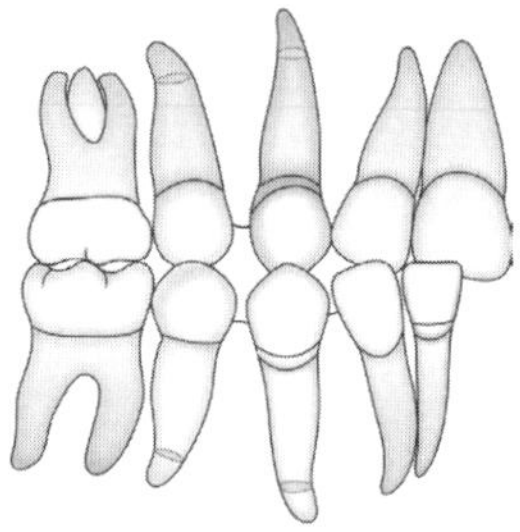

- Step 5.

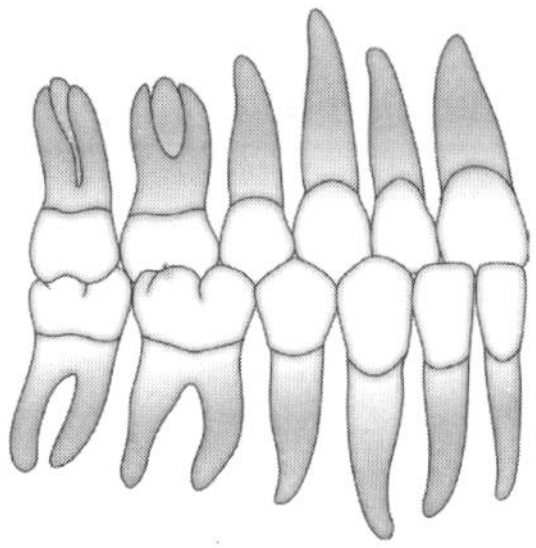

Group B: Class I Dentoalveolar Protrusion

- Step 1

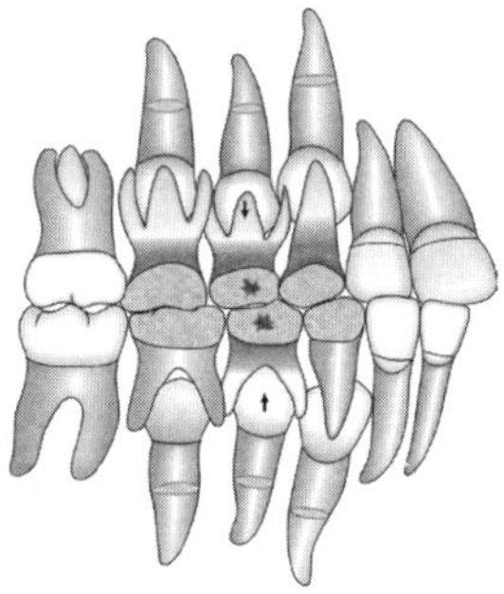

- Step 2

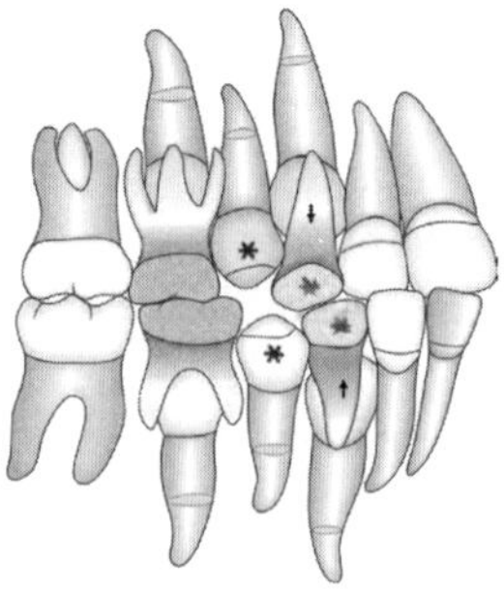

- Step 3

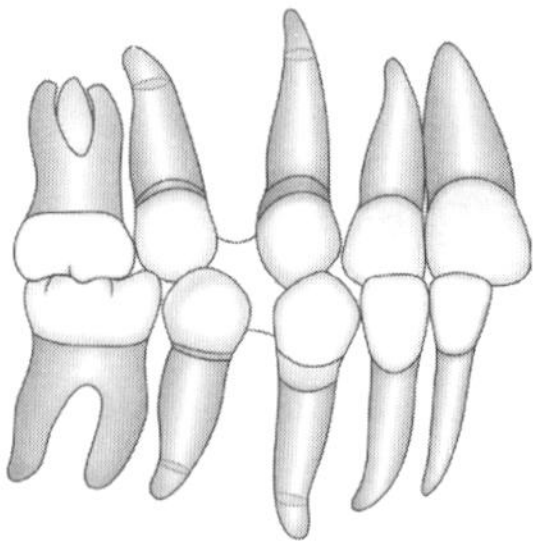

- Step 4

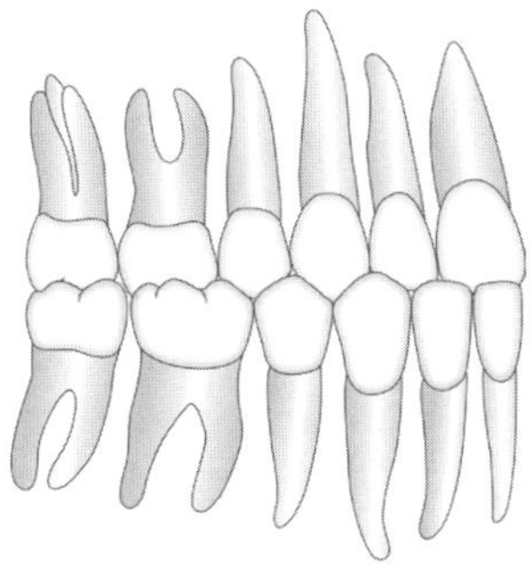

Developing Anterior Crossbite

Anterior crossbite can be classified into:
- Dental crossbite
- Functional
- Skeletal.

Dental

- The most common etiologic factor of nonskeletal anterior crossbites is lack of space for the permanent incisors
- If the developing crossbite is discovered before eruption is complete, the adjacent primary teeth can be extracted to provide the necessary space
- A tongue blade therapy can be used
- Anterior crossbites diagnosed after the incisors have erupted require appliance therapy for correction
- Bilateral disking of extraction of adjacent primary teeth is done for space. Finger spring of Z-spring is used in an appliance with multiple clasps for retention
- Anterior or posterior bite plate can be used to reduce overbite while the cross bite is being corrected
- Fixed appliance like maxillary lingual arch with finger springs can also be used
- Fixed appliance using posterior bands and anterior bonded attachments with round wires can be used as well.

Functional

- Due to occlusal prematurities or other reasons because of which mandible is positioned forward
- This can be treated by removing the occlusal prematurities or the aetiological factor.

Skeletal

These are best treated during growth by growth modification procedures by the use of myofunctional or orthopaedic appliances.

Habits

- Most children indulge in non-nutritive sucking habits
- Intervention is not usually indicated until 5 years of age. As long as the habits stop before eruption of permanent incisors, most of the dental changes resolve spontaneously
- "Adult" approach of straight forward discussion between the child and dentist can be very beneficial. If this approach fails, an inward system can be implemented
- Pleasure of sucking can be removed by placing a cotton glove on the hand or a bandaid on thumb or finger. A maxillary lingual arch, especially quad-helix has the reminder effect when used for maxillary expansion
- A cemented reminder appliance comprising of a maxillary lingual arch and a crib can be used
- An oral screen can be given for patients with mouth breathing
- Tongue thrusting habit should be intercepted using habit breakers. The patient should be trained and educated on the correct technique of swallowing.

Space Regainers

It is the process of gaining space lost by drifting of adjacent teeth following premature loss of deciduous tooth/teeth

Space regainer is a fixed or removable appliance capable of moving a displaced permanent tooth into its proper position in dental arch.

Indications

- One or more primary teeth have been lost
- Some space in the arch has been lost due to mesial drift of the first permanent molar.
    - Loss of arch perimeter usually is the result of caries or premature loss of primary teeth.

The most frequent cause of arch perimeter loss in the mixed dentition is caries of the primary molars.

A carious lesion on the distal surface of the second primary molar, in particular allows the first permanent molar to tip mesially.

Usually when several primary teeth are lost, the arch perimeter is shortened and space regaining is indicated.

Appliances for Space Regaining

Gerber Space Regainer

- A seamless orthodontic band or a crown is selected for the tooth to be distalised
- This space regainer consists of a "U" shaped hollow tubing and a "U" shaped rod that enters the tubing
- The tube is soldered or welded on the mesial aspect of the first molar to be moved distally

- The "U" shaped wire or rod is fitted into the tube, in such a way that the base of the "U" rod contacts the tooth mesial to the edentulous area
- Open coil springs of adequate length are placed around the free ends of the "U" shaped rod and inserted into the tubing assembly **(Fig. 20.1)**
- The forces generated by the compressed open coil springs bring about a distal movement of the first molar.

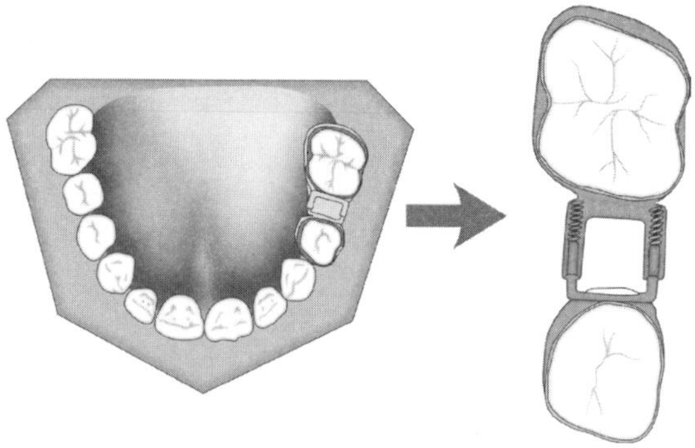

Fig. 20:1 Gerber space regainer

Jack Screw

- Space regaining can be brought about using jack screws placed in such a way that an increase in arch length is obtained by distalisation of the molar **(Fig. 20.2)**
- The appliance consists of a split acrylic plate with a jack screw in relation to the edentulous space and is retained using Adam's clasps.

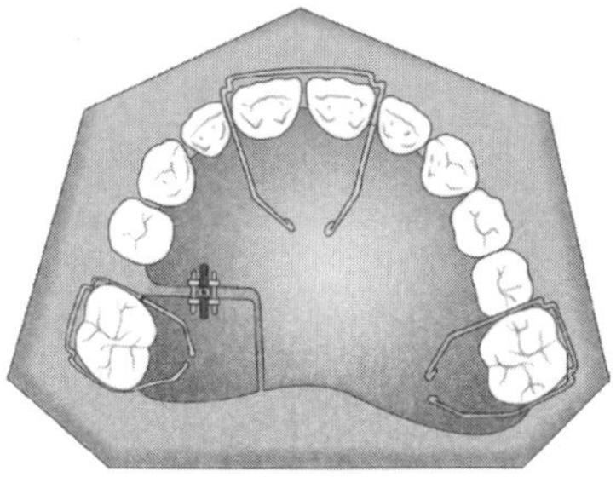

Fig. 20.2: Jack screw

Recurved Helical Spring

- The upper or lower hawley appliance with recurved helical spring against the mesial surface of a molar that has drifted forward is effective in molar distalisation
- A removable appliance retained with Adam's clasps and incorporating a helical finger spring adjacent to the tooth to be moved is very effective **(Fig. 20.3)**
- This appliance is the ideal design for tipping one molar. One posterior tooth can be moved up to 3 mm distally during 3-4 months of full time appliance wear
- The spring is activated approximately 2 mm to produce 1 mm of movement per month. The molar generally will derotate spontaneously as it is tipped distally.

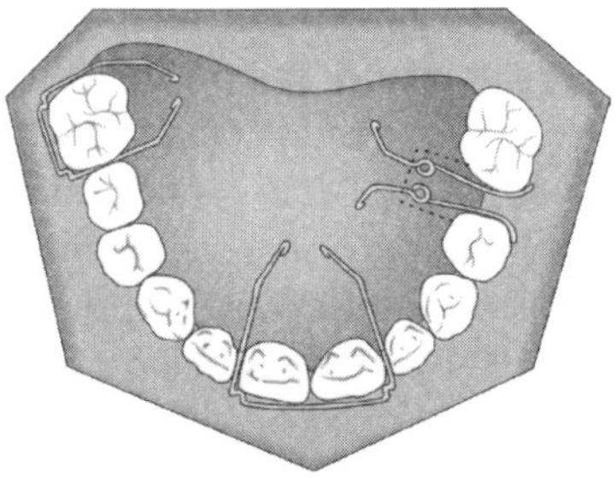

Fig. 20.3: Recurved helical spring

Muscle Exercises

It helps in developing improving aberrant muscle functions.

Masseter

Clenching of teeth while counting till ten. Process should be repeated ten times.

Lips

Stretching of upper lip to maintain lip seal (paper may be held between lips)—for hypotonic lip patients.

- Stretch upper lip downwards towards chin
- Hold and pump water back and forth behind lips
- Massaging of the lips.

Button pull exercise: Take 1½ inch diameter button, pass a thread through buttonhole, place the button behind lips and pull thread, while restricting it from being pulled by using lip pressure.

Tongue

- One elastic swallow: 5/16 inch intra oral elastic is placed on the tip of the tongue and patient is asked to raise the tongue and hold the elastic against rugae area and swallow
- Tongue hold exercise: 5/16 inch intraoral elastic is placed on a designated spot on the tongue for a prescribed time with lip closed and then the patient is asked to swallow keeping elastic in place and lips apart
- Two elastic swallow: Two 5/16 inch elastics are placed over the tongue. One in the midline and the other on the tip and the patient is asked to swallow with the elastics in place

- The hold pull exercise: The tip and the midpoint of tongue are made to contact the palate and the mandible is gradually opened. This helps in stretching of lingual frenum.

Removal of Soft Tissue or Bonny Barriers

- Surgically exposing the crown
- Tissue removal
- Removal of bony barriers.

Interception of Skeletal Malrelations

Class II: Promoting growth of mandible—myofunctional appliances. Restricting growth of maxilla using head gear and facebow combination

Class III: Restricting growth of mandible or promoting growth of maxilla or both.

CHAPTER 21

Methods of Gaining Space

LONG ESSAYS

Question 1

What are the different methods of gaining space? Explain in detail about Proximal stripping/Tooth Reproximation/ Slenderization/Disking/Proximal Slicing/Enamel Stripping?

Answer

Different methods of gaining space are:
- Proximal stripping
- Expansion
- Extraction
- Distalisation
- Molar uprighting
- Derotation of posterior teeth
- Proclination of anterior teeth.

Proximal Stripping

According to Peck and Peck Proximal stripping or Tooth Reproximation is a clinical procedure involving the reduction, anatomic recontouring, and protection of the mesial and/or distal enamel surfaces of a permanent tooth".

Indications

- Class I arch length discrepancies with orthognathic profiles
- Minor Class II dental malocclusions (particularly non-growing patients)
- Bolton tooth size discrepancies
- Arch length discrepancies less than the size of two premolars
- Peck and Peck ratio indicating need for slenderization.

Amount of Proximal Stripping

- Various studies have reported that approximately 50% of the enamel can be safely removed
- Premolars–0.5 mm
- Canines–0.4 mm
- Incisors–0.3 mm.

Advantages of Proximal Stripping

- With the help of this procedure in borderline cases, extraction can be avoided which is especially beneficial when treating adult non-growing patients
- A more favourable overbite and overjet can be established by eliminating tooth material excess in either of the arches conforming with the Bolton's tooth size discrepancy, which improves anterior function in the mutually protected occlusion
- Reduction of the widths of the upper and lower incisors and canines for orthodontic purposes conforms more closely to basic biologic requirements than does orthodontic tooth extraction
- Prevention of relapse: Williams gave six keys for elimination of lower incisor retention. The sixth key was slenderization as needed after treatment to achieve broad flat contacts which helps to resist labio-lingual crown displacement in comparison to rounded point contacts of unattachted enamel
- Areas of inter-proximal gingival recession can be improved
- Removal of cracked enamel after treatment.

Diagnostic Procedures to Determine Need for Proximal Stripping

- Bolton tooth size discrepancies: Proximal stripping is utilized to remove the excess tooth material in anterior or posterior teeth
- Arch length discrepancies less than the size of two premolars; determined by Carey's and arch perimeter analysis
- Peck and Peck ratio indicating need for slenderization.

Procedure

There are two steps:
1. Initial reduction
2. Polishing.

Methods of Reduction

- Mechanical
  - Abrasive strips (hand held/motor driven)
    - Abrasive linen strips **(Fig. 21.1)**
    - Diamond coated metal.
  - Abrasive discs
    - Safe sided carborundum discs (mounted on contra-angle handpiece) **(Fig. 21.2)**
    - Perforated diamond coated disc (in an oscillating handpiece). Thin double sided diamond disc **(Fig. 21.3)**.
    - Ultrasonic unit using an aluminium hydroxide paste and special reducing tips
    - Long thin burs **(Fig. 21.4)**.
- Chemical
- Combination techniques.

Fig. 21.1: Abrasive linen strips

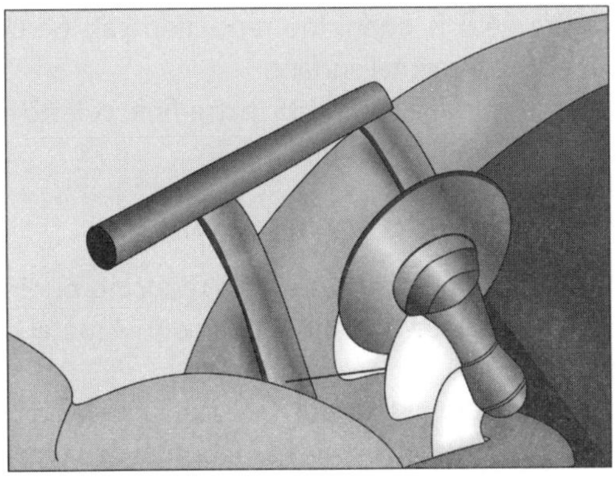

Fig. 21.2: Carborundum disc

Polishing

- Tungsten carbide burs
- Oscillating Elastrips (fine/ultrafine)
- Sof-Lex XT discs (fine/ultrafine).

Technique of Proximal Stripping

- Air-rotor stripping (ARS)
- Modified ARS (for anterior teeth)
- Combination technique (mechanical and chemical).

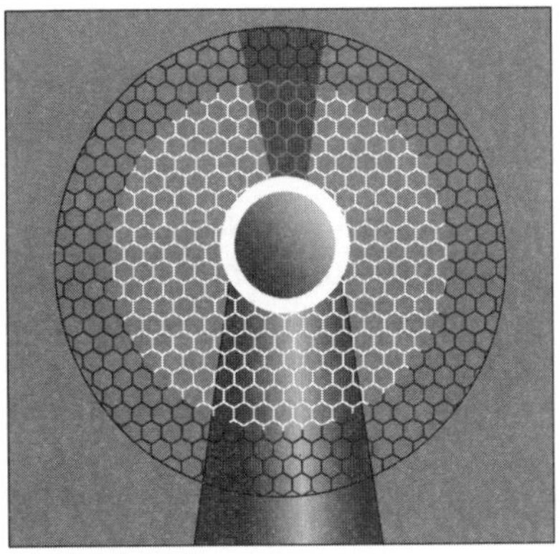

Fig. 21.3: Diamond coated disc

Air-Rotor Stripping (John Sheridan)

- This technique is used primarily in buccal segment in order to retract anterior teeth **(Fig. 21.5** and **21.6)**
- It enables the operator to eliminate precise amount of tooth material
- Up to 8–9 mm space can be obtained per arch
- Align all the teeth
- Gain visual access in the desired area preferably by placing a separator for a couple of days prior to the procedure
- To prevent injury to the gingiva, a brass wire (0.20") is placed between tissue and bur, this wire also act as indicator wire
- Removal of enamel:
  - The bur of choice for the initial reduction is a 699L, a small, tapered crosscut fissure carbide bur with an extended cutting area
  - Water spray.
- The above bur is fitted in an air-rotor and then the handpiece is placed on the indicator wire and moved parallel to the plane of the wire occlusally or incisally with a light wiping motion

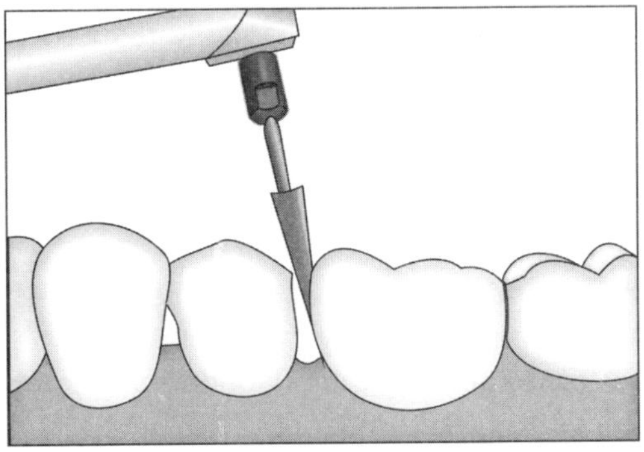

Fig. 21.4: Diamond coated Tungsten carbide

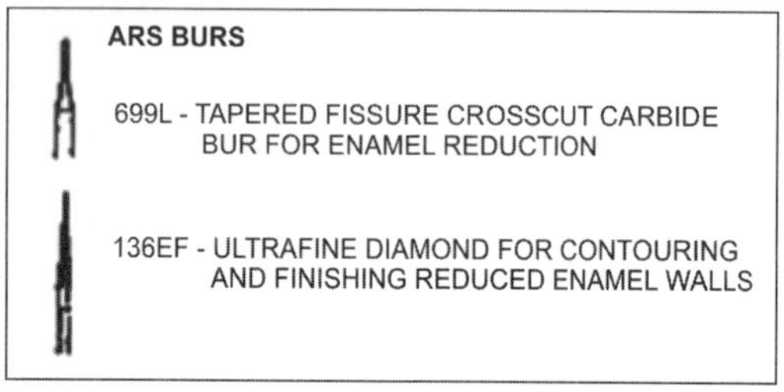

Fig. 21.5: Types of air-rotor stripping (ARS)

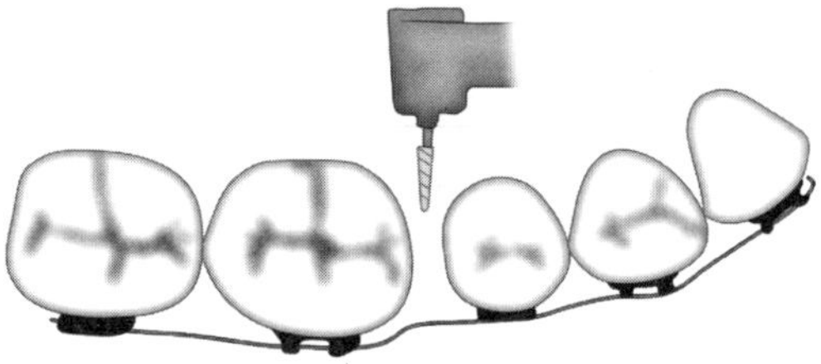

Fig. 21.6: Air-rotor stripping in open field

- Since the field is open, the reduction can be done on either of the proximal surface
- Finish the surface with 135 extra-fine stiletto shaped ultra-fine finishing diamond bur.

Modified Air-Rotor Stripping (ARS)

- A modified ARS procedure uses a reducing bur in an air-turbine handpiece in combination with a metal abrasive strip
- This modification is useful for the removal of smaller amounts of inter-proximal enamel and is usually reserved for the lower anterior teeth, where thin inter-proximal enamel permits less mesiodistal reduction
- The inter-proximal enamel is reduced with a 699L stripping bur on the lingual and facial surfaces until the contact area is a knife-edge of enamel
- This enamel is then removed with the handheld abrasive strip
- The advantage of this two-stage procedure is that the air-rotor reduces the bulk of the enamel so that less force is required with the handheld abrasive strip
- This procedure is most efficient before or after treatment, when the teeth are not mobile.

Combined Technique

- It is advocated by V.P. Joseph, P.E. Rossouw and N.J. Basson which Combined mechanical and chemical stripping method
- In this technique, the mechanically reduced proximal surface is treated with 37% orthophosphoric acid
- The furrows created by the mechanical reduction are more or less flattened by this acid etch procedure producing a surface which can better "heal itself" by re-mineralization
- Artificial re-mineralization of the etched enamel surface is possible as shown by crystal growth
- A low concentrate calcium-fluoride solution produced this growth in a time dependent fashion.

Fluoride Application for Re-mineralisation of Enamel Surface

Any stripping procedure removes the caries-resistant, fluoride-rich layer of surface enamel. This can readily be re-established with commercially available, office-applied fluoride rinses.

Precautions

- Utmost care must be taken in performing this procedure in teeth of young individuals as they have larger pulp horns and might develop sensitivity
- The teeth which have undergone the procedure should be recorded and charted carefully to avoid repetition of procedure again in the same tooth
- Improper slicing may cause ledging of enamel which should be avoided
- The procedure must not be performed without achieving adequate separation of teeth as this causing slicing of teeth and results in unstable arch form.

Advantages

- Removal of precise amount of inter-proximal enamel to create space, primarily in the buccal quadrants, for aligning or retracting teeth
- In selected cases, ARS can resolve significant differences in ratios of tooth size to arch length, and the technique can become an alternative to extraction or expansion. Up to 8.9 mm of space can be obtained in an arch using ARS
- Air-rotor stripping can create substantially more space than is usually obtained by conventional inter-proximal reduction procedures
- The lower incisors have less proximal enamel than posterior teeth, and lower incisor irregularity generally increases naturally at an age when most orthodontic cases are in retention
- Anterior inter-proximal reduction of more than 2–3 mm would virtually eliminate the option of further reduction to eliminate post-treatment crowding, simply because there would be little if any enamel remaining on the lower incisors

- In lower incisor extraction cases, a tooth material disproportion is created between upper and lower anteriors leading to unfavourable overjet
- Stripping in the upper anteriors only can lead to unaesthetic shapes. ARS helps in redistributing the tooth material reduction.

Disadvantages

- The technical concern in reproximation procedure is the precised removal of substantial inter-proximal enamel, following which the complete reduction site should have smoothly finished enamel walls without undercuts and the reduced surfaces should be reshaped to resemble the original inter-proximal morphology
- Space opening occurs infrequently in an ARS site, and the majority of the space closes during retention, but it is a possible long-term effect of the ARS procedure
- Irreversible, hence should be done with utmost caution and responsibility
- The technique should be selectively used on patients with good oral hygiene and low caries susceptibility.

Question 2

What is molar distalisation?

Answer

"Molar distalisation" in orthodontics is defined as the backward movement of dental units to gain space for the sagittal correction of malocclusion. As with other dental movements along the arch, distalisation can be a simple tipping of the molar crown or a bodily movement of crown and root complex.

Classification

Classifications of the various molar distalising appliances are as follows:

Intra-oral

Appliances for Maxillary Arch

Fixed Appliances

- Buccally acting
- Palatally acting
- Both buccally and palatal acting
- Implant supported appliance.

Buccally acting appliances:

- Jones Jig
- Nickel-titanium (NiTi) double loop system
- Repelling magnets
- Carriere distaliser
- Super elastic NiTi
- Wilson's rapid molar distaliser
- Lokar appliance
- K-Loop.

Palatally acting appliances:

- Distal jet appliance
- Nance appliance
- Titanium-molybdenum alloy (TMA) transpalatal arch
- Pendulum appliance
- Simplified molar distaliser
- Green field lingual distaliser.

Palatally and buccally acting:

- First class appliance
- Fixed piston appliance
- Intra-oral bodily distaliser.

Implant supported appliances:

- Mid palatal screw
- Implant supported distal jet
- Skeletal anchorage system (SAS).

Removable Appliances

- Tube plates
- Cetlin appliance
- Acrylic cervical occipital appliance (ACCO)
- Removable molar distalising splint
- C-space regainer
- Cricket appliance
- Essix-based molar distalisation.

Appliances for Mandibular Arch

- Franzulum appliance
- Unilateral Crozat appliance.

Inter Arch

- Herbst appliance
- Lip bumper
- Klapper superspring
- Jasper Jumper.

Indications

- Class-II molar relationship due to maxillary dento-alveolar protrusion
- Class-II molar relationship due to impacted or high labially placed cuspids
- Class-II subdivision cases requiring unilateral distal molar movement
- Class-II molar relationship due to ectopic eruption of either first or second bicuspid

- Midline discrepancy cases
- Regaining the space loss due to mesial drift of first molars, following premature loss of deciduous teeth
- Anchorage loss during active orthodontic treatment.

The indications of molar distalisation can be summarised under the following headings:

Profile

Straight profile.

Functional

- Normal, healthy temporomandibular joint
- Correct mandible to maxillary relationship.

Skeletal

- Class I skeletal
- Normal, short lower face height
- Maxilla/normal transverse width
- Brachycephalic growth pattern
- Skeletal closed bite.

Dental

- Class II molar relationship
- Deep overbite
- Permanent dentition
- Maxillary first molar mesially inclined
- Prior to eruption of second molar
- Maxillary cuspids labially displaced
- Loss of arch length due to premature loss of second deciduous molar.

Contraindications

- An end on or full Class II molar relationship due to mandibular retrognathism
- Retrognathic profile (Class II skeletal with orthognathic maxilla and retrognathic mandible)
- Skeletal and dental open bite
- Excessive lower anterior facial height (dolichofacial form)
- Constricted maxilla
- Patients with Class-II or Class-III molar relation.

The contraindications of molar distalisation can be summarised under the following headings:

Profile

Retrognathic profile.

Functional

- Numerous signs and symptoms of temporomandibular joint
- Posteriorly and superiorly displaced condyles.

Skeletal

- Class II skeletal
- Skeletal open bite
- Excess lower face height
- Constricted maxillary arch
- Dolichocephalic growth pattern.

Dental

- Class I or Class III molar relation
- Dental open bite
- Maxillary first molar distally inclined.

Extra-oral

Extraoral forces are used through headgears to carry out molar distalisation.

Cervical Pull Headgear

Effects (Fig. 21.7)

- Extrusion of upper jaw
- Distal movement of maxilla
- Steepening of occlusal plane
- Expansion of the upper dental arch.

Advantages

The direction of pull is advantageous in treatment of short face, Class II maxillary protrusive cases with low mandibular plane angle and deep bites.

Disadvantages

- It normally causes extrusion of the upper molars
- This movement is seldom desirable except in patients with reduced lower anterior facial height
- It is contraindicated in patients with steep mandibular plane and in open bite cases.

Occipital Pull Headgear

Effects (Fig. 21.8)

- Distalising and intrusive forces since the force is exerted above the occlusal plane
- Distalises the molar without any unwanted extrusion
- A high pull headgear can decrease the vertical development of the maxilla, thereby allowing for autorotation of the mandible and maximizing the horizontal expression of mandibular growth.

Advantages

These headgears can be used in patients with steep mandibular planes and in cases where in mandibular growth is more vertical than horizontal.

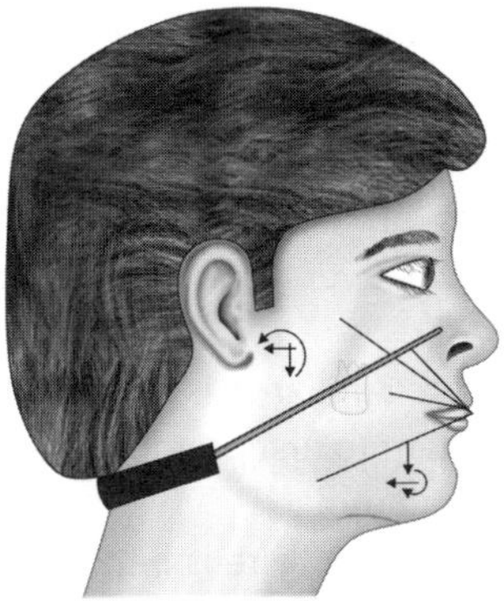

Fig. 21.7: Cervical pull headgear

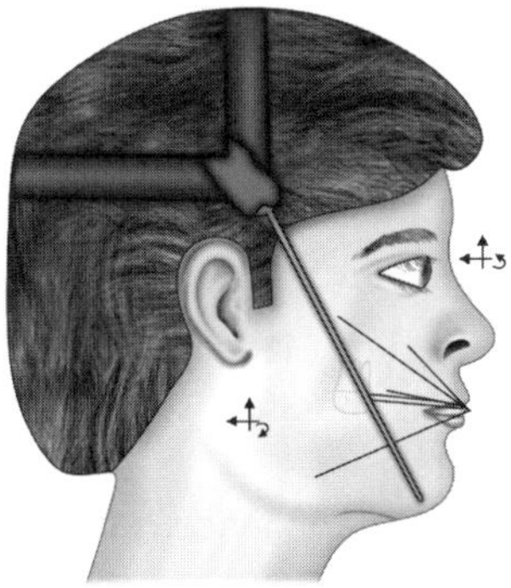

Fig. 21.8: Occipital pull headgear

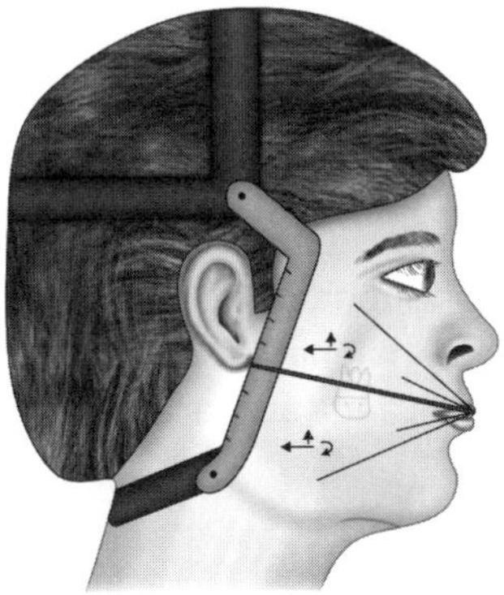

Fig. 21.9: Combination headgear

Combination Headgear

- Combination headgear has both occipital and cervical traction springs **(Fig. 21.9)**
- For distal translation of the upper posteriors, a distal traction is needed that passes through the Cres (centre of resistance), neither above nor below
- Based on occlusal plane requirements
    - To obtain a distal force and to flatten the occlusal plane, the outer bow should be adjusted above Cres
    - To obtain a distal force and to steepen the occlusal plane, the outer bow should be adjusted below the Cres
    - To obtain a distal force with no moment, the outer bow should be adjusted at the Cres.

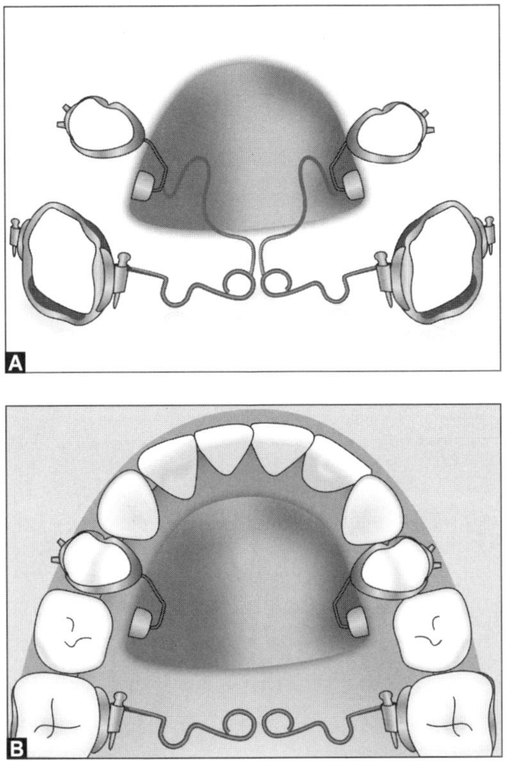

Figs. 21.10A and B: Pendulum appliance

Intraoral Methods

Pendulum Appliance

- It is developed by James Hilgers **(Figs. 21.10A and B)**
    - It is a hybrid appliance that uses a large Nance acrylic button in the palate for anchorage, along with 0.032" titanium molybedenum alloy (TMA) spring that deliver continuous force to the inner first molar without affecting the palatal button
- Thus the appliance produces a broad swinging or pendulum of force from the midline of palate to the upper molars
- Since appliance drives molar distally, it has the tendency to open the bite anteriorly, hence it is not advised in dolichofacial type
- Distal movement of first molars appears most efficiently before the eruption of second molars hence the appliance should be used before the second molars have erupted
- Almost 5 mm of distal molar movement is obtained in 3–4 months.

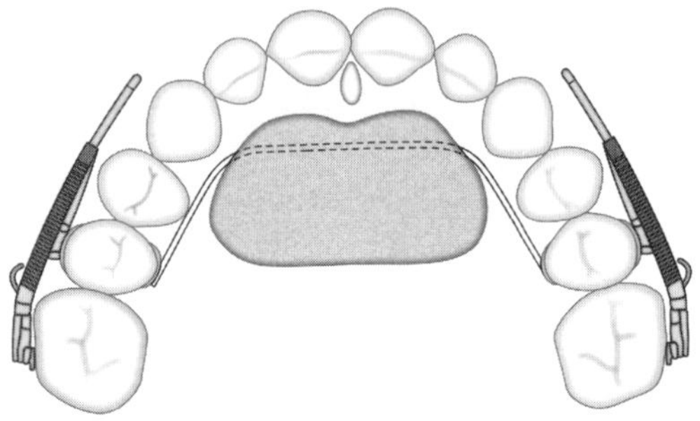

Fig. 21.11: Jones Jig appliance

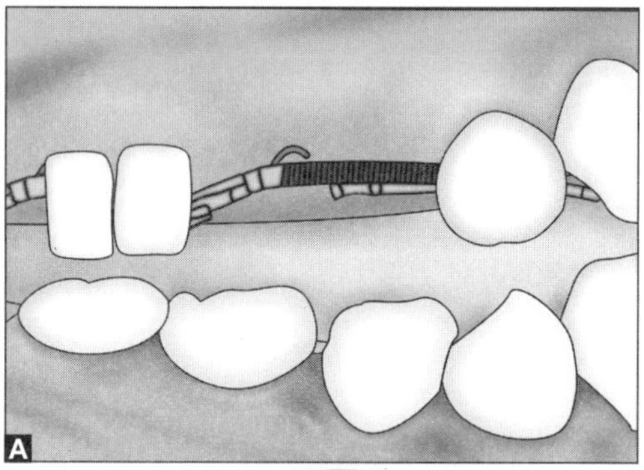

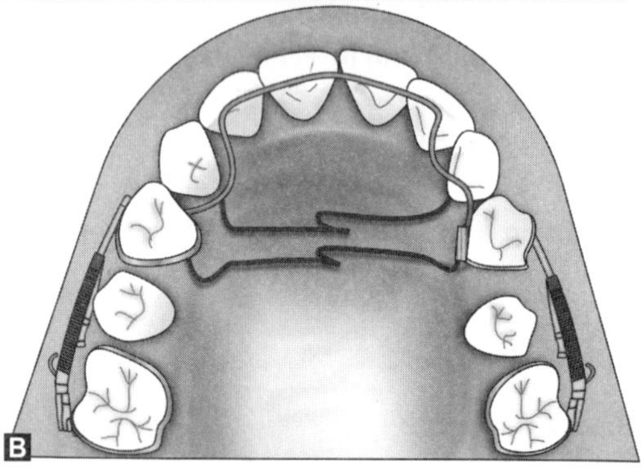

Figs. 21.12A and B: Repelling magnets

Jones Jig Appliance

- Jones Jig was developed by Richard D Jones and J Michael White **(Fig. 21.11)**
- Jones Jig uses an open coil spring NiTi to deliver 70–75 mg of force over a compression range of 1–5 mm to the molars
- A modified Nance appliance is used with the Jones Jig for ease of attachment to first premolar, second premolar, or deciduous second molar
- A 0.036" stainless steel wire is bent to the palate on the cast extending it as far as the canines, and it is soldered to the anchor bands
- Acrylic button is fabricated about half inch in diameter
- The Nance appliance is cemented and the Jones Jig is laid in place on both sides
- Reactivation is done after every 4-5 weeks interval.

Repelling Magnets

- This was developed by Gianelly **(Figs. 21.12A and B)**
- Nance appliance is modified with the incorporation of repelling magnets
- The modified Nance appliance is cemented on the first premolar; this is to encourage the distal drift of the second premolar that occurs normally as first molars are moved posteriorly
- Activation of magnets is done by tying a 0.014 inch ligature wire through the loop and extended anteriorly to encircle a tie back hook mesial to the magnets
- When tightened, the magnets are held in contact to contain the reaction force arising from the magnets
- The reactivation shoud be done once a week
- Force exerted by magnet is 200–225 g
- This drops significantly as space gets opened.

CHAPTER 22 Arch Expansion

LONG ESSAYS

Question 1

What is rapid maxillary expansion/ rapid palatal expansion?

Answer

Rapid maxillary expansion is essentially a dentofacial orthopaedic therapy. The forces employed range from 10 to 20 pounds per day and the active phase is of around 4 weeks followed by a retention phase of 4 months.

Indications

- Cases of real and relative maxillary deficiency with posterior crossbite
- All type of Class III cases, i.e., pseudo-dental and skeletal Class III
- Cases of nasal stenosis—(Usually characterized by full time mouth breathing and a constricted nasal aperture with the conchae laterally compressed against the septum)
- Mature cleft lip and cleft palate patients with collapsed maxilla
- Anteroposterior maxillary deficiency cases.

Contraindications

- Poor patient cooperation
- Single tooth in crossbite
- Patient who have anterior open bites, steep mandibular plane, and convex profile
- Patient with skeletal asymmetry of maxilla or mandible and adults with severe anter-posterior and unilateral skeletal discrepancies. RME can be done if it is to be followed with orthognathic surgery.
- Some operators set an upper age limit, i.e., the age when synostosis has occurred. But with adjunctive surgery this is surmounte
- Normal buccal occlusion
- However if there are overriding medical reasons of a respiratory nature for RME, we have to give priority to this and correct
- If there is a medical reason for RME but with "cover bite" (i.e., maxillary teeth completely outside mandibular teeth) then it is a definite contradiction
- Periodontally weak teeth.

Types of Appliance

Removable

Fixed:

- Tooth born
  - Bande
  - Splints.
- Tooth and tissue borne:
  - Banded
  - Splints.

Removable Expansion Plates

- Removable expansion plates are not recommended if significant skeletal changes are required
- Midpalatal splitting with such appliances is possible, but not predictable
- For these appliances to be effective, they must be used in the deciduous or early mixed dentition and must have sufficient retention to be stable during the expansion phase (Ivanovsky)
- Retention is often difficult and the forces created tend to dislodge the appliance before sufficient force is created to cause a palatal split.
- Though, fabrication and maintenance of oral hygiene is much easier, removable RME appliances are not recommended
- Various designs of removable RME appliances have been tried.

Examples

- Expansion screw with palatal acrylic coverage and retentive clasp components
- Acrylic embedding the screw and covering the palate and extending onto the anchor teeth up to facial aspect designed by Ivanovsky.

Fixed type of RME Appliances

The appliance is attached to the teeth with bands cemented on the anchor teeth or by means of bonded splints.

Splints are basically of two type:

1. Cast cap splints
2. Acrylic splint

Cap splints are usually cast in silver/copper alloy and incorporate palatal extensions to recieve the acrylic components.

Acrylic splints are made using polymethyl methacrylate with or without a wire support framework adapted around the cervical third of the anchor teeth. The expansion screw can be spring-loaded or non-spring-loaded jackscrew.

Fixed Tooth Borne Appliance

Isaacson Type

- This appliance uses a special spring-loaded screw called a Minne expander, which is adapted and soldered directly to the bands without the use of acrylic
- The screw may be reduced in length to suit narrow arches by shortening the spring, tube and rod.

Biedermann Type

- Here special screws like the Hyrax (Dentaurum 602–813, leone 620 or Unitek 44 0–160) are used
- These have extensions of heavy gauge wire from the screw or splints.

Fixed Tooth and Tissue Borne Appliance

- Here the screw is embedded in acrylic which appraises the palatal vault and the alveolar ridges
- Usually the first premolars and first permanent molars are banded with bands of a slightly loose fit as it is extremely difficult to seat four tightly fitting bands simultaneously
- Wires (1 mm diameter) can be soldered to the buccal aspects of the bands to increase rigidity; or brackets may be welded and used to attach arch wires for connection of teeth not covered by the RME device.

Derichsweiler Type

Wire lags are welded and soldered to the palatal aspect or the bands to facilitate attachment for the acrylic, which is extended to the palatal aspect of all nonbanded teeth except incisors.

Haas Type

- A length of 0.045 inches (1.15 mm) stainless steel wire is welded and soldered along the buccal and palatal aspects of the bands
- The free ends are turned back and embedded in the acrylic base, which stops short of the bands and teeth
- A proprietary screw is set in the midline of the split acrylic base
- The screw is mounted in the midline of the vault with the thread axis in line with the anterior border of the first permanent molars
- The thread axis must be at right angles to the sagittal plane if there is mesial migration of one of the molars
- To facilitate easier turning of the screw by the patient, it is mounted so that the thread is rotated from front to back for expansion.

Effects of RME

- Maxillary complex: Rapid maxillary expansion occurs when the force applied to the teeth and the maxillary alveolar processes exceed the limits needed for orthodontic tooth movement. The applied pressure acts as an orthopaedic force that opens the mid-palatal suture. The appliance compresses the periodontal ligament, bends the alveolar processes, tips the anchor teeth, and gradually opens the mid-palatal suture
- Palatal vault: The palatine processes of the maxilla were lowered as a result of the outward tilting of the maxillary halves
- Alveolar process: Lateral bending of the alveolar processes occurs early during RME
- Maxillary anterior teeth: Opening of a diastema between the maxillary central incisors. The incisors separate approximately half the distance the expansion screw has been opened.

Maxillary Posterior Teeth

The posterior teeth/molar tip buccally due to both alveolar bone bending and tipping of the molar.

Mandible

The mandible autorotates downwards and backwards making the profile convex and increasing vertical height of lower face.

SHORT ESSAYS

Question 1

What is expansion screw?

Answer

Expansion screws are devices incorporated in appliance to carry out expansion of maxilla.

Types of expansion screw broadly classified into:

- Skeleton screws: Part of the spiral embedded in the acrylic, more superior and more preferred. It is available in various sizes, broader for maxilla and narrower for the mandible. The smaller size is also effective for distal movement of teeth
- Encased screws are sturdy and resist stress. The spiral part may sometimes turn back
- Special screw like:
  - Pull screws here an expanded encased screw is inserted and subsequently closed to effect the desired tooth movement
  - Bertoni screw for expansion in three dimensions
  - Articulated screw.
- Eccentric screws, e.g., for fan wise expansion with hinge axis with omega spring:
  - Two stage expansion screw: Widening of the maxillary arch by palatal expansion technique often necessitates using, two different expansion screw appliance an initial one, small enough to fit in an extremely narrow arch and produce, preliminary expansion and a subsequent larger appliance with which to achieve desired arch width
  - Hyrax expansion screw: For mid palatal suture separation by means of fixed appliance without the need for acrylic plates. Metal frame work used in combination with performed band which are soldered to the retention arm.

Protocol for Expansion

- Young growing patients two turns each day for the first 5 days, one turn each day for the remainder of rapid maxillary expansion (RME) treatment
- Adult (non-growing) patient—because of increased skeletal resistance, two turns each day for the first 2 days, one turn each day for the next 7 days, and one turn every other day for the remainder of RME treatment.

CHAPTER 23 Extractions

LONG ESSAYS

Question 1

Discuss extraction planning in orthodontic treatment?

Answer

Extraction of teeth is a common method of gaining space during orthodontic treatment protocol. The choice of teeth for extraction depends on following factors:

- Treatment objectives
- Type of malocclusion
- Aesthetics (large chin button, prominent nose)
- Growth pattern
- Conditions of teeth (caries, multi-filled teeth, impacted, ectopic and severe rotation)
- Health of supporting tissues.

Extraction of First Premolars

Advantages

- Strategically located close to the incisors, therefore, help in resolving anterior crowding or proclination
- Centre of each half of arch, thus, can help in resolving both anterior and posterior defects
- Adequate anchorage for retraction of six anterior teeth
- Contact between canine and second premolar satisfactory, therefore, chances of food impaction below the contact point are less.
- Indications for first premolar extraction are:
  - Convex profile with severe crowding
  - Class II, division I with deep anterior bite
  - Class I with severe crowding
  - Class I with bimaxillary protrusion.

Second Premolar Extraction

Advantages

- Lesser tendency for extraction space to open in mandibular arch
- First premolar are more aesthetic along with canine
- Less possibility of formation of buccal/lingual furrow in extraction space
- Easy correction of Class II molar relation to Class I molar relation
- Original facial contours retained without reduction of lip profile.

Indications

- Good profile with mild crowding cases
- Cases with flat profile and moderate crowding
- Class II, division I malocclusion with skeletal Class I and mild crowding
- Mild Class III malocclusion with mild crowding in U-arch
- Impacted second premolar
- Grossly destructed/heavily restored
- Abnormal root morphology
- Open bite.

Extraction of First Molar

Extractions of first molars for orthodontic treatment are avoided for following reasons:

- Do not provide adequate space in the anterior region
- Second molar or second premolar may tip into the extraction space
- Deepening of bite occurs
- Masticatory efficiency is reduced.

Indications

- Grossly decayed teeth that cannot be preserved with restoration
- Root canal treated, than a perfectly good premolar
- Multiple fillings in the crown
- Facial considerations: Large chin buttons and prominent nose
- Open bite cases.

Extraction of Second Molar

Indications

- Disimpaction of third molars
- Prevention of late incisor crowding
- Facilitation of first molar distalisation
- Distal movement only as needed to correct the overjet.

Advantages

- Fewer "residual"spaces at the end of treatment
- Less likelihood of relapse
- Good functional occlusion
- Good mandibular arch form
- Good overbite reduction.

Third Molar Extraction

Indications

- When first and second molar have to be distalised
- When third molar is impacted
- When it is grossly decayed
- When it interferes with normal occlusion
- To prevent late mandibular anterior crowding.

Contraindications

In cases, where first and second molar are extracted.

Extraction of Incisor

Indications

For mandibular incisors:

- Extreme crowding/protrusion
- Gingival recession and loss of overlying bone on labial surface
- Lateral incisors severely fractured in young children
- Rare-discrepancy in sizes of upper and lower incisors themselves; central incisor can be removed
- Angles Class III malocclusion with anterior crowding.

Advantages

- Maintains or reduces inter-canine width
- General arch form is maintained leading to greater stability
- Retention period is less
- Anterior segments can be retracted readily, if need be
- Mechanotherapy is simplified. Space closure is quick.

For Maxillary Incisors

- Rarely indicated
- Unfavourable impaction of U-incisor
- Buccally or lingually blocked out lateral with good contact between central and canine
- Congenital missing one lateral incisor
- Dilacerated tooth
- Grossly decayed incisor which cannot be salvaged
- Malformation that cannot be restored by prosthesis
- Fractured or traumatised tooth
- Dilacerated tooth or ankylosed tooth that cannot be moved with orthodontic therapy
- Extraction of Canines.

Indications

- Unfavourable impaction
- Ectopically erupted with a good contact between premolar and incisor
- Deciduous canine are extracted as part of serial extractions.

CHAPTER 24 Orthodontic Appliance: General Concepts

LONG ESSAYS

Question 1

Classify orthodontic appliances. What are the advantages and disadvantages of removable and fixed appliances?

Answer

Orthodontic appliances can be classified as:

- Mechanical appliances
  - Removable appliances
  - Fixed appliances.
- Myofunctional appliances
  - Removable appliances
  - Fixed appliances.

Advantages of Removable Appliances

- Patient can maintain good oral hygiene during orthodontic therapy
- Appliance can be kept clean by the patient
- Tipping type of tooth movement can be carried out by removable appliances
- Most of the tooth movements like tipping, overbite reduction can be carried out
- These are fabricated in laboratory thus, chair side time is reduced
- Orthodontist can handle more number of patients, since, these appliances takes less chair side time
- Lesser forces are used for these appliances than those needed for bodily tooth movement thus, putting less strain on anchorage
- It can be used by general dental practitioners who have received adequate training
- Less inventory is required for the fabrication of removable appliances
- They are less expensive than fixed appliances
- They can be used in community based programmes, wherein a large number of patient are treated, since they are less expensive and require very less chair side time
- They are less conspicuous than multi-banded fixed appliances
- Appliances that are damaged and apply undesirable forces can be removed by the patient.

Disadvantages of Removable Appliances

- Patient cooperation is important for the success of the treatment since the appliance can be removed
- Only tipping movement is possible
- In case of multiple tooth movements, it should be done one at a time
- Therefore, the treatment duration is prolonged in case of severe malocclusion
- It is difficult to treat multiple rotation
- In cases which require extraction, it is very difficult to close residual space by forward movement of posterior teeth
- There is a greater chance of patient misplacing or damaging the appliances
- Patient should have enough skill of removing and replacing the appliance without distorting them
- They cannot be used to treat severe cases of Class II and Class III malocclusion with unfavourable growth pattern.

Advantages of Fixed Appliances

- Patient cooperation is dispensed with to a large extent in the use of fixed appliances. The orthodontist does not depend on the patient for timely wear and management of the appliance
- It is possible to bring about various types of tooth movements, such as tipping, bodily movement, rotation, intrusion and extrusion
- Multiple tooth movements are possible simultaneously. As many tooth movements are undertaken at the same time, the treatment duration is considerably reduced

- More precise tooth movements and detailing of occlusion is possible using fixed appliances
- Fixed appliances can be used to treat most malocclusions including very complicated ones
- Fixed appliances offer better control over anchorage.

Disadvantages of Fixed Appliances

- Oral hygiene maintenance is difficult
- Fixed appliances are more time consuming to fix and adjust
- They are more conspicuous than removable appliances
- They require special training of the operator and are handled by specialized orthodontist
- Damaged appliances that apply misdirected forces cannot be removed by the patient
- Patient has to visit the orthodontist at regular intervals
- Fixed appliances are by far more expensive than removable appliances
- Unless the treatment is done by skilled operator who has been trained to use fixed appliances, there is a greater possibility of producing adverse tooth movements.

Question 2

What are the ideal requirements of an orthodontic appliance?

Answer

There are four ideal requirements of an orthodontic appliance which are as follows:

1. Biologic requirements
2. Mechanical requirements
3. Aesthetic requirements
4. Hygienic requirements.

Biologic Requirements

- The appliance should bring about the desired tooth movements
- The appliance should not produce pathologic changes such as root resorption
- The appliance should not interfere with normal growth
- It should not interfere with the normal function
- The appliance should not bring about sudden changes
- It should not bring about unwanted tooth movement
- The material used in its fabrication should be biocompatible and should not produce toxic effects
- The appliance should not disintegrate in oral fluids.

Mechanical Requirements

- The appliance should be simple to fabricate
- It should not be bulky
- The patient should be comfortable using them
- The appliance should be strong enough to withstand masticatory forces
- The appliances should be universally applicable, i.e., it must be able to handle various malocclusions.

Hygienic Requirements

- The orthodontic appliance should ideally be self-cleansing
- If not, it should be easy to clean them
- The appliance should not interfere with oral hygiene maintenance.

Aesthetic Requirements

- Orthodontic appliance should be aesthetically acceptable
- It is desired to have an appliance that is as inconspicuous as possible.

CHAPTER 25 Removable Appliances

LONG ESSAYS

Question 1

What is removable orthodontics? How does a removable appliance work? Explain in detail about the component of removables appliances?

Answer

Removable orthodontic appliances are the devices which can be inserted into and removed from the oral cavity by the patient at his will.

Action of Removable Appliances

- Removable appliances act by tipping the tooth around its centre of resistance, since they work by applying a single force on to the crown of the teeth
- Tipping can be brought about in the mesio-distal or bucco-lingual direction
- Position of the root apex is considered very important before the beginning of the treatment
- Teeth which have their apex at the correct position are best suited for treatment with removable appliances
- In such patients, the irregularity is usually due to the crown being tipped from its correct position and therefore, a removable orthodontic appliance responds well to tipping and make tooth movement possible
- These appliances do not bring about bodily changes, derotation and uprighting of teeth because of single point contact of these appliances.

Components of Removable Appliances

There are three basic component of removable appliances:

1. Retentive components.
2. Active component.
3. Base plate.

Retentive Components

- These components keep the appliance in place and also resist displacement of the appliance
- A good retention of an appliance leads to the success of removable appliance
- Necessary tooth movements are not possible, if the appliance is loosely fitting or do not have adequate intra-oral anchorage
- Certain wire components which engage undercuts on the teeth provide adequate retention of a removable appliance
- These wire components that aid in retention of a removable appliance are known as clasps.

Mode of Action of Clasps

- Clasps are those components of a removable appliance, which help in stabilising the appliances in the oral cavity by engaging the undercuts found on the teeth
- The wire components are fabricated in a manner so that they engage the following undercuts:
    - **Buccal and lingual cervical undercuts**: These are seen, on the buccal and lingual cervical margins of the molars and premolars
    - Mesial and distal proximal undercuts: These anatomy of molar show that they are widest mesio-distally and become thinner towards cervical margin, thus forming undercuts
- These are utilized by clasps to engage the appliance.

Requisites of an Ideal Clasp

- They should provide adequate retention
- They should be able to be used in both fully and partially erupted teeth
- They should be passive and not apply any force onto the tooth
- Should be easy to fabricate
- Should not impinge on the soft tissue
- Should not interfere in growth
- Should not interfere in occlusion.

Circumferential Clasp or Three-quarter Clasp

- This clasp is fabricated in a manner so that it engages bucco-cervical undercuts
- It is made from 0.8 mm wire (21-gauge)
- It is designed to engage, one proximal undercut along the cervical margin and then carried over the occlusal embrassure across the teeth with the palatal/lingual side (Retentive arm) which get embedded into the acrylic base plate **(Fig. 25.1)**.

Advantage

Simple design, easy to fabricate.

Disadvantage

It cannot be used in partially erupted teeth.

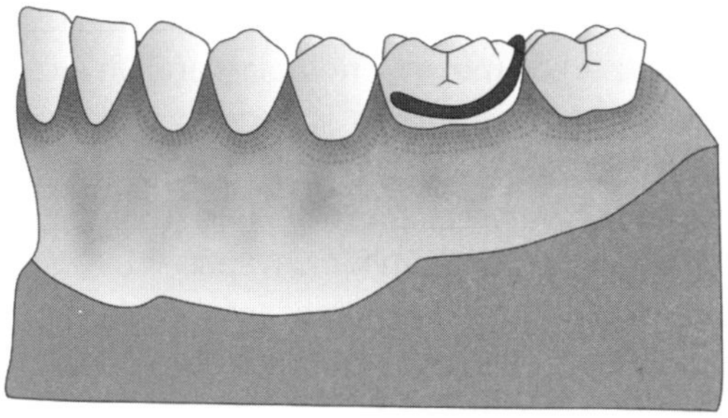

Fig. 25.1: C Clasp

Jackson's Clasp/Full Clasp/U-Clasp

- Fabricated from two guage wire
- Engages bucco-cervical, mesial and distal proximal undercut
- Wire is adapted along bucco-cervical margins and mesial and distal proximal undercuts and is then carried across both the occlusal embrassure of the molar as a retentive arm **(Fig. 25.2)**.

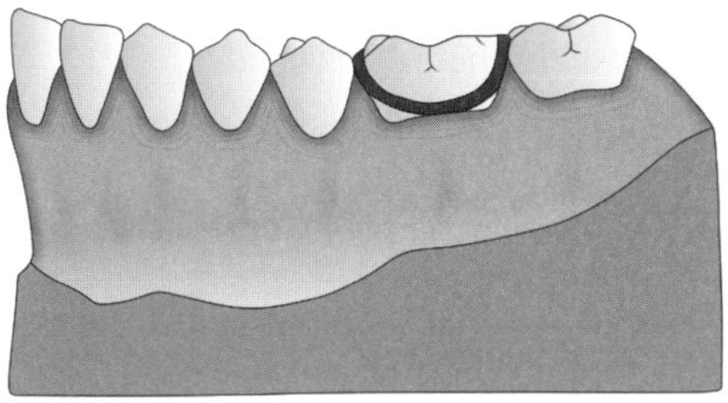

Fig. 25.2: Jackson's Clasp/Full Clasp/U-Clasp

Advantages

- Easy to construct
- Provides adequate retention.

Disadvantage

Does not offer good retention for partially erupted teeth.

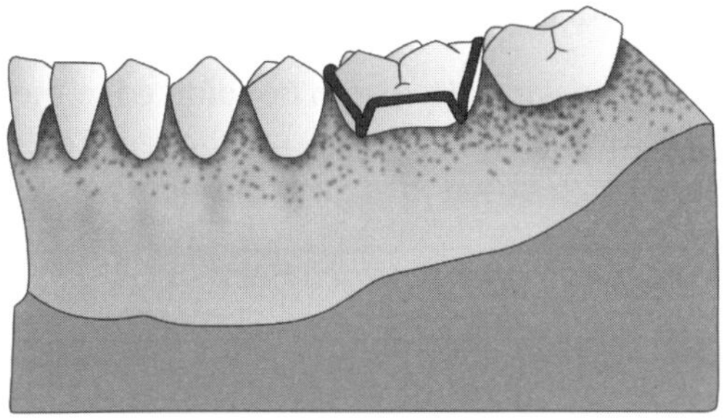

Fig. 25.3: Adam's clasp buccal view

Adam's Clasp

- Professor Philip Adam first described the Adam's clasp
- Other names for Adam's clasp are namely; Liverpool clasp, universal clasp and modified arrowhead clasp
- This clasp provides maximum retention, when constructed properly
- 0.7 mm hard round stainless steel wire is used for the construction of clasp
- Adam's clasp is made up of following parts:
  - Two arrowheads
  - Bridge
  - Two retentive arms.
- The two arrowheads engage the mesial and the distal proximal undercuts
- These arrowheads are connected to each other by a bridge which is at 45° angle to the long axis of the tooth **(Figs 25.3 and 25.4)**.

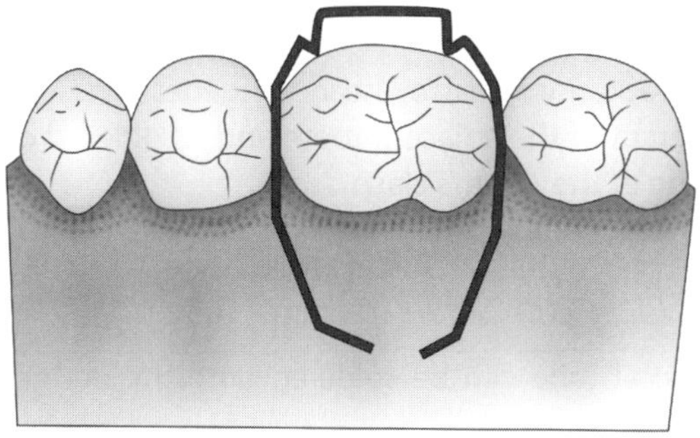

Fig. 25.4: Adam's clasp occlusal view

Advantages

- It is rigid and offer excellent retention
- It can be fabricated on deciduous as well as permanent teeth

- They can be used on partially or fully erupted teeth
- It can be used on molars, pre-molars and on incisors
- No specialised instrument is needed to fabricate the clasp
  - Young's universal plier can be used
- It is small and occupies minimum space
- Clasp can be modified in number of ways.

Modifications of Adam's Clasp

Modifications provide enhanced retention.
Modification are as follows:

Adam's Clasp with Single Arrowhead

- Adam's clasp can be fabricated so that it can have single arrowhead
- This is fabricated for partially erupted tooth, mostly last erupted molar
- Single arrowhead engages the mesio-proximal undercut of the last erupted molar
- Bridge encircles the tooth distally and ends on the palatal aspect as a retentive arm.

Adam's Clasp with J-Hook

- Adam's Clasp with J-Hook can be soldered to the bridge of the Adam's clasp
- These hooks are used to engage the elastics.

Adam's Clasp with Incorporated Helix

A helix can also be incorporated onto the bridge of the Adam's clasp to engage the elastic.

Adam's Clasp with Additional Arrowhead

- An additional arrowhead can be fabricated in an Adam's clasp
- This additional arrowhead engages the proximal undercut of the adjacent tooth and is soldered onto the bridge of the Adam's clasp
- This feature provides additional retention.

Adam's Clasp with Soldered Buccal Tube

- A buccal tube can be soldered onto the bridge of the Adam's clasp
- This modification permits the use of extra-oral anchorage using face-bow-headgear assembly.

Adam's Clasp with Distal Extension

- In this modification, the distal arrowhead has a small extension incorporated distally
- This distal extension engages the elastics.

Adam's Clasp on Incisors and Premolars

- When retention in incisor and premolars are required then the Adam's clasp is fabricated on these areas
- They can be fabricated to span a single tooth or two teeth.

Southend Clasp

- When retention is needed in anterior regions, then the southend clasp is fabricated
- The wire is adapted along the cervical margin of both the central incisors
- The distal ends are carried over the occlusal embrasures to end as retentive arms on the palatal side.

Triangular Clasp

- These are small triangular shaped clasps that are used between two adjacent posterior teeth
- They engage the proximal undercuts of two adjacent teeth
- When additional retention is required, these clasps are preferred.

Ball-end Clasp

- They are constructed using stainless steel wires having a knob or a ball-like structure on one end
- The ball can be made at the end of the wire using silver solder
- Pre-formed wires having a ball at one end are also available
- Ball engages the proximal undercut between two adjacent posterior teeth, as in a triangular clasp
- The distal end of the wire is carried over the occlusal embrasure to end on the palatal aspect as a retentive arm
- The ball-end clasp is used where additional retention is needed.

Schwarz Clasp

- It is also known as arrowhead clasp
- It is the predecessor of Adam's clasp
- In this clasp, a number of arrowheads engage the inter-proximal undercuts between the molars and between premolars and molars

Disadvantages

- Needs special arrowhead forming pliers to fabricate
- Occupies a large amount of space in the buccal vestibule
- The arrowhead can injure the interdental soft tissues
- It is difficult and time consuming to fabricate. Because of so many drawbacks, the clasp is not frequently used.

Crozat Clasp

- It resembles a few clasps but has an additional piece of wire soldered, which engages into the mesial and distal proximal undercuts
- Thus it offers better retention than the full clasp.

Active Components of Removable Orthodontic Appliances

- These components exert forces to bring about necessary tooth movement
- Active components are as follows:
  - Bows
  - Springs
  - Screws
  - Elastics
  - Bows: It is mainly used for incisor retraction.
- Commonly used labial bows are as follows:
  - Short labial bow
  - Long labial bow
  - Split labial bow
  - Reverse labial bow
  - Robert's retractor
  - Mill's retractor
  - High labial bow with apron springs
  - Fitted labial bow.

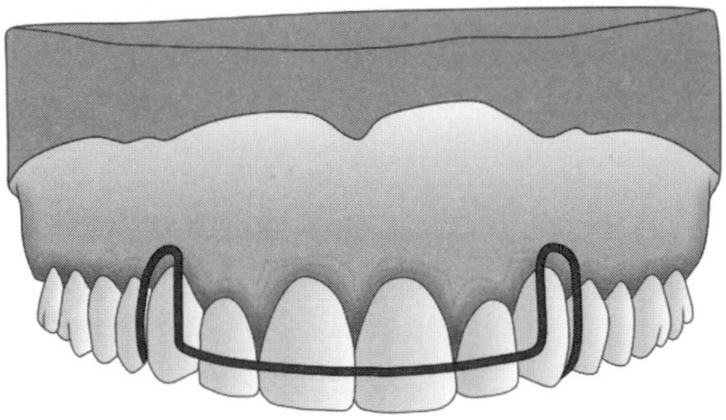

Fig. 25.5: Short labial bow

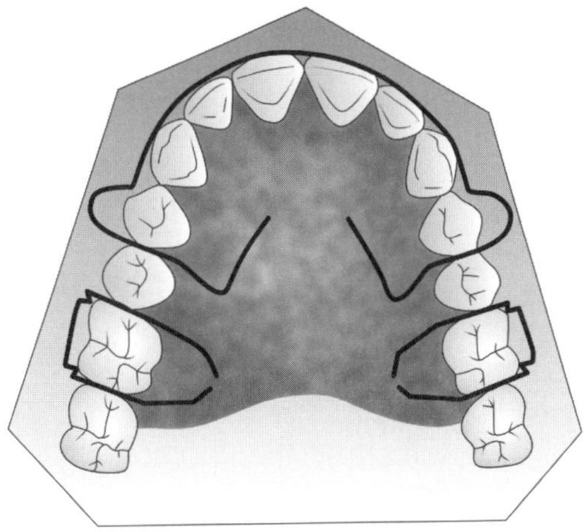

Fig. 25.6: Long labial bow

Short Labial Bow

- It is fabricated using 0.7 mm hard round stainless steel wire
- It consists of a bow that makes contact with the most prominent labial teeth and two U loops that end as retentive arms, distal to canines **(Fig. 25.5)**
- It is stiff and has low flexibility
- Because of this stiffness, they are indicated in cases of minor overjet reduction and anterior space closure
- It can also be used for retention at the end of treatment of fixed orthodontic therapy
- They are activated by compressing the U loops, such that the labial bow is displaced palatally by 1 mm.

Long Labial Bow

- It is similar to short labial bow, but it extends from one first premolar to the opposite first premolar
- The distal arms of the U loop are adapted over the occlusal embrasure between the two premolars to get embedded in the acrylic plate **(Fig. 25.6)**
- Indications of long labial bow are as follows:
  - Minor overjet reduction
  - Minor anterior space closure
  - Closure of space distal to canine
  - Guidance of canine during canine retraction using palatal retractor
  - As a retaining device at the termination of fixed orthodontic treatment.
- It is activated in the similar manner as the short labial bow
- Long labial bow can be modified by soldering the distal arm of the U loop on to the bridge of the Adams clasp.

Split Labial Bow

- There is a split in the middle of this labial bow
- Because of this split, there are two separate buccal arms having a U loop each
- It exhibits more flexibility as compared to the conventional short labial bows
- This labial bow is used for anterior retraction
- It can also be modified for usage in closure of midline spacing
- In the modified form, the free ends of the buccal arms are made to hook on to the distal surface of the opposite central incisor **(Fig. 25.7)**
- It can be activated by compressing the U loop 1–2 mm at a time.

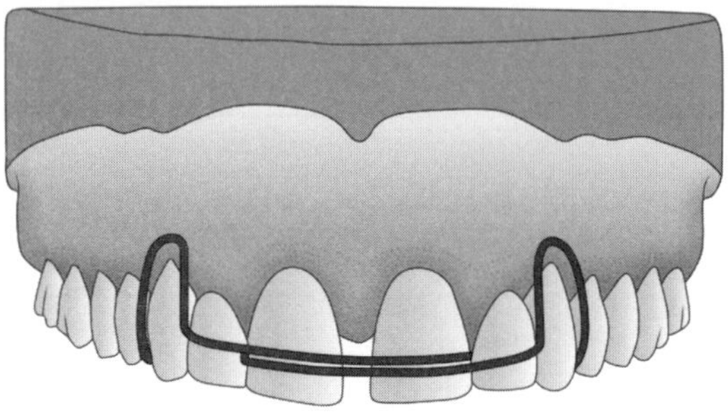

Fig. 25.7: Split labial bow

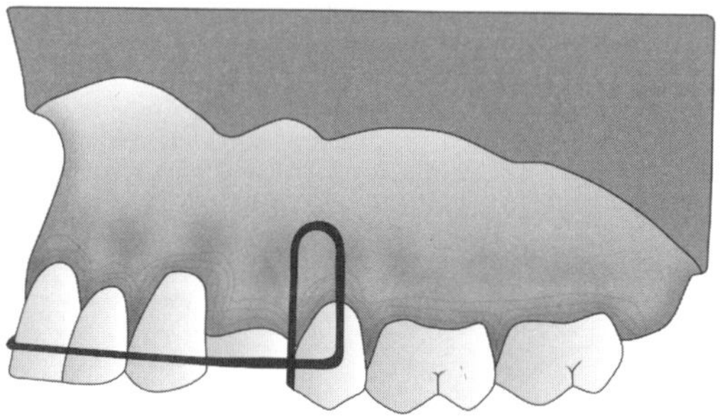

Fig. 25.8: Reverse labial bow

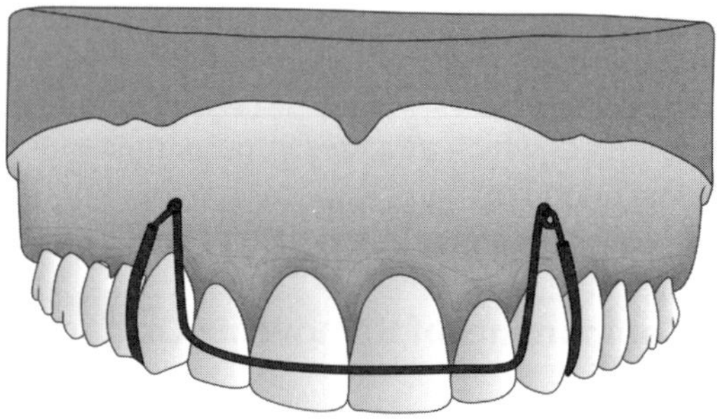

Fig. 25.9: Robert's Retractors

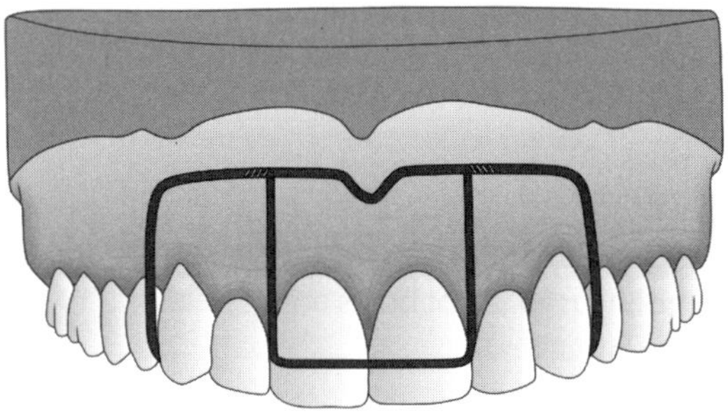

Fig. 25.10: High labial bow with apron springs

Reverse Labial Bow

- It is also known as loop labial bow
- In this labial bow, the U loops are placed distal to the canine and the free ends of the U loops are adapted occlusally between the first premolar and canine **(Fig. 25.8)**
- The flexibility of the bow can be increased by incorporating a longer span of the wire
- Its indications are similar to that of short labial bow

It can be activated in two steps:

1. In the first step, the U loop is opened, which result in lowering of the labial bow in the incisors regions
2. In the second step, a compensatory bend is given at the base of the U loop to maintain proper level of the bow.

Robert's Retractors

- It is made up of thin gauze stainless steel wire which has a coil of 3 mm internal diameter, mesial to the canine
- Its fabrication requires thin 0.5 mm diameter wire along with increased wire length because of incorporation of coil **(Fig. 25.9)**
- This bow lacks adequate stability in the vertical plane
- Therefore, a stainless steel tubing of 0.5 mm internal diameter is used to support the distal part of the retractor
- It is given in those patients who have a severe anterior proclination with overjet of over 4 mm
- Light forces are generated by this bow, therefore, it can be used in adult patients in whom lighter forces are required.

Mill's Retractors

- Extensive looping is present in this labial bow so as to increase the flexibility and range of action
- Indicated in patients with large overjets
- Its cosntruction is difficult and patients acceptance is poor because of the complex design of the bow. This is the disadvantage of this bow.

High Labial Bow with Apron Springs

- It consists of heavy wire bow of 0.9 mm thickness
- It extends into the buccal vestibule
- 0.4 mm wire is used for the construction of apron spring and is attached to the high labial bow **(Fig. 25.10)**
- It is highly flexible and is therefore used in cases of large overjet
- It can be used in adult patients as very light forces are generated by them
- Apron spring can be activated by bending towards the teeth
- Activation of up to 3 mm at a time can be done, as it is highly flexible
- It is difficult to construct and can cause soft tissue injuries.

Fitted Labial Bow

- The wire is adapted to confirm the contours of the labial surface **(Fig. 25.11)**
- U loops are small usually
- They cannot be used to bring active tooth movements
- They can be used as retainers at the termination of fixed orthodontic therapy.

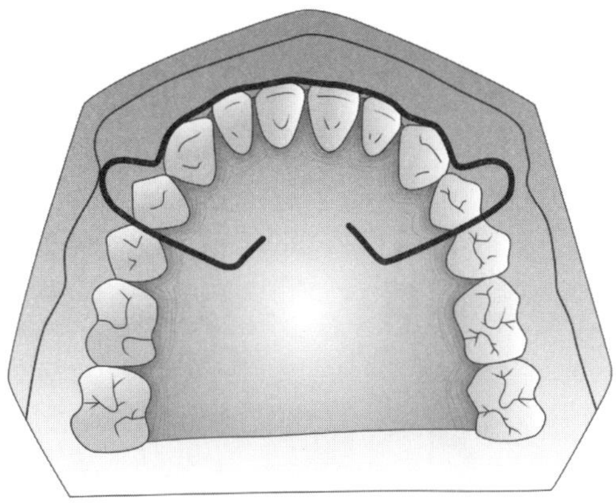

Fig. 25.11: Fitted labial bow

Springs

- Springs are one of the components of removable orthodontic appliances
- They are used to effect various tooth movements
- Classification of springs are as follows:
  - Based on the presence or absence of helix:
    - Simple—without helix
    - Compound—with helix.
  - Based on the presence of loops or helix
    - Helical spring- with helix
    - Looped spring- with loop.
  - Based on the nature of stability of the spring
    - Self-supported spring: It is made up of thick gauge wire and therefore, they can support themselves.
    - Supported spring: It is made up of thin gauge wire and therefore lacks adequate stability.
- Therefore, a metal tubing in used to encase a section of spring to provide an adequate support.

Ideal Requirements

- It should be easy and simple to fabricate
- It should be easy to adjust
- It should fit into the available space without discomfort to the patient
- It should be easy to clean
- It should not slip or dislodge when placed over a sloping tooth surface
- It should apply forces of required magnitude and directions
- It should be robust.
- There are certain factors which should be kept in mind during designing a spring. They are as follows:
  - Diameter of wire: Flexibility of the spring depends to a large extent, on the diameter of wire used. The force generated is $F = \frac{D^4}{L_3}$
    Where f = force, D = diameter of wire and L = length of wire.
    - If thick diameter wires are used, it would lead to application of greater force and flexibility is decreased
    - If thinner diameter wires are used, force applied is lesser and there is greater flexibility
- The spring can remain active for a longer period of time.
  - Length of wire: If the length of the wire is increased, forces generated are reduced
    - Therefore, longer springs generate less force and are more flexible, and remain active for longer durations
    - They make the springs more active, helices and loops can be incorporated into the springs.
  - Force to be applied: The amount of force that should be generated by this spring can be evaluated depending upon the number of teeth to be moved, root surface area and patient comfort. In an average, recommended forces for most of the tooth movements of about 20 gm/cm^2 of root area
  - Patient comfort: The spring should be comfortable for the patient in term of its design, size and its force generation.
    - It should be comfortable for the patient to insert the appliance with the spring in the proper position so as to bring about the desired movement.
  - Direction of tooth movement:
    - It is an important aspect in designing a spring
    - The direction of tooth movement is determined by the point of contact between the spring and the tooth
    - For labial mesio-distal tooth movements, palatally placed spring are used
    - When tooth is to be moved palatally and in a mesio-distal direction, then bucally placed springs should be used.

Finger Springs

- It is also known as single cantilever spring because its one end is fixed in acrylic and the other end is free
- It is fabricated by 0.5 mm or 0.6 mm hard round stainless steel wire

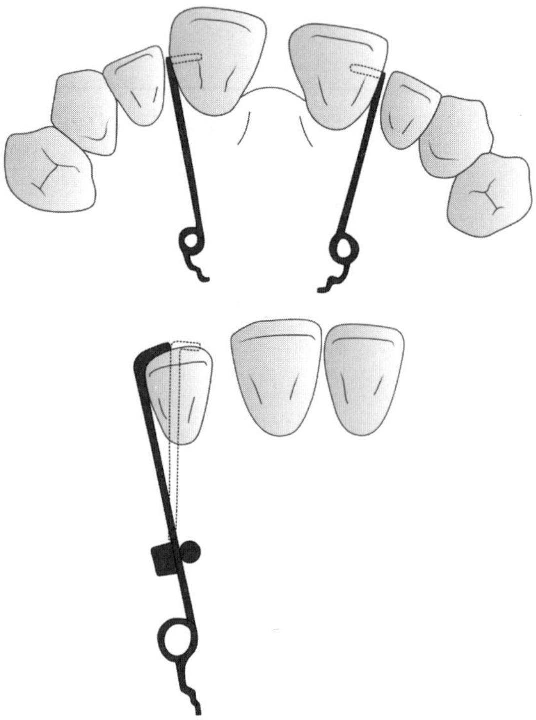

Fig. 25.12: Finger Spring

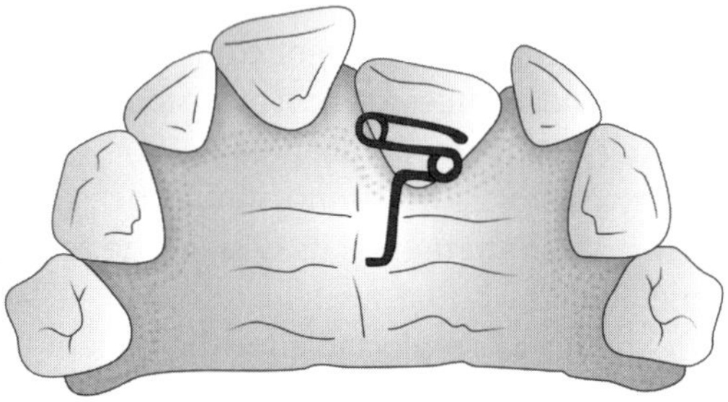

Fig. 25.13: Z Spring

- Finger springs are used for teeth to be moved in mesio-distal direction **(Fig. 25.12)**
- They are used for teeth which are in the line of arch, i.e., those teeth which are located exactly in the buccolingual direction
- Finger spring contains an—
  - Active arm of about 12–15 mm is length which faces towards the tissue;
  - A helix of an internal diameter of 3 mm;
  - Retentive arm is of 4–5 mm length, which is away from the tissue and ends in a small retentive tag.
- The coil of the finger spring should lie along the long axis of the tooth to be moved and perpendicular to the direction of movement
- The direction of the coil is opposite to that of intended tooth movement
- It should be made sure that the spring lies is a recess between the mucosa and the base plate therefore, before acrylisation, the helix and the active arm are boxed in wax
- Spring can be activated by moving the active arm towards the teeth intended to be moved
- This is done as close to the coil as possible
- Activation of up to 3 mm is considered to be ideal, when 0.5 mm wire is used for its construction
- When 0.6 mm wire has been used, the activation should be half of that recommended for 0.5 mm.

Cranked Single Cantilever Spring

- 0.5 mm hard stainless steel wire is used for the construction of this spring
- This spring is used to move teeth labially
- This spring contains a coil close to its emergence from the base plate
- This spring is cranked to keep it clear off the other teeth
- The coil is designed in such a manner that the spring is activated by unwinding the coil

Z-spring

- It is also known as double-cantilever spring **(Fig. 25.13)**
- It is used for labial movement of incisor
- They can also be used for minor rotation of incisor
- It is fabricated from 0.5 mm hard round stainless steel wire
- Spring consist of two coils of very small internal diameter
- The spring should be perpendicular to the palatal surface of the tooth
- It has a retentive arm of 10–12 mm length that gets embedded in acrylic
- Before acrylisation, z spring should be boxed in wax
- Z spring can be activated by opening both the helices by 2–3 mm at a time
- In minor rotation correction, one of the helices is opened.

T-spring

- T-spring is used for buccal movement of premolars and occasionally canines **(Fig. 25.14)**
- It is fabricated using 0.5 mm hard round stainless steel wire
- T-spring consists of a T-shaped arm whose ends are embedded in acrylic
- T-spring is activated by pulling the free end of the T towards the intended direction of tooth movement.

Coffin Spring

- It was introduced by Walter Coffin. It is a removable type of arch expansion spring **(Fig. 25.15)**
- It brings about slow dento-alveolar arch expansion in patient where the upper arch is constricted or there is a unilateral cross-bite
- It is constructed using 1.2 mm hard round stainless steel wire
- It has a omega or U shaped wire placed in the mid palatal region with the retentive arms incorporated into base plates
- Adams clasps on first molars and the first premolars or deciduous molars provides retention to the appliance
- It can be activated by holding both ends at the region of the clasps and pulling the sides apart gently.

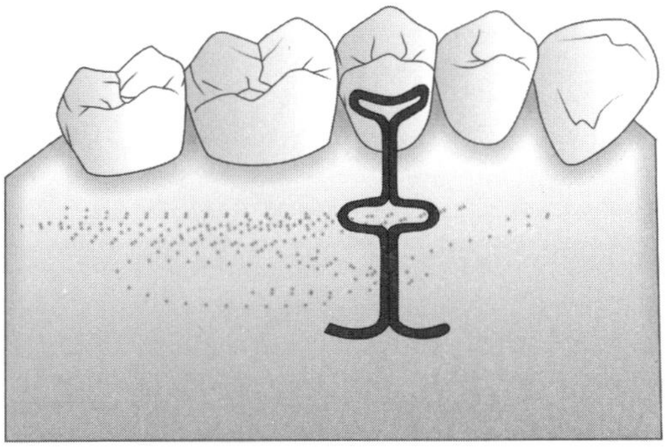

Fig. 25.14: T Spring

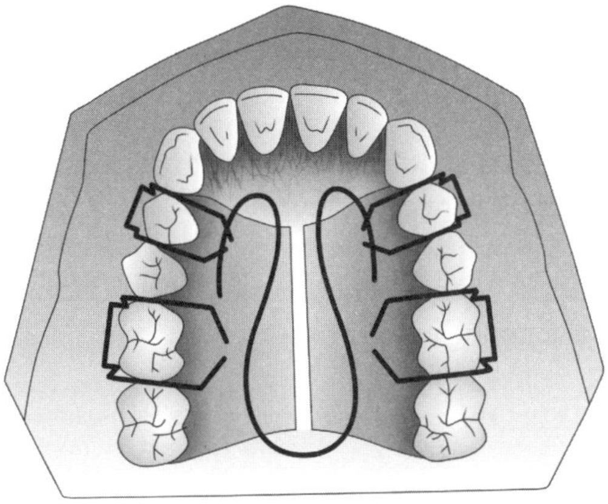

Fig. 25.15: Coffin Spring

Canine Retractors

- These are the spring which are used to move canines in a distal direction
- Canine retractors can be classified as following:
  - Based on their location:
    - Buccal—buccally placed
    - Palatal—palatally placed.
  - Based on the presence of helix or loop:
    - Canine retracter with helix
    - Canine retractor with loop.
  - Based on their modes of action:
    - Push type
    - Pull type.

U-Loop Canine Retractor

- It is fabricated from a 0.6 mm or a 0.7 mm wire
- Contains a U loop, an active arm and a retentive arm
- The base of U loop should be 2–3 mm below the cervical margin **(Fig. 25.16)**
- It is less effective and is used where minimum retraction of around 1–2 mm is needed
- It can be activated by closing the loops by 1–2 mm or cutting the free end of the active arm by 2 mm and readapting it
- It is less bulky and easy to construct.

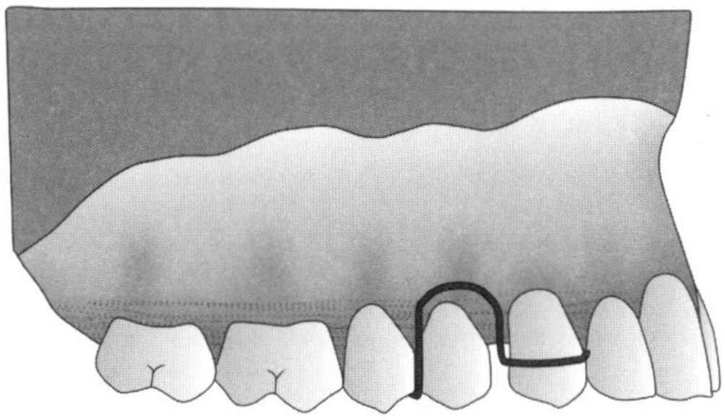

Fig. 25.16: U loop Canine Retractor

Helical Canine Retractor

- It is also knows as reverse loop canine retractor
- It is made up of 0.6 mm wire **(Fig. 25.17)**
- Parts: 3 mm diameter coil, active arm (towards the tissue), and a retentive arm

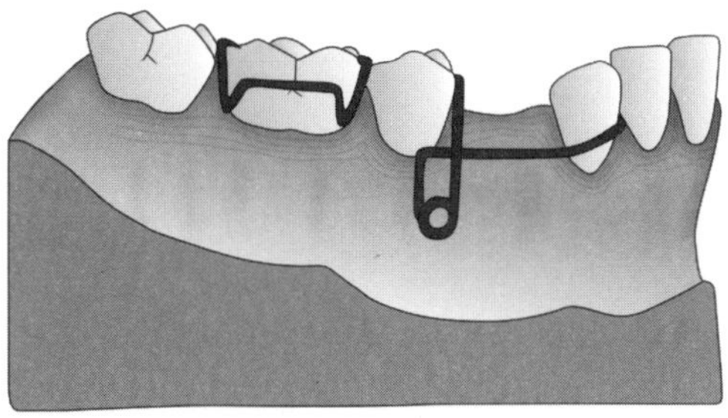

Fig. 25.17: Helical Canine Retractor

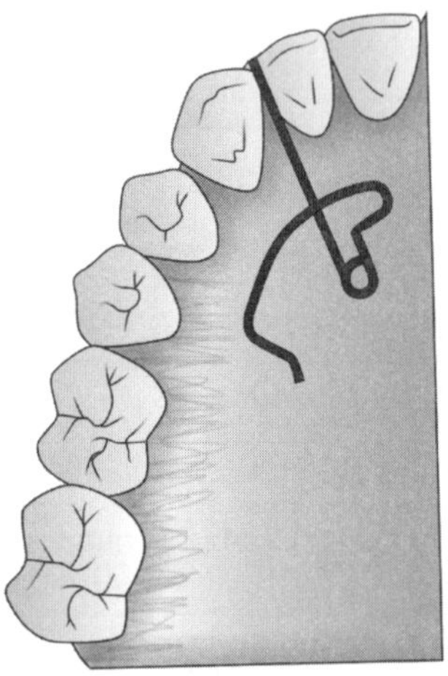

Fig. 25.18: Palatal Canine Retractor

- Active arm is bent at right angles to engage the canine, below the height of contour
- Coil is 3–4 mm below the gingival arm
- Activation: Opening the helix by 1 mm or cutting the free and readapting around the canine.

Palatal Canine Retractor

- Wire—0.6 mm stainless steel wire components
  - 3 mm coil
  - Active arm
  - Guide arm
- Active arm is place mesial to canine. Helix is along the long axis of the canine on the palatal side **(Fig. 25.18)**
- Indication: Retractor of palatally placed canines
- Activation: Opening the helix by 2 mm at a time.

Buccal Canine Retractors

- Self supported (0.7 mm SS wire)
- Supported (0.5 mm SS wire)

The three components are

1. Coil of 3 mm diameter
2. Active arm away from tissue
3. Retentive arm

Indication: Retraction of highly placed canines in buccal vestibule.

Screws: Refer Chapter Expansions.

CHAPTER 26 Fixed Appliances

LONG ESSAYS

Question 1

Discuss in detail about the component of fixed appliances? Also discuss about the methods of fixing attachment onto the teeth?

Answer

Components of fixed appliances are as follows:

- Active components
  - Arch wires
  - Springs
  - Elastics
  - Separators.
- Passive components.
  - Bands
  - Brackets
  - Buccal tubes
  - Lingual attachment
  - Lock pins
  - Ligature wires.

Passive Components

- **Bands**: They are used on teeth which receive excessive forces / large restorations or crowns
  - They are the passive component that help in fixing the various attachment to the tooth
  - They are available in various size for various teeth
  - They are made up of stainless steel.
- **Brackets**: They help in transmitting the force from the active components to the teeth
  - Brackets have one or more slots that accept the arch wire
  - There are a various of bracket designs. They are as follows:
    - Edgewise type of bracket
    - Ribbon arch bracket
    - Weldable and bondable brackets
    - Metallic brackets
    - Ceramic brackets
    - Plastic brackets.
- **Buccal tubes**: Brackets are generally fixed on the anterior teeth and premolars, whereas buccal tube or the molar tubes are used on the molars
  - Buccal tube can be weldable, i.e., welded directly to bands which are cemented around the teeth or they can be bonded, i.e., attached directly to teeth by using bonding adhesives.
- **Lingual attachment**: In some cases, it may be necessary to have attachment on the lingual side as well
  - They are generally required for engaging elastics
  - Examples of lingual attachments are lingual cleats, lingual buttons, eyelets, and ball and hook.
- **Lock pins**: They are small pins that are used to secure the arch wire to brackets with vertical slots such as ribbon arch brackets
  - They are generally made-up of brass.
- **Ligature wires**: They are soft stainless steel wires of 0.009 to 0.011 inches diameter and are used to secure the arch wire to the brackets
  - The process of securing the arch wire to the brackets is known as ligation.

Active Components

Arch Wires

They bring about various tooth movement through the medium of brackets and buccal tubes, which act as handles on the teeth.

Classification of Arch Wires

- Based on material used:
  - Gold and gold alloys
  - Stainless steel

- Nickel titanium alloys
- Beta titanium
- Cobalt chromium nickel alloys
- Optiflex arch wires.

- Based on cross section:
  - Round
  - Square
  - Rectangular
  - Multi-standard.

Ideal Requirements of Orthodontic Arch Wires

- **Spring back**: It is the measure of how far a wire can be deflected without causing permanent deformations
  - It is also known as elastic deflection
  - An arch wire should have high spring back, which results in an increase in its range of action.
- **Stiffness**: Low stiffness provides the ability to apply lower forces and a more constant force over time
- **Formability**: Wire should have high formability as to bend the arch wire into desired configuration, such as coils and loops, without fracturing the wire
- **Resilience**: Wires should be highly resilient in order to increase the working range of the appliance
- **Biocompatibility and environmental stability**: Wires should be resistant to tarnish and corrosion and should be non-toxic
- **Friction**: The wire should provide least friction at the wire bracket interface, as high friction causes high strain on the anchorage and causes limitation of tooth movement
- **Joinability**: Wire should be amenable to soldering and welding.

Elastics and Elastomerics

- Elastic resembles a rubber band
- They can be simple elastic, elastic chain, elastic thread and elastic modules
- They are made-up of latex rubber and are available in various diameters
- They are used for space closure, to correct open bites, treatment of crossbite and to correct inter-arch relationship
- There are various types of elastic like:
  - Class I elastics
  - Class II elastics
  - Class III elastics
  - Crossbite elastics
  - Box elastics.
- Elastic chain (E-chain): The elastics which are available as long chains of inter-connected rings are referred to as E-chain
  - They are used to close the space between teeth by stretching the rings between them.
- Elastic threads: They are made up of a core of latex rubber surrounded by a sleeve of woven silk and is available in a spool
  - It is used to close the space and to derotate the tooth.
- Elastic modules: They are made up of two elastic rings separated by a variable distance
  - They are used to close the space and for derotation of teeth.
- Ligating rings: They are small elastomeric rings which are used to secure the arch wires to the brackets.

Springs

- They are used to bring about various tooth movements
- The springs used in orthodontics are as follows:
  - Uprighting springs: They move the root in a mesial or distal direction
  - Torquing springs: They move the root in a lingual or palatal direction
  - Open coil springs: They are compressed between two teeth to open up space between them
  - Closed coil springs: They are stretched between teeth to close the space.

Separators

- To break the tight interdental contacts, separators are used
- There are many types of separators available like:
  - Brass wire separators
  - Ring separators
  - Dumbell separators
  - Keslying's spring separators.

Methods of Fixing Attachments on to the Teeth

There are two methods of fixing the attachment on to the teeth:

1. Bonding: It is the method of fixing the attachment directly to the teeth
2. Banding: When the attachments are fixed to bands which are cemented around the teeth, this technique is referred to as banding.

Banding

It involves use of thin stainless steel strips known as bands that are pinched tightly around the teeth and then cemented to the teeth.

Indications

- Banding is preferred in posterior teeth since banded attachments are better capable of resisting occlusal forces than bonded attachment
- It is better to band a tooth that requires buccal as well as lingual attachment
- Bands efficiently resist the heavy forces
- Banding is preferred on teeth that have procelain or gold restorations or crowns
- The teeth that show recurrent breakage of the bonded attachments, are preferred to bond those teeth
- It is preferable to use banded attachments whenever they are likely to contact the opposing dentition in closed jaw position.

Steps in Banding

- Separation of teeth
- Selection of band material
- Pinching of the band
- Fixing the attachment
- Cementation of the band.

Bonding

It is the method of fixing attachments directly over the enamel using adhesive resins is known as bonding.

Advantages

- It is more esthetic
- It is faster than banding
- Maintenance of oral hygiene is better
- It is possible to bond on teeth that have aberrant shapes or forms. It might be impossible to band such teeth
- In cases of partially erupted teeth and fractured teeth, it is easier to bond than band
- The risk of caries under loose bands is eliminated
- Interproximal areas are accessible for restoration and proximal stripping.

Disadvantages

- Bonded attachment are weaker than banded attachments
- It involves etching of enamel with an acid, which may lead to enamel loss and an increased risk of demineralization
- During debonding, enamel fracture may occur.

Steps in Bonding

- Cleaning of the teeth should be done, which are to be bonded
- Then teeth are washed and dried, adequate moisture control should be maintained by using suction and cotton rolls
- Then 30–50% phosphoric acid should be used to etch the enamel for at least 45–60 seconds, after which the etchant is washed off with water
- The teeth are then again dried and the appearance of the etched enamel should be white and frosted
- Then primer is applied on the etched enamel
- Then bonding adhesive is placed on the base of the bracket
- The bracket is placed on the tooth and is firmly pushed into the position
- Excessive adhesive should be removed
- The bond is allowed to strengthen for some time (self-cure) or is light cured before placing the arch wires.

SHORT ESSAYS

Question 1

What are the various tooth movements possible using fixed appliance?

Answer

Various tooth movements possible using fixed appliances are as follows:

- Tipping
- Bodily movement
- Torqueing
- Uprighting
- Derotations
- Extrusion and intrusion.

Tipping

- It is the simplest types of tooth movement, produced by the application of a single force on the tooth crown
- As a result, the crown moves in the direction of the force around a fulcrum in the apical region of the root.

Bodily Movement

In this movement, there is an equal movement of both, crown as well as the root in the same direction.

Torquing

It is the root movements in the labial or lingual direction.

Uprighting

It is the mesio-distal movement of the roots.

Rotations

Teeth which are rotated around their long axis can be derotated using fixed appliances.

Extrusion and Intrusion

It is the vertical movement of teeth along their long axis.

Question 2

What are the stages in fixed orthodontic treatment?

Answer

Stages of fixed orthodontic treatment are:

- Levelling and aligning
- Overbite reduction
- Space closure
- Detailing and settling
- Retainer delivery.

Levelling and Aligning

In this stage, the teeth are aligned in vertical and horizontal planes of space.

- Rotations of teeth are corrected
- Mesial and distal tipping of tooth / teeth are achieved
- Arch wires used during this stage are nickel titanium wires followed by stainless steel wires with progressively increasing size.

Overbite Reduction

- This stage involves correction of deep overbite by either intrusion of anterior teeth or extrusion of posterior teeth
- Growth pattern, lip position, gummy smile and inter-occlusal clearance should be kept in mind while correcting deep overbite
- Anterior bite plane or intrusion arches can be used to carry out required tooth movement.

Space Closure

- During this stage, the extraction space / space between teeth are closed
- It is carried out using two mechanics:
  - Friction mechanics or sliding mechanics
  - Frictionless mechanics or loop mechanics.

Settling and Detailing

- During this stage, the intercuspation of maxillary and mandibular teeth is carried out
- Minor tooth corrections like tipping or torquing of individual tooth are carried out
- Tooth movements of achieving root parallelism are done.

Retainer Delivery

- During this stage, the retainers are delivered after debonding of orthodontic appliance
- Removable retainer or fixed retainers can be given to the patient.

CHAPTER 27 Myofunctional Appliances

LONG ESSAYS

Question 1

What are myofunctional or functional appliances? Explain activator in detail?

Answer

The term functional appliance refers to "a variety of removable appliances designed to alter the arrangement of various muscle groups that influence the function and position of mandible in order to transmit forces to dentition and basal bone". These muscular forces are generated by altering mandibular position sagittally and vertically resulting in orthodontic and orthopaedic changes.

According to Linden "functional appliance can be defined as removable or fixed appliance that alters the position of the mandible and transmits the forces created by the resulting stretch of muscles and soft tissues and by the change of neuromuscular environment to the dental and skeletal tissues to produce movement of teeth and modification of growth".

The theoretical basis of functional treatment in general is "a new pattern" of function dictated by the appliance which leads to development of corresponding new morphologic pattern. "The new pattern" of function refers to different functional components of orofacial systems: tongue, lips, facial, masticatory muscles, ligaments and periosteum.

Classification of Myofunctional Appliances

I. Myotonic Appliances

They are functional appliances that depend on the muscle mass for their action.

Myodynamic Appliances

They are functional appliances that depend on the muscle activity for their function.

II. Removable Functional Appliances

They are myofunctional appliances that can be removed and inserted into the mouth by the patient.

For example: Activator and Bionator.

Fixed Functional Appliances

They are functional appliances that are fitted on the teeth by the operator and cannot be removed by the patient at all.

For example: Herbst appliance, Jasper jumper.

III. Passive Tooth Borne Appliances

These appliances have no intrinsic force generating capacity from springs or screws and depend only on the soft tissue stretch and muscular activity to produce treatment effects.

For example: Andresen activator, Bionator, Herbst appliance, Twin block, Oral screen, Inclined planes.

Active Tooth Borne Appliances

These appliances transmit forces to the teeth, e.g., modification of activators and bionators that include expansion screws or spring to move teeth.

Tissue Borne Appliances

These appliances main area of function is the vestibule, e.g., Frankel appliance.

IV. Group I Appliances

They consist of appliances that transmit the muscle force directly to the teeth for purpose of correction of the malocclusion.

For example: Oral screen, inclined plane.

Group II Appliances

These appliances reposition the mandible and the resultant force is transmitted to the teeth and other structure.

For example: Activator and bionator.

Group III Appliances

These appliances also reposition the mandible but their area of operation is the vestibule, outside the dental arch, e.g., Frankel appliance, vestibular screen.

Treatment Principle

- **Force application**: Compressive stress and strain act on the structures involved and result in primary alteration in form with a secondary adaptation in function
- **Force elimination**: These act by elimination of abnormal and restrictive environmental influences on the dentition thereby allowing optimal development.

Advantages

- Eliminate abnormal muscle function
- Treatment at early age
- Less chairside time
- Oral hygiene maintenance easy
- Mostly worn at night.

Disadvantages

- Not for adult patients
- Not bring about individual tooth movement
- Depend on patient for timely wear

Activator

The activator was originally used by Viggo Andresen in 1908 in Denmark, which was developed as a loose fitting appliance.

He made a modified Hawley type of retainer on the maxillary arch to which he added a lower lingual horseshoe shaped flange, which helped in positioning the mandible forward for his daughter who was going on a 3-month summer vacation. Upon her return after 3 months, he observed a marked anteroposterior correction and improvement in facial profile.

He along with Karl Haupl improved the design and the appliance came to be known as "Andresen-Haupl activator or Norwegian appliance".

Indications

- It is used actively in growing individuals with favourable growth pattern
- The maxillary and mandibular teeth should be well aligned; the mandibular incisors should be upright over the basal bone
  - Partial or total correction of Class II division I cases
  - Partial or total correction of Class II division 2 cases
  - Correction of Class I open bite (dental/non-skeletal)
  - Correction of Class I deep bite cases
  - As a preliminary treatment before major fixed appliance therapy to improve skeletal jaw relation
  - Post-treatment anterior retention
  - Children with lack of vertical development
  - Partial or total correction of Class III cases (mild cases-reverse activator)
    - Retrognathic mandible
    - Decreased lower facial height
    - Low mandibular facial height [Frankfort-mandibular plane angle (FMA)] and a horizontal growth pattern
    - Class II cases with mild early extraction of first permanent molars.

Contraindications

- This appliance is not used in correction of Class I problems of crowded teeth caused by disharmony between tooth size and jaw size
- Contraindicated in increased lower facial height and extreme vertical mandibular growth
- This appliance cannot be used in children whose lower incisors are severely proclined
- Appliance cannot be used in children with nasal stenosis caused by structural problem within nose or chronic untreated allergy
- Limited application in non-growing individuals
- Extreme hypodivergent and hyperdivergent skeletal patterns.

Objectives

- To achieve major changes in facial aesthetics
- To achieve major occlusal changes in the mesiodistal, vertical and transverse planes of space and to remodel arch form
- To achieve moderate changes in apical base dysplasia
- To increase the vertical dimensions and hence assist in mandibular prognathism.

Limitations

- It can slip the mandibular anchorage unless care is taken in appliance construction and manipulation
- Active intrusion of teeth is difficult
- It cannot be used by itself to correct crowding
- Ideally, it should be used in growing individual
- It tends to produce moderate mandibular rotations and hence increase lower face height. This is undesirable in patients with excess face height at the initiation of treatment.

Mechanism of Action

According to the concept of Andresen and Haupl, the activator is effective in exploiting the interrelationship between function and changes in the internal bone structure.

During the growth period there is an interrelationship between function and external bone form.

- Activator induces musculoskeletal adaptation by inducing "new pattern" of mandibular closure
- The neuromuscular adaptation to the increased distance and the change in direction is the basic requirement for re-educating the orofacial musculature
- The condylar adaptation to the anterior position of the mandible consists of growth in an upward and backward direction to maintain the integrity of temporomandibular joint (TMJ)
- In construction bite, mandible is not opened beyond postural rest position (maximum 4 mm). Myotactic reflex activity is stimulated causing isometric muscle contraction
- It is this muscle force being transmitted by the appliance that moves the teeth (it works on kinetic energy)

However if the construction bite is opened more than 4 mm, the activator works in a different manner as explained by Harvold and Woodside.

- They stated that activators with high construction bite separated the jaws wide apart. The effect was stretching of elevators and retractors. He recommended forward positioning of the mandible by 3 mm distal to most protrusive position. Vertically extreme separation of jaws to the extent of opening the bite 8–10 mm beyond the freeway space. According to this hypothesis, more the muscles were stretched, greater force was delivered. It is possible that forces are generated by swallowing, biting, activation of myostatic reflex in the stretched muscle of mastication and the force delivered through viscoelastic properties of stretched muscle, tendon and skin
- The basis for such severe increase in the displacement of mandible is the clasp knife reflex or lengthening reaction according to this reflex
- Harvold and Woodside, by increasing the vertical height construction doubled the actual contraction taking place, when the patient is sleeping. They recommend wide open construction bite, so that appliance does not fall off during sleep
- They opened the mandible with construction bite of 15 mm beyond postural rest position
- Muscle tension arises, as a consequence of stretching of tissues over extended activator stretches the soft tissue like a splint. The appliance induced no myotactic reflex activity but instead a rigid stretch and build-up potential energy
- Stretching of muscles give rise to stretch reflex which is either tonic or phasic type. A maintained stretch elicits a long lasting tonic stretch contraction
- A momentary stretch gives rise to a transient phasic stretch contraction. Stretch reflex elicited by activator displacing mandible beyond rest position is tonic type. The tonic activity of the muscles varies with level of wakefulness or sleep
- In working state, tonic activity is increased. In sleeping state, tonic activity is depressed and in deep sleep it is completely abolished
- When worn during the day the activator increases frequency of swallowing movement. Also as the activator is squeezed between the teeth, it elicits passive tension in the stretched muscles and transfers continuous forces from the muscle to the teeth
- During sleep when muscles are at tonic state, myotonic twitch of tongue push the activator against the teeth. Those intermittent forces are transferred through the appliance to the teeth.

Construction Bite

- In a forward positioning of the mandible of 7–8 mm, vertical opening must be moderate 2–4 mm
- If forward positioning is no more than 3–5 mm than vertical opening should be 4–6 mm
- Upper and lower midlines should be matched unless a dental midline shift exists before the activator therapy. In such cases the midlines are corrected during fixed therapy phase.

The following steps are undertaken to record construction bite: Impressions of the upper and lower arches are made to construct two pairs of models.

1. Study models
2. Working models.

Maximum forward movement of mandible:

- Correct occlusal clearance of postural rest is determined when a functional lateral shift is observed
- Midline is marked on labial surfaces of upper and lower incisors in patient's mouth and on the casts.
    - Amount of horizontal and vertical displacement of the mandible is determined.
    - Mark the amount of horizontal shift on the buccal surfaces of first molars.
    - Show the patient the cast and the mirror, in which direction the mandible should move.

- Practice the movement by guiding the mandible in the desired direction
- Advice patients to move according to the verbal direction and stop when asked to do so.
  - The patient is made to sit in an upright position, relaxed and non-strained
  - The mandible is guided to the desired sagittal position. The operator should merely guide the mandible using thumb and forefinger. He should not use pressure of force
  - A horseshoe wax block is prepared for insertion between the upper and lower teeth. It should be 2–3 mm thicker than planned vertical opening
  - Soften the wax with hot water, chill it and place it on lower dental cast.
- Press the roll, so that only buccal teeth are covered
- In anterior region wax lies lingual to the incisors
- Make groove to indicate midline
- Remove the excess wax from the distal half of the lost erupted molars and retromolar region.
  - When the operator is relatively sure that patient can replicate the exercise the softened wax bite rim is placed in the mouth
  - Wax should not be too soft
  - During the closing movement the operator controls the edge-to-edge incisal relationship and the midline registration
  - The wax should be cut away from the labial of the central incisors so the midline can be visualized and a correct reproduction of incisal relationship is established
  - In final step the wax is carefully removed and is checked on Upper and Lower (U/L) models.

Margins are trimmed with scissors, remove excess wax till occlusal surfaces of molars are visible, and also wax contacting interproximally and on palate should be removed.

- Check whether the mandible has moved in all three planes
- If incorrect wax bite should be repeated. Replace hard wax bite in patient's mouth to check for a proper fit.

A softened wax bite placed on upper arch, the mandible can be moved easily into a retruded position for Class III malocclusion.

Articulation of Model

The wax bite registration is placed on the occlusal surface between the U/L models. The models are articulated in a reverse direction such that an anterior tooth faces the hinges.

It assures sufficient access to the palatal surface of upper and lingual surface of lower models during the fabrication of the appliance.

Preparation of the Wire Elements

As discussed earlier casts have been mounted, the pencils marking are done to known the extension of the acrylic body and flanges. It also helps to draw the wire elements on the models. The usual design requires the upper and lower labial bow.

Labial Bow

They consist of a horizontal middle section, two vertical loops and wire extensions through the canine-deciduous first molar embrasure into the acrylic body.

Horizontal portion contacts the labial surfaces of the four incisors. Depending on the vertical dimension (deep bite or anterior open bite) the wire crosses the incisors above or below the area of their greatest convexity.

The bow can be active or passive:

- The passive labial bow influences the soft tissues without touching the teeth
- The gauge of wire for active labial bow is 0.9 mm thick passive—0.8 mm thick
- Additional elements or screws can be added according to requirement

Fabrication of Acrylic Portions

The appliance consists of upper, lower and interocclusal parts:

- In the upper and lower parts the dental and gingival portion can be differentiated. (In lower cast the gingival part can be extended posteriorly)
- If the construction bite is high as for vertical activator, the extension of the flanges is greater than for a horizontal type of activator which positions mandible more anteriorly
- This extension is important to enhance the retention of the appliance particularly for vertical activator, because the patient habitually has an open mouth posture
- The flanges for the upper part are 8–12 mm high on the gingival area covering alveolar crest. The palate is free
- If the acrylic plate is thin, it does not encroach on the tongue space, but this may cause too much appliance flexibility
- To increase the rigidity, a palatal bar is used which is –2 mm thicker for stabilisation
- Lower acrylic plate is 5–10 mm wide on an average although in the molar area is sometimes greater with flanges of 10–15 mm.

After the polymerisation the appliance is polished and it is carefully checked for a proper fit in the mouth.

- Exact plan of needed tooth movement is developed
- Approximate trimming can be done.
- Final grinding must be done in the mouth
- Any undercut acrylic surface that might interfere in planned tooth guidance must be removed.

Trimming of Activator

In order to stimulate the functional activity of the perioral musculature with the loose appliances so that the movement and eruption of selected teeth can be guided, certain areas of the acrylic which contact the teeth should be ground away.

Vertical Plane

Intrusion

Only limited intrusion is possible. Relative intrusion is one of the objectives.

- Incisor Intrusion
  - Loading the incisal edge
  - Labial bow placed in the incisal third.
- Molar Intrusion
  - Acrylic plate touching only the cusps
  - Acrylic plate ground away from fissures and grooves. If larger occlusal surfaces are loaded, reflex opening occurs frequently resulting in less depressing action by the appliance.

Extrusion

Indicated in open bite problems.

- Incisor Extrusion
  - Labial bow is placed in the gingival one-third
  - Loading the gingival one-third on the lingual surface.
- Molar Extrusion
  - Enhancing eruption by grinding the acrylic plate from the occlusal surface
  - Acrylic contacting the gingival one-third on the lingual surface.

Sagittal Plane

Protrusion

- Loading the lingual surface with acrylic contacts
- Screening away lip strains with passive labial bow or lip pads. Auxiliaries used are
  - Protrusion springs (0.8 mm)
  - Wooden pegs
  - Guttapercha may be added to the lingual acrylic.

Retrusion

- Acrylic trimmed away from behind the incisors
- Active labial bow.

For distal movement of the posteriors:

- Guide planes should be on the mesiolingual surfaces
- Stabilising wires or spurs can be used
- Active open springs
- In Class II division 1 malocclusion with deep-bite, acrylic contacts the mesio-gingival surfaces of upper posterior and distogingival surface of lower posteriors. The upper teeth are hence guided in downward and backward directions and lower teeth in an upward and forward direction to establish the proper sagittal and vertical relations. Acrylic on the lingual surface of the upper incisors is ground away and labial bow made active if they are to be retracted.

Transverse Plane

To achieve transverse movement lingual acrylic surface opposite the posterior should be in contact with the teeth. Higher level of force can be obtained by adding a thin layer of self-cure soft acrylic. More effective expansion can be achieved with use of jack screws.

Selective Trimming of the Activator

During selective trimming only the upper or lower molars are extruded. After erupting, eruption of antagonist can be controlled. Thus both sagittal and vertical relationship can be influenced.

Eruption pathway of the molars should be considered. *Controlled Differential Eruption Guidance* must be employed for the best interdental and occlusal plane relationship, particularly in case of flush terminal plane relationships, proper selective grinding can convert an impending Class II or Class III malocclusion into class I interdigitation.

- Here only upper and lower molars are extruded
- The path of eruption of the molars must be taken into consideration
  - The lower molars erupt in an upward and slightly forward direction
  - The upper molars move downward and forward, with a greater mesial migration component if left unattended.

In Class II

- Eruption of maxillary molars is inhibited while that of mandibular molars is stimulated
- Upper molars remain in their mesiodistal position with the basal structures, but the lower molars will improve their sagittal relationship
- It is favourable in cases with horizontal mandibular growth direction and deep overbite.

Patient Instructions

- Patient should be sufficiently convinced about the benefits of using the activator
- The patient is taught how to use, place and remove the appliance by himself
- Usually the patient is asked to wear the appliance 2–3 hours a day during the day time for the 1st week. During the 2nd week the patient is asked to wear it for 3 hours during the day as well as while sleeping. In case he has difficulty in using it whole night, more day time use is prescribed till he can use it for the entire night
- A trimming plan should be developed based on the individual needs of the patient.

Question 2

What is functional regulator?

Answer

Functional regulator (FR) of Frankel was developed by Rolf Frankel in 1966.

The FR appliances are orthopaedic exercise devices that aid in the maturation, training and reprogramming of the orofacial neuromuscular system.

Philosophy of Functional Regulator

This appliance system was developed to the basic principles of Roux (1895) concerning "Functional Orthopaedics". According to Roux, an aberrant postural behaviour does play a primary role in causing skeletal deformities.

Whatever mechanical or surgical procedures are employed, muscle exercises and training are required parts of such orthopaedic treatment. So the primary aim of the treatment is to identify a faulty postural performance of the musculature and to correct it by a functional therapy. The same principles are followed in the functional approach to orofacial orthopaedics.

Frankel states that the FR appliances are not orthodontic appliances intended to move teeth rather treatment with this appliance is directed towards the correction of functional disorders associated with skeletodental malformations (**Table 27.1**).

This can be achieved by training the associated muscles like the muscles of cheeks, lips, tongue and mastication to re-establish physiologic conditions within the orofacial complex. The Frankel appliances are constructed to prevent faulty muscular function and to stimulate normal postural activity of circular and radial muscles arranged around the oral cavity to establish a proper competent oral seal.

Evidence has shown that postural disorders of the orofacial musculature play a significant role in the causation of dentofacial disharmony. Therefore the aim of functional therapy is to identify the faulty performance of the orofacial musculature and to correct it by orthopaedic exercises. Therefore, functional appliances have to be effective as "muscle trainers" of orofacial musculature, the functional environment to correct poor postural behaviour. This is the basis of the Frankel functional philosophy.

The Frankel philosophy is to induce a stepwise alteration of the postural position of the mandible. This is accomplished through a construction bite, which permits the protractor muscles to physiologically position the mandible forward. The necessary neural input for such a postural maintenance is afforded through the appliance design of the function regulator, i.e., the lingual shields that contact only the lingual gingival mucosa.

Frankel states, that the pressure sensation provoked by the lingual shield as the mandible falls back activate the nociceptors in the gingival and as a feedback, the protractors are signalled to maintain the forward posture, to eliminate the painful input.

Frankel philosophy acknowledges the potential restraining influence of the orbicularis-buccinator mechanism on the outward development of the dental arches, thus majority of the functional regulator is placed in the vestibular area.

The buccal shields and the lip pads effectively hold the buccal and labial musculature away from the dentoalveolar complex thus warding off the restrictive effect of these structures on the normal growth and development of the dental arches. The buccal shields establish a framework for the exercising of the buccal and labial musculature and prevent the cheeks from invaginating into the interocclusal space.

Table 27.1: Types of Frankel functional regulator (FR) and its indications

	According to Frankel	Current use
FR I	Class I, Class II division 1	Case II (rarely used)
FR II	Class II division 2	Class II division 1 and Class II division 2
FR III	Class III	Class III Retention appliance (according to Petit)
FR IV	Skeletal open bite	Skeletal open bite
FR V	Not used	Class I, Class II high angle cases with increased lower LFH (according to Austin Owen)

Abbreviation: LFH, lower facial height

The role of the tongue is also stressed in the establishment of proper arch form and intra- and extraoral muscle balance.

Frankel has used the buccal shields to exert a positive tension at the depth of the buccal sulcus, inducing periosteal tension and thereby bone deposition. Combined with the tongue force, and blocking out of the buccal musculature pressure, bodily movement of the posterior teeth can be accomplished for effective increase in the transverse dimension.

Presence of an anterior lip seal and posterior oral seal between the dorsum of the tongue and the soft palate is essential to the postural performance of the mandible because of the interplay of intraoral, gravitational and atmospheric forces.

Indications of Functional Regulator

Indication of the FR I

Class I

Early treatment: Discrepancy between tooth-size and arch-size and in cases with normal overbite.

Late treatment:

- Mild crowding in presence of an adequate apical base where an expansion of the dental arch may be expected to take place as the result of a spontaneous uprighting of the permanent teeth
- Malocclusions associated with arch-size deficiency require mechanotherapy and removal of permanent teeth if necessary.

Class II, division 1

Early treatment:

- Mandibular retrusion with normal overbite particularly when associated with apical base inadequacy
- In the presence of a large overjet (7 mm. or more), retrusion of the maxillary incisors is advisable as pre-treatment mechanotherapy.

Late treatment:

- Mandibular retrusion associated with normal overbite and an overjet no more than 7 mm. The dental arches should be approximately normal
- Mandibular retrusion associated with crowding and a marked arch-size deficiency requires a pretreatment mechanotherapy and removal of permanent teeth if necessary. After the irregularities of the dental arches are corrected, the FR-I is used for correction of the basal malrelationship. A stimulation of mandibular development may be expected to occur as long as the FR is inserted not later than in the age of 16 years
- Mandibular retrusion associated with open bite, particularly in presence of backward rotation of the mandible.

Indication of the FR II

Class I

Early treatment: Deep bite, particularly when accompanied by arch-size deficiency and a forward rotational pattern.

Late treatment:

- Deep bite without irregularities of the dental arches, particularly when associated with a forward rotational pattern
- Cases with severe crowding and apical base inadequacy require pretreatment mechanotherapy and extraction of permanent teeth if necessary.

Class II, division 1

Early treatment: Mandibular retrusion with deep-bite and excessive overjet, particularly indicated when accompanied with apical base inadequacy. In presence of severely proclined maxillary incisors, pretreatment mechanotherapy for reducing and excessive overjet is advisable.

Late treatment: Mandibular retrusion with deep-bite and excessive overjet. Retrusion of severely proclined maxillary incisors as pretreatment mechanotherapy is advisable.

Class II, division 2

Early treatment: Mandibular retrusion with deep-bite particularly when associated with mandibular forward rotation and arch-size deficiency. As a necessary pretreatment mechanotherapy, the retroinclination of the maxillary incisor has to be corrected.

Late treatment:

- Mandibular retrusion with deep-bite without irregularities in the dental arches, particularly when accompanied with mandibular backward rotation. Correction of the retroinclination of the maxillary incisors is as pretreatment mechanotherapy necessity.
- Mandibular retrusion, accompanied by irregularities of the dental arches due to space deficiency require pretreatment mechanotherapy possibly combined with removal of teeth in order to restore normal dental arches.

Indication of the FR III

Class I

Early treatment: Maxillary retrusion and/or mandibular protrusion possibly accompanied by space deficiency in the dental arches.

Late treatment: Maxillary retrusion and/or mandibular protrusion without irregularities in the dental arches. The presence of severe arch-size deficiency requires a pretreatment mechanotherapy and sacrifice of permanent teeth if necessary.

Skeletal Open Bite

Early and late treatment: Cases of skeletal open bite associated with Class III.

Indication of the FR IV:

Early treatment: Skeletal open bite and bi-maxillary protrusion.

Visual Treatment Objective Diagnostic Test

- Visualised treatment objective (VTO) is a term coined by Holdaway, to indicate the facial aesthetic alteration an operator has in mind to be affected and achieved by a given treatment procedure or appliance
- It is a functional test that also helps establish whether a patient can tolerate a protrusive bite as well as whether satisfactory aesthetic improvement occurs
- It is important that the patient be relaxed at the commencement of this test
- The patient is instructed to gently move the mandible forward, reducing the overjet to the point where aesthetics becomes optimal. The mandible should be held in this position for 3–4 minutes
- Patient should be comfortable exhibiting no signs of fatigue at the end of this period. Sometimes these exercises cause the profiles to have a "bimax" look, indicating dental procumbency. A mirror could be used to explain and convince the patient at this stage of the potential benefit of FR and add to the motivational process
- If the outcome of VTO test is positive, the candidate can be judged suitable for FR therapy.

Clinical Procedures and Fabrication of the Frankel Appliance

- Impression taking
- Model preparation
- Bite registration
- Trimming of the models
- Articulation and waxing up
- Preparation of the wire elements
- Finishing and polishing the appliance.

Impression Procedure

- Prior to the impression appointment, separators are placed in the maxillary deciduous second molar- first permanent molar area. This is for the proper seating of the palatal bow, and to ensure a proper fit of the appliance
- Impression is then recorded about 5–7 days later post placement of separators
- Care should be taken to record the vestibule in full depth
- Two sets are required, one for records and the other for appliance fabrication.

Bite Registration

- The mandible may be moved to an edge to edge incisal relationship if the overjet is less than 5 mm
- Care should be taken to see that there is no obvious strain on the facial muscles and that no fatigue occurs in this position
- It is necessary to train the patient to consistently bite in the desired forward posture
- If the overjet is greater than 5 mm it is better to move it in steps
- The vertical opening should be just adequate to permit the cross-over wires through the interocclusal space.

In Class III cases, the bite is to be registered by clinically retruding the mandible as much as possible. The vertical opening should be only to the extent, to allow the maxillary incisors to move labially over the mandibular incisors for crossbite correction.

The bite may be taken using semi-soft modelling wax, preferably softened, with moist heat. It should be rolled into a horseshoe shape and placed on the maxillary arch. The mandible should then be gently guided to establish the construction bite. Care should be taken to check the dental midlines. Sometimes migration of teeth causes a synchrony between the skeletal and dental midlines. In such instances, the skeletal midlines should be aligned with the option to correct the dental midlines with full bands later. The bite should be cut away adequately to reveal the occlusal interrelationship. The bite should then be removed from the mouth, chilled in cold water and placed on the models to verify that proper registration has been achieved.

Preparation of Working Models

- The base of the models should extend outward away from the alveolar base by at least 5 mm. This thickness is required for proper carving of the model and placement of wax relief and acrylic at later stage.
- The work model along with the construction bite is mounted on an articulator.
- Trimming of the models is done by the patient chairside, so that extensions may be checked properly, particularly the anatomic dictates of each case.
- A proper extension of the vestibular shields is best achieved when carving is done in the presence of the

patient allowing for inspection and palpation of the anatomical condition of the sulcus. A gauge can be used to measure correct depth of the buccal sulcus especially in area of maxillary tuberosity, maxillary first premolar, and first deciduous molar and anterior to the buccal frenum

- The basic principle of model trimming is to ensure, that the shields exert a positive tension on the periosteum to stimulate bone deposition, but also not ulcerate the mucosa by over extension
- Under extension will cause the cheek to invaginate into the space negating the stimulatory activity
- Trimming can be done with on oblong acrylic trimmer, in a hand piece and fine derailing done with a plaster knife or carver.
- For FR II, trimming is done in the maxillary premolar and mandibular labial regions. The carving should be to the extent of 5 mm only. In the lower labial region, proper trimming results in a nearly vertical alveolar surface. The depth of the labial sulcus, after trimming should be a minimum of 12 mm from the gingival margin. This permits the superior margin of the lip pads to be about 7 mm from the gingival margin
- In the maxilla, the trimming is done in the apical region of the deciduous molars to the extent for 5 mm. The sulcular depth at the end of trimming should be at least 10–12 mm above the gingival margin. Care should be taken not to trim the buccal frenum.
- In FR III, trimming for labial pads is done in maxilla instead of mandible. The sulcular depth at the end of trimming should be 7–8 mm from the incisor gingival margin.

Seating grooves (FR II): Notching of deciduous canine and first deciduous molar for seating of canine loop and notching of distal aspect of deciduous second molar for seating of palatal bow is done in the cast and replicated in the patient's mouth before appliance insertion **(Fig. 27.1)**.

Notching of permanent teeth is never done for this purpose. Space between the teeth can be created with separators for seating of the interproximal wires.

Articulation and Wax Relief

Since the shields should remain away from the alveolus, towards the pernicious muscular influence, adequate wax relief should be given. The areas for wax relief can be outlined on the models.

FR II: The thickness of wax relief is 2.5 mm in maxillary alveolar region, 3 mm in tooth area, and thinning out to a knife-edge in the mandibular alveolar region.

- The wax relief is important in the region of maxillary first premolar or first deciduous molar because this is the region of maximum narrowing in most Class II division 1 cases
- The wax relief should never exceed 4 mm because buccal shields standing away discourage cooperation and make lip seal exercises impossible.

FR III: If crossbite exists, thickness of wax relief may exceed 3 mm in maxilla. No wax relief is given in mandible. The inferior border of the wax relief should coincide with the maxillary occlusal surface the buccal and the inferior surface should meet at 90 degrees to permit tooth movement for lateral expansion.

Wire Fabrication

The wire elements basic to the FR series are:

- Palatal bow
- Labial bow
- Lip pads connecting wires
- Canine rests.

In general the stainless steel wire used for the wire elements which are stabilising and or connecting wires are of thicker gauge, i.e., 0.980 "(1.0 mm) and 0.051" (1.3 mm) respectively.

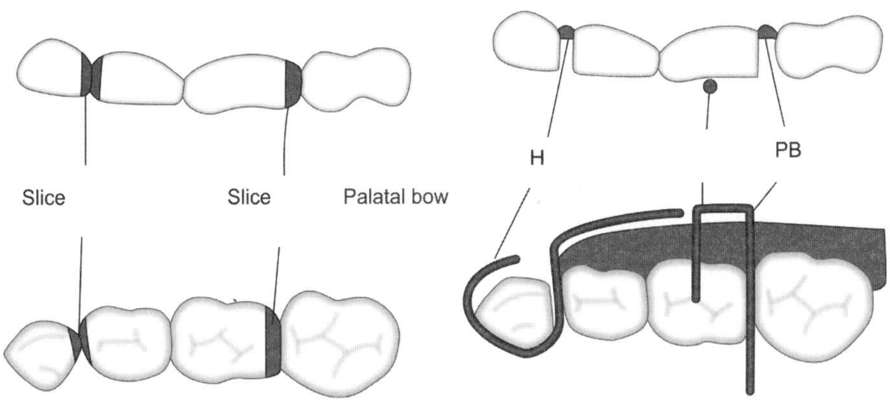

Fig. 27.1: Seating grooves

Tooth moving wires may be made of 0.028" (0.7 mm). As a general rule, wire elements not incorporated into the acrylic should be placed 1.5–2 mm from the alveolar mucosa to prevent mucosal abrasions. Wires to be embedded in the acrylic shield should have 1.00 mm clearance from the wax relief.

- **FR I**: There are three versions of the FR I; FR Ia, Ib and FR Ic. The differences are minor, among these three types:
  - **FR Ia:** FR Ia is recommended for Class I deep-bite cases with protruded maxillary incisors. It is seldom used in Class II division 1 cases where the overjet does not exceed 5 mm
  - **FR Ib:** FR Ib is recommended in Class II division 1 malocclusions with a deep-bite and where the overjet does not exceed 7 mm. This has become the most popular of the FR series, and the patients readily adapt to the lingual acrylic pads. FR Ia has a lingual bow which is replaced in FR Ib with a lingual acrylic pad. There are also two passive lingual springs resting on the cingula of the mandibular incisors
  - **FR Ic:** FR Ic is recommended by Frankel for severe Class II division 1 malocclusions with an overjet greater than 7 mm in such instances the mandibular advancement is to be done in steps and the design of the appliance permits such advancements.
- **FR II**: Differs from FR I only by an upper lingual loop and by a modified canine loop **(Fig. 27.3)**.

Upper Lingual Loop

- Runs on the lingual surface of maxillary incisors and between the maxillary canine and first premolar
- Function: The interproximal portion stabilizes the appliance against maxilla
- In Class II division 2 cases the lingual portion of the wire prevents the maxillary incisors from tipping lingually.

FR III (Figs. 27.2)

Acrylic Components

Buccal shields:

- Buccal shields stand away from the maxillary alveolus by 2.5 mm and 3 mm from the dentition thus aiding in lateral expansion of circumoral capsule.
- The mandibular part of shield lies against the buccal aspect of the dentoalveolar process in order to restrict any mandibular development in lateral direction.

Upper Lip Pads

They are larger than those of FR I and FR II should be parallel and stand away from the alveolus by 2.5 mm.

Initial Treatment Phase

Delivery of the Appliance

- The appliance should be inserted into the mouth with a slight rotatory motion. No attempt should be made to forcefully stretch the lips at the commissures for introducing the appliance into the mouth. It should be given to the patient and asked to be put in
- At the appliance delivery appointment, check out whether the heavy wire maxillary separators are in place the palatal bow
- Care should be taken to avoid injury to the enamel of the first molars. Assure adequate seating of the appliance so that the cross-over wire seats completely in the embrasure or in the seating grooves
- The peripheral portion of the shield should contact the sulcus properly without producing any blanching
- The appliance should be first seated on the maxilla, check the palatal bow for proper seating between the permanent molar and deciduous second molar and stability of the appliance
- Check the labial bow for proper fit on the incisors and any impingement from the 'U' loops. The procedure is then repeated for the lower arch
- The lingual pad, lip pad and peripheral extensions of the buccal shields are checked for any tissue impingement and proper extension
- The position of the lip pads should also be checked for parallelism to the gingival wall, so that no tissue impingement occurs on insertion, removal and mandibular movements.

Once it has been made sure that the appliance is comfortable instructions may be given:

- A little discomfort is to be expected initially
- Salivation may be increased but it should not be a problem
- Outline the breaking period and the duration of near problem
- Give instructions on appliance care, oral hygiene maintenance and sports activities
- Demonstrate the lip seal exercise. A small piece of paper may be given to the patient for this purpose
- Make the patient speak a few words and reassure that speech would normalise.

Lip Seal Exercises

To keep the lip closed all the times to keep a coin or tongue blade in between the lips at least for 30 minutes a day. Swallowing and speaking with the appliance. Tightly grasping the appliance in the vestibule. Motivation by asking the child to perform the lip seal exercise in front of the mirror.

Wearing of appliance:

- 1–3 hours for first 2 weeks
- 4–6 hours for next 3 weeks.
  - It normally takes 3–4 months before the patient has fully adapted to wear the appliance whole day
  - Then the patient is instructed to wear the appliance whole night
  - FR-III can be worn at night after first 4 weeks except in cases with a tendency to skeletal hyperdivergency.
    - Treatment progress checked every 3–4 weeks.

Retention Phase

- The FR as a retention appliance is worn for few hours in the afternoon and at night for 6 months and only at night for next 12 months
- The appliance itself can be worn at night only up to 6 months.

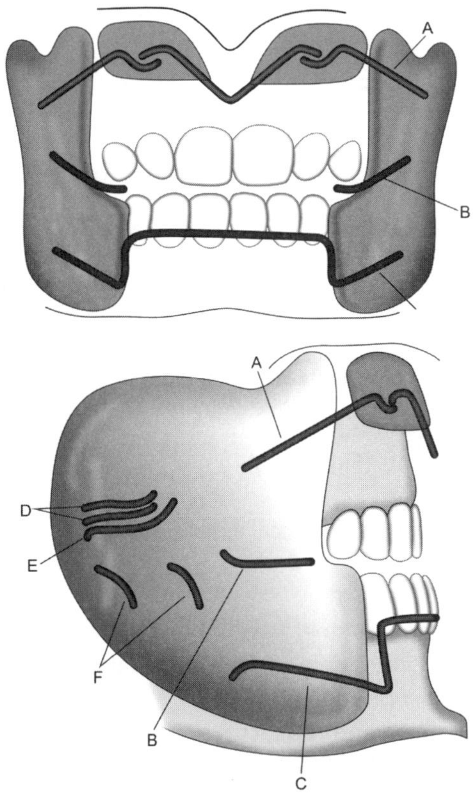

Fig. 27.2: Upper lip pads: The wire components of the appliance [A—upper labial wires (three-wire design)]; (B—upper lingual wire); (C—lower labial support wire); (D—upper occlusal rest); (E—palatal wire); (F—Lower occlusal rest)

Question 3

What is bionator?

Answer

- Bionator is a functional appliance introduced by Balters in 1956
- Balters worked on the principles established by Robin, Andresen and Haupl and designed his appliance.

According to Balters

- The equilibrium, between the tongue and cheeks, especially between the tongue and lips in height, breadth and depth in an oral space of maximum size and optimal limits, providing functional space for the tongue, is essential for the natural health of the dental arches and their relation to each other **(Fig. 27.4)**
- The tongue as the centre of the reflex activity was the most important factor
- The functional space for the tongue is essential for normal development of the orofacial system
- The equilibrium between the tongue and circumoral muscles is responsible for the shape of the dental arches and intercuspation
- A discoordination of its function could lead to abnormal growth and actual deformities.

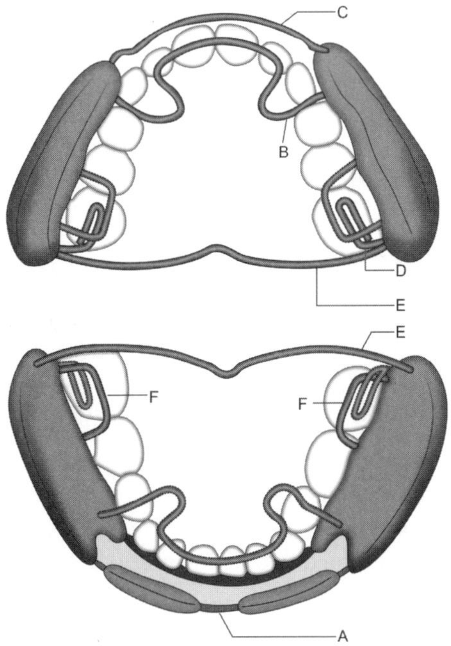

Fig. 27.3: (A) Maxillary view with upper lingual wire; (B) Lower labial support wire; (C) Upper occlusal rest; (D) palatal wire; (E) B, Mandibular view with upper labial support wire (A) palatal wire (E), and lower occlusal rest (F)

Balters constructed his appliance to achieve the following:

- Accomplish lip seal and bring dorsum of tongue into contact with soft palate
- Bring incisors into edge to edge relationship
- Enlarge oral space and train tongue functions
- Improve relationships of jaws, tongue and teeth
- Designed to help patients learn normal functional patterns.

The principle of the bionator is not to activate the muscles but to:

- Modulate muscle activity
- Enhance normal development of the inherent growth pattern
- Eliminate abnormal and deforming environmental factors.

Bionator is of three types:

1. The standard appliance
2. The open bite appliance
3. The reverse [or] Class III appliance.

Standard Appliance

This appliance was primarily designed for use in Class II cases with retrognathic mandible.

Indications

Actively growing children with the following malocclusions:

- Class II/I in mixed dentition
- Class I malocclusion with Class II/I symptoms with lip trap
- In well aligned Class II/I dental arches
- The mandible in posterior position when the skeletal discrepancy is not very severe.

Contraindications

- Class II due to prognathic maxilla
- Labially tipped lower incisors
- Vertical growth pattern
- Not used in deep-bite cases with strong horizontal growth pattern.

Construction Bite

- Horizontal plane: It can tolerate 7–8 mm advancement
- Lateral plane: The condyles on both the sides should move symmetrically
- Vertical plane: The bite opening is about 2–3 mm.

Parts

- Acrylic part **(Fig. 27.5A)**
  - Horse shoe shaped lower lingual plate
  - Upper arch has lingual extensions to cover the molars and premolars.

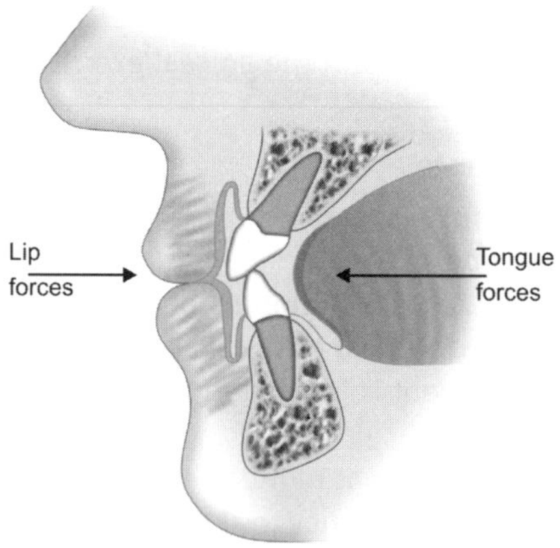

Fig. 27.4: Equilibrium between tongue-cheeks and tongue-lips

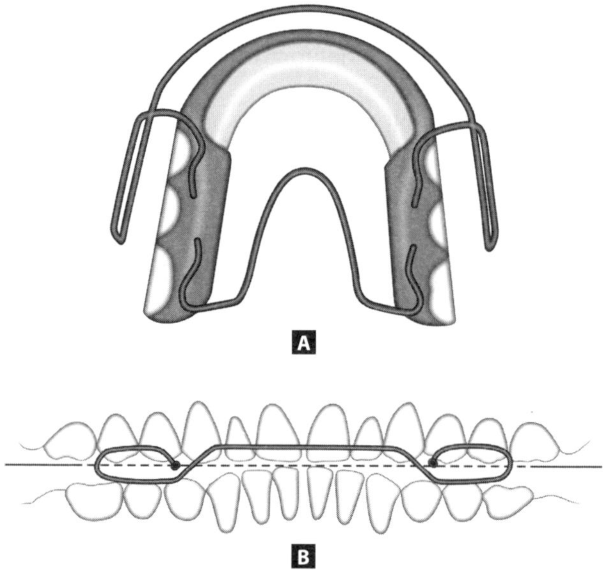

Figs. 27. 5A and B: Parts of bionator (A) Acrylic; (B) Wire elements

- Wire elements **(Fig. 27.5B)**.
  - Palatal bar
  - Labial bow with buccal extensions.

Palatal Bar

- 1.2 mm stainless steel wire
- Extends from middle of first premolar to a line joining distal of first premolars
- Egg shaped and the curve is directed distally to stimulate the distal part of the tongue and effect forward orientation of the tongue and mandible.

The vestibular wire:

- 0.9 mm stainless steel wire
- Anterior part-labial wire.

Lateral part-buccinator bends:

- Keep the cheeks away thus levelling the bite and allows eruption to proceed in this region
- Favours expansion/transverse development of maxillary dentition.

Skeletal changes:

- Mandible-point B is moved forward
- Length of mandible (Ar-Go) is increased.

Dentition:

Overjet and overbite is decreased.

Soft tissues:

- Facial convexity is decreased
- Uncurling of the lower lip.

The Open Bite Appliance

Construction Bite

It is kept as low as possible with a slight opening for interposition of posterior bite blocks to prevent their eruption.

Acrylic Part

The lower lingual part extends into the upper incisor region as a lingual shield, closing the anterior space without touching the upper teeth.

Wire Elements

Labial bow runs between the upper and lower incisors at the height of correct lip closure **(Fig. 27.6)**.

Class III or Reverse Bionator

- It is used to encourage development of the maxilla
- Construction bite—recorded in the most retruded position possible to allow labial movement of the maxillary incisors and simultaneously exert a slight restrictive influence on mandible
- Bite is opened slightly, 2 mm between incisal edges.

Acrylic Part

- Lower acrylic part extended incisally from canine to canine behind the upper incisors. Acrylic is trimmed away by 1 mm behind the lower incisors **(Figs. 27.7A and B)**
- Palatal bar only flattens the dorsum of the tongue but does not move it forward
- Reverse appliance only tips the maxillary incisors labially and does not stimulate basal bone forward

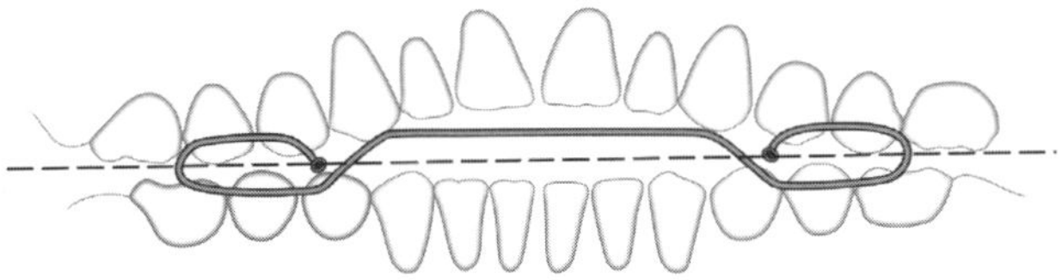

Fig. 27.6: Labial bow for the open bite appliance. It crosses the interincisal area

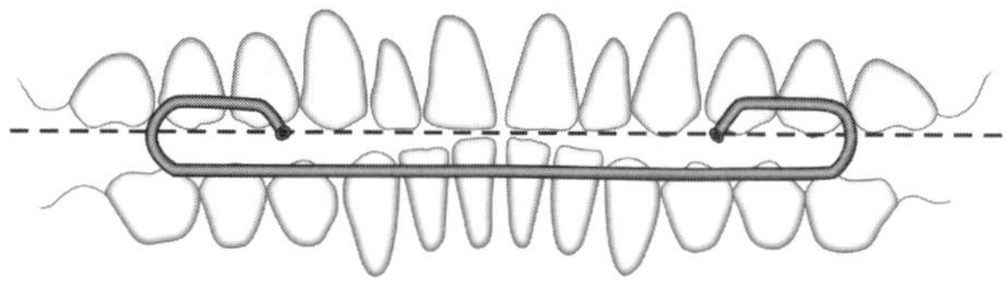

A

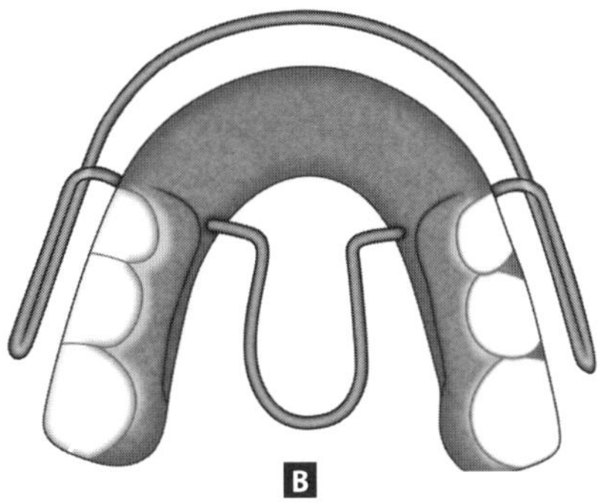

B

Figs. 27.7A and B: Labial bow for the Class III reversed appliance

- It is indicated in pseudo-class III problems with the upper incisors tipped lingually causing anterior mandibular displacement on closure from postural rest to habitual occlusion.

Question 4

What is twin block?

Answer

The twin block appliance was developed by William Clark in 1977.

- The name twin block originates from the fact that unlike other functional appliances, the twin block comprises of separate upper and lower units which are not joined together
- Twin block appliances are simple bite blocks designed to be worn 24 hours a day to take full advantage of all functional forces applied to the dentition including the forces of mastication
- They achieve rapid functional correction of malocclusions by transmitting favourable occlusal forces to occlusal inclined planes that cover all posterior teeth.

Indications

- Angle's Class II division 1 with proper arch form
- Upper arch which is aligned or can be easily aligned
- Lower arch which is decrowded or uncrowded and aligned
- An overjet of 10–14 mm with a deep overbite
- A full unit distal occlusion in the buccal segments
- Skeletal Class II case with a combination of an orthognathic maxilla and a retrognathic mandible.

Basic Twin Block Design

It is made up of the following parts:

- Base plates
- Bite blocks
- Inclined planes
- Wire components (the delta clasp and ball end clasp)

Base Plate

It can be either from:

- Heat cure acrylic
- Cold cure acrylic

Heat cure acrylic has the advantage of additional strength and good accuracy. Cold cure acrylic has the advantage of speed and easier manipulation.

Bite Blocks

- It consists of two bite blocks—maxillary and mandibular, on to which the inclined planes are incorporated
- The upper bite block extends distally from the mesial surface of the first molar to the remaining posterior teeth in a wedge shape
- The lower bite block runs from the mesial marginal ridge of the lower first premolar and does not extend distally to the marginal ridge on the lower second premolar or deciduous second molar.

Inclined Planes

- The position and angulation of the occlusal inclined planes are a very crucial parameter for the efficiency in correcting arch relationships
- The inclined planes are mostly angled at 70° to the occlusal plane, although the angulation may be reduced to 45° if the patient fails to posture forwards consistently
- The position of the inclined plane is determined by the lower block
- The upper inclined plane is angled from the mesial surfaces of the upper second premolar to the upper first molar, passing distally over the remaining posterior teeth in a wedge shape.

Wire Components

- Delta clasp was designed by Clarke
- It is similar to the Adam's clasp but has got the added advantage of improved retention, reduced metal fatigue and minimal requirement for adjustment
- The delta clasp retains all the basic elements of the Adam's clasp, the crucial difference being that the retentive loops are shaped as a closed triangle or a circle
- Advantage being that the clasp does not open with repeated insertion and removal, thereby maintaining its shape and requiring less frequent adjustment
- It gives excellent retention on lower premolars
- Ball end clasps are routinely placed mesial to lower canines and in the upper premolar or deciduous molar regions for "interdental retention" from adjacent teeth.

Construction Bite

- In Class II division I malocclusion, a protrusive bite is registered to reduce the overjet and distal occlusion by 5–10 mm on initial activation depending on the freedom of movement in protrusive function
- The maximal forward positioning of the mandible should not exceed 70% of the total protrusive path of the patient
- Generally horizontally growing young patients have a maximal protrusive path of about 13 mm and hence, up to 10 mm of forward positioning can be done for these patients. If overjet is greater than 10 mm, initial activation of 7–8 mm is done followed by reactivation later
- The vertical activation is determined by two factors:
  - Firstly adequate vertical clearance must be available between upper and lower teeth to accommodate blocks of sufficient thickness to activate the appliance
  - Secondly, the vertical activation must open the bite beyond the freeway space to ensure that the patient cannot drop the mandible into rest position and negate the proprioceptive functional response to inclined planes.
- In Class II division 2 malocclusion, edge to edge bite may be sufficient to achieve 6 mm of opening in premolar region. While in anterior open bite, generally incisal clearance of 4–5 mm is required
- In Class III malocclusion, bite registration is done with 2 mm interincisal clearance and mandible in fully retruded position. The inclined plane direction is reversed.

Progressive Activation

This is indicated in the following conditions:

- If overjet is greater than 10 mm, initial activation is 7–8 mm

- The second activation brings the incisors in edge to edge relationship
- If full correction is not achieved by initial activation
- If the direction of growth is vertical, gradual advancement is preferred to allow adequate time for compensatory mandibular growth
- In adult patients in whom muscles and ligaments are less responsive to a sudden large displacement of the mandible
- In the treatment of TMJ dysfunction, activation should not be beyond the level of tolerance of injured tissue.

Reactivation

- Reactivation of the twin block can be done as a simple chairside procedure by the addition of cold cure acrylic to extend the anterior incline of the upper twin block mesially as the clinician inserts the appliance to record a new protrusive bite before the acrylic is fully set
- No acrylic should be added to the distal incline of the lower twin block. This is especially pertinent in deep-bite cases as extending the occlusal acrylic of the lower block distally will prevent eruption of lower first molar.

Stages of Treatment

Twin block functional therapy is divided into three stages:

1. Active phase
2. Support phase
3. Retention.

Active Phase

- During the active phase, twin blocks are worn full time
- The objective is to correct the arch relationship in the sagittal, vertical and transverse dimensions
- Overjet and overbite are corrected within 6 months and the lower molars erupt into occlusion in 9 months
- The average wear time for twin blocks is 6–9 months although sagittal correction may be obtained in 2–6 months
- At the end of the active phase, there should be a three point contact in the incisor and molar region and the sagittal relationship should be in a slightly overcorrected position to compensate for the mild relapse.

Support Phase

- The objective of the support phase is to retain the corrected incisor relationship until the buccal segment occlusion is fully established
- The lower twin block is left out at this stage and posterior bite blocks are removed
- Patient is given a removable steep anterior inclined plane in this phase. The inclined plane has an angulation of 70–80 degrees to the occlusal plane and a thickness of 6–8 mm
- The anterior inclined plane without interfering with occlusion, should engage the lower incisors and canines which should occlude at the base point of the upper incisors and canines
- If the molars have fully settled, an upper Hawley type of retainer with clasps on molars can be used to bear the inclined planes. If the molars still requires some settling, the inclined plane can be borne on a Begg wraparound type retainer
- If fixed appliance therapy is to be instituted after the twin block stage, a simple "clip-over" removable retainer or a fixed anterior bite plane can be used
- The upper and lower buccal teeth usually settle into occlusion within 4–6 months. Full time wear is continued for another 3–6 months to allow time for internal bony remodelling to support the corrected occlusion

Retention Phase

- The same appliance used during the support phase is used, where in appliance wear is gradually reduced to night time wear
- Support phase and retainers are vital to ensure stability of results achieved with twin blocks. For stable changes, the total treatment time should not be less than 15–18 months
- Support phase and retention are especially prolonged if twin blocks have been used for correction in the mixed dentition and final detailing of the occlusion is to be done in the permanent dentition.

Instructions to the Patient

- With the twin block, 24 hours wear is recommended for optimal results and should not interfere with normal movements of the tongue, lips and lower jaw even though your teeth will not be touching
- The twin block should only be removed while brushing
- Patient should be strongly advised to eat food while wearing the twin block
- Patient should be educated about the screw activation regimen
- Patient should be told that there will be difficulty in speech and there will be excessive salivation for first few days. Both of these subside with time
- Care of the twin block should consist of brushing the upper and lower appliance every time you brush your teeth and a denture cleaner should be used a minimum of three times a week

- Appointments—follow all appointments. The upper plate needs to be adjusted once a month
- Breakages—are costly in both time and money. Do not fiddle with your plate or try to alter or repair it yourself.

Question 5

What is Herbst appliance?

Answer

The Herbst appliance is a fixed bite-jumping device for treatment of Class II malocclusion. It was first introduced by Emil Herbst in 1930s and then reintroduced by Hans Pancherz in 1979 after years of obscurity.

Description of the Herbst Appliance

It is a telescopic device which consists of: a tube, a plunger, two pivots, and two screws **(Fig. 27.8)**.

- The length of the tube determines the amount of bite jumping. Usually the mandible is retained in an incisal end-to-end relationship
- The length of "the plunger" is kept at maximum in order to prevent it from slipping out of the tube when the mouth is opened wide
- If too short—plunger disengages from the tube on mouth opening and may get stuck in the tube opening and on subsequent mouth closure damages the appliance
- If too long—protrudes far behind tube and injures buccal mucosa distal to the maxillary permanent first molar
- Two pivots: The pivot for the tube is soldered to the maxillary permanent first molar band, the pivot for the plunger to the mandibular first premolar band. The upper and lower pivots on each side—placed parallel to each other, provide correct and smooth function of the telescope mechanism
- Two screws—prevent the telescoping parts from slipping off the pivots
- The bilateral telescopic mechanism is attached to orthodontic bands to keep the mandible mechanically in a continuous anterior jumped position
- The mechanism permits—vertical opening movements and limited lateral movements of the mandible. Widening pivot openings on tube and plunger—provides increased lateral movement capacity of the mandible and reduces load on anchorage teeth during mandibular lateral excursions.

Indications

- To "stimulate mandibular condylar growth", in growing patients with Class II malocclusions due to a retrognathic mandible

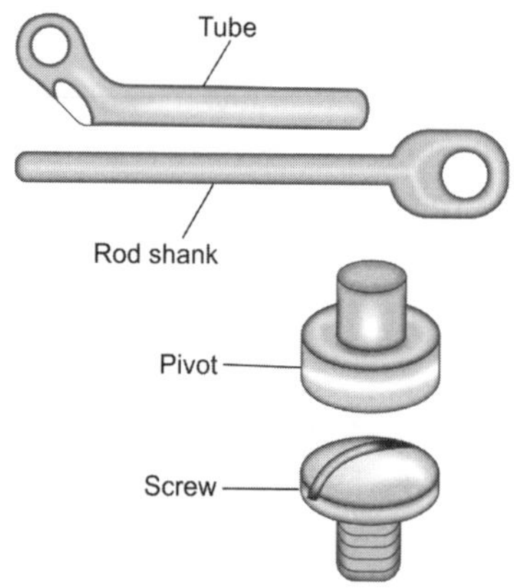

Fig. 27.8: Herbst Appliance consists of a tube, a plunger, two pivots, and two screws

- "Post-adolescent patients past the maximal pubertal growth"—treatment finished within 6–8 months, using the residual growth left
- Mouth breathers with nasal airway obstructions that prevent proper use of removable appliances
- Uncooperative patients: The Herbst appliance is fixed to the teeth and works continuously 24 hours a day without any assistance from the patient
- Patients unresponsive to removable functional appliances, which are worn part time and may not reach the optimal threshold for adaptive growth changes in the condylar region.

Contraindications for Herbst Treatment

- Dental and skeletal open bites
- Vertical growth with high mandibular plane angle
- Excessive lower facial height
- Cases prone to root resorption
- Contraindicated in non-growing patients
- Hyperdivergent facial pattern
- A patient with negative VTO.

Modifications of Herbst Appliance Design

- In Class II cases with transverse maxillary deficiency, Herbst appliance combined with expansion devices, e.g., Quadhelix/rapid-palatal expansion appliance
- In the deciduous or early mixed dentition—bonded type of Herbst appliance is used
- In Class II cases with maxillary prognathism and mandibular deficiency, Herbst appliance with headgear is used
- Langford introduced Herbst appliance with stainless steel crowns instead of bands, reduces failure rate due to band breakage at the solder joint

- Modified Herbst appliance by Larry White uses stainless steel crowns on the maxillary first molars and a removable mandibular occlusal coverage acrylic splint, which allows temporary removal of mandibular component to facilitate oral hygiene and adjustments for erupting teeth.

Treatment Effects

Skeletal Changes

- Restraining effect on maxillary growth and a stimulating effect on mandibular growth
- Sagittal condylar growth is increased but vertical growth is unaffected.

Dental Changes

- Proclination of mandibular incisors
- Maxillary molars moved posteriorly and intruded
- The effect of this appliance on upper molar is same as high pull headgear.

Vertical Changes

- Reduction of overbite
- Increase in lower anterior facial height.

On Facial Profile

- Reduction in soft tissue and hard tissue convexity
- In relation to E line upper lip becomes retrusive while lower lip remains same.

Advantages

- Used in uncooperative patient, i.e., patients compliance is not required
- Action is continuous for 24 hours of the day
- Achieve the results in around 6–8 months
- Advantageous in mouth breathers
- Does not interfere with speech or mastication
- Used successfully in post-adolescent patients in whom very little growth is remaining to work with
- Procedures such as rapid maxillary expansion, fixed appliance or headgear can be given with appliance in place
- The appliance is fixed to teeth
- Patient cooperation is not required
- Appliance works 24 hours a day
- Treatment time is short (6–8 months).

Disadvantages

- Appliance is prone to breakage
- Lateral movement is restricted

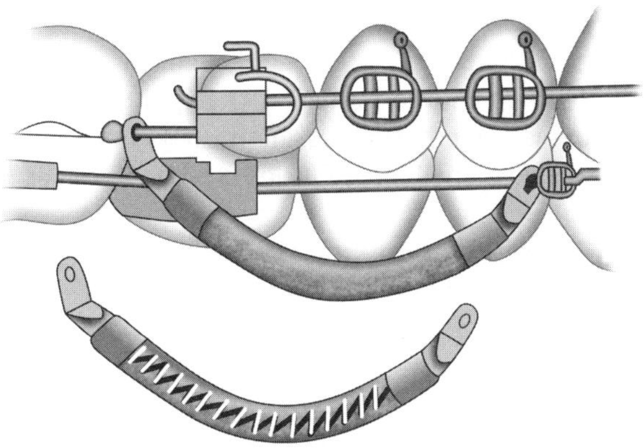

Fig. 27.9: Jasper jumper

- Though treatment can achieved within 6–8 months, retention of the result has to maintain using removable functional appliance
- Risk of development of dual bite
- Masticatory efficiency is reduced
- High incidence of breakage and loosening of the appliance
- May restrict lateral mandibular movements
- It is expensive
- Plaque accumulation and enamel decalcification occur, especially in the splint type of appliance.

Jasper Jumper

Jasper jumper is a modification of Herbst appliance consisting of an interarch flexible force module that allows patient greater freedom of mandibular movement than with original bite jumping mechanism of Herbst **(Fig. 27.9)**.

Parts of the Appliance

The modular system is composed of two parts:

1. The force module
2. The anchor units.

Force Module

- The flexible force module—analogous to tube and plunger parts of Herbst appliance
- Consists of stainless steel coil or spring attached at both ends to stainless steel end caps, which have holes drilled in the flanges to accommodate the anchoring unit
- It is surrounded by an opaque polyurethane covering for hygiene and comfort
- Available in seven lengths, ranging from 26 mm to 38 mm in 2 mm increments
- Designed for use on either side of the dental arch.

Mechanism of Action

- When straight, the force module remains passive. As the teeth come into occlusion, the spring of the force module is curved axially as the muscles of mastication elevate the mandible, producing a range of forces from 1 to 16 ounces
- This kinetic energy is captured when the force module is curved and the force is converted to potential energy to be used for a variety of clinical effects
- For orthopaedic effects, the spring mechanism is curved or activated 4 mm relative to its resting length, storing 8 ounces (250 g) of potential energy for force delivery
- Increasing the activation beyond 4 mm does not yield more force from the module, but only builds excessive internal stress in the module.

Anchor Units

- A number of methods be used—to anchor the force modules in the permanent or mixed dentition
- In permanent dentition—attached to the dental arches with fixed orthodontic appliances
- Attachment to the main arch wire: In Class II malocclusions—attached posteriorly to the maxillary arch distally into the face-bow tube of molar band
- Anteriorly, the module is anchored to the lower arch wire in the canine region
- The removal of the brackets on the lower first and second premolars allows patient greater freedom of movement.

In the mixed dentition: Patient's premolars and permanent canines are unerupted therefore.

- The maxillary attachment—by means of ball pin to the maxillary first molars
- The mandibular attachment—through arch wire that extends from brackets on lower incisors posteriorly to first permanent molars, bypassing deciduous canines and molars
- In mixed dentition, use of a transpalatal arch and fixed lower lingual arch is mandatory to control potential unfavourable side effects produced by the appliance (e.g., molar and incisor tipping and flaring).

Treatment Effects

Jasper's "theory of two's"—Class II corrections with Jasper jumper therapy equally partitioned between five components, as follows:

- 20% due to maxillary basal bone restraint
- 20% due to posterior maxillary dentoalveolar movement
- 20% due to mandibular dentoalveolar movement anteriorly
- 20% due to stimulation condylar growth
- 20% due to remodelling of glenoid fossa in the downward and forward direction.
  - The maxilla underwent significant posterior displacement
  - The maxillary incisor retroclined and the maxillary molars tipped distally
  - Clockwise or backward rotation was evident for the mandible
  - The mandibular incisors proclined significantly and the mandibular molars translated and tipped mesially.

Maxillary Adaptations

- Headgear effect: The distalisation of the upper posterior segment (i.e., the headgear effect) is achieved by not cinching or tying back the maxillary arch wire but rather by allowing the arch wire to remain straight and slightly extended past the buccal tubes. Light forces (e.g., 2–4 ounces) then can be expressed by the modules to distalise the upper molars
- Retraction of anterior teeth: Canines can be retracted in both extraction and non-extraction patients with the posterior maxillary dentition supported by the force module
- A NiTi coil or an intramaxillary elastic attached to the pin through the face-bow tube can be used to retract upper canines or the six anterior teeth en masse
- The force module system also can be used in patients who have sagittal dental asymmetries. In a Class II subdivision-type patient, the maxillary arch wire can be tied back on the side of the existing Class I molar relationship.

Mandibular Adaptations

- For mandibular advancement greater force levels required (i.e., 6–8 ounces)
- When attempting to produce mandibular advancement: The arch wire should be cinched or tied back.
- By maximizing the force values produced by the module, patients tend to posture their jaw in a forward position.

Indications

Treatment of Class II Malocclusions

- Enhance anchorage for retraction of maxillary anterior teeth in Class I occlusions
- It can be used in conjunction with rapid maxillary expansion. Forces generated are light (e.g., 2–4 g)
- The post-surgical stabilisation of Class II malocclusion
- Pre-surgical muscle conditioning of patients with Class II malocclusions.

SHORT ESSAYS

Question 1

What is vestibular screen or oral screen?

Answer

Vestibular screen or oral screens was first introduced by Newell in 1912. It is a simple functional appliance that takes the form of labial vestibule formed by acrylic.

Indications

- Patients with mouth breathing habit
- Patients with thumb sucking, lip biting and tongue trusting habit
- In patients with mild disto-occlusions
- For helping in performing lip exercises for correction of hypotonic lips
- In patients with flaccid musculature
- To correct mild proclinations.

Fabrications

- Maxillary and mandibular impressions are made. The impression to record the vestibular depth
- Working models are poured reproducing the impression
- The maxillary and mandibular models are occluded in normal occlusion and sealed
- In cases of mild disto-occlusion, construction bite should be recorded into the desired position
- The models are covered with 2–3 mm of wax over the labial surface of maxillary and mandibular teeth and alveolar process. In cases requiring correction of mild proclination, wax relief is not provided in the incisal one-third of the concerned teeth
- The wax extends posteriorly up to the last erupted molar
- The appliance is then fabricated over the wax using self-cure acrylic
- Appliance is then finished and delivered to the patient.

Management

- In patients with mouth breathing habit, four to five holes are made in the anterior region of the oral screen initially. These holes are gradually closed with acrylic during the course of the treatment
- The patient is instructed to wear appliance full time in nights and 2–3 hours in day time
- Patient is advised to maintain the lip seal
- In case patient complains of soft tissue irritation, the concerned areas in the oral screen should be trimmed and smoothened with sand paper and polished.

Modifications

- Hotz modification: Oral screen is formed with a metal ring projecting outward between the upper and lower lip. This ring helps in performing muscle exercises.
- Kraus modification: In this modification a small lingual screen running in the incisor area is placed which is attached to the vestibular screen with two 0.036" wire. This modification helps in eliminating tongue thrusting habit.

CHAPTER 28 Orthopaedic Appliances

LONG ESSAYS

Question 1

What are different orthopaedic appliances? Describe each of them briefly?

Answer

Orthopaedic appliances are of three types:
- Headgear
- Face mask
- Chin cup.

Headgear

The main components of headgear are **(Fig. 28.1)**:
- Force delivering unit
  - Face bow
  - J hook.
- Force generating unit
- Anchor unit.
  - Head cap
  - Neck strap.

Face Bow

- Outer bow/whisker bow—0.051″ or 0.062″
- Contoured around the face
- Short, medium and long **(Figs. 28.2A and B)**.

Inner Bow

- 0.045″ or 0.052″
- Insertion in the buccal tube of molar
- Adapted according to shape of arch
- it has Ssops, bayonet bends or U loop.

Junction

- Soldered or welded
- Centred/shifted **(Fig. 28.2C)**.

Force Generating Unit

- Connects face bow to anchor unit
- Springs/elastics.

Anchor Unit

- Head cap/neck strap
- Skull/back of neck
- Combination.

Classification

According to location of anchor unit:
- Cervical pull **(Fig. 28.1A)**
- Occipital pull **(Fig. 28.1B)**

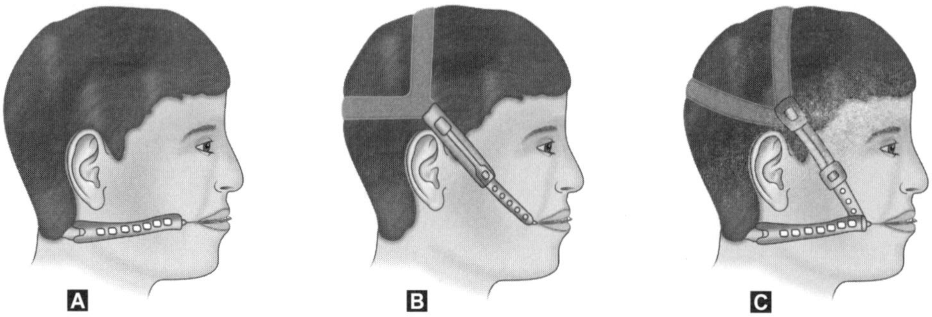

Figs. 28.1A to C: (A) Cervical headgear; (B) Occipital headgear; (C) Combination headgear

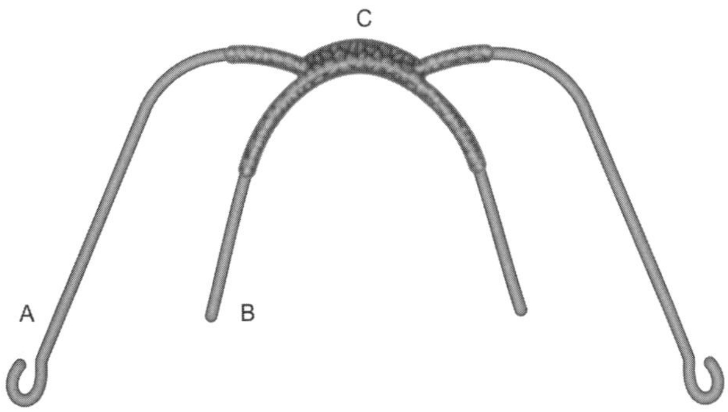

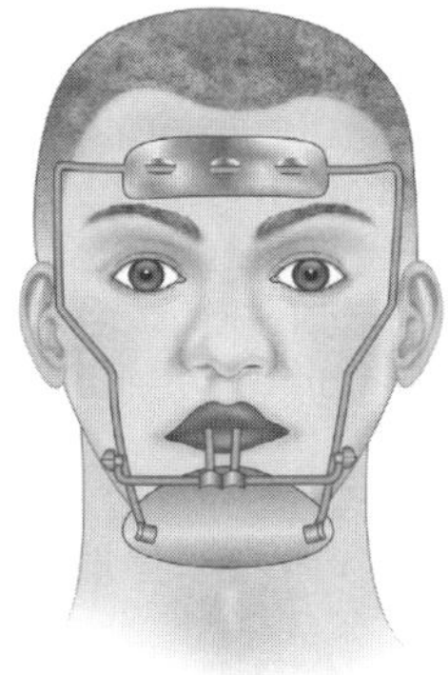

Figs. 28.2A to C: (A) Face bow; (B) Outer bow; (C) Junction—Delaire type of face mask

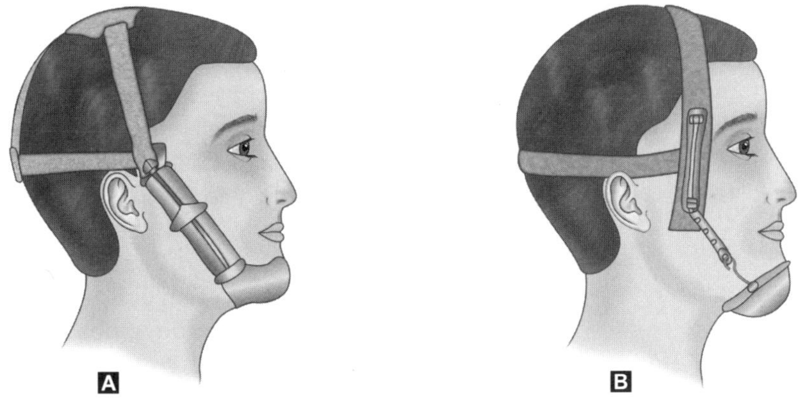

Figs. 28.3A and B: (A) Occipital pull chin cup; (B) Vertical pull chin cup

- High pull
- Combination pull (**Fig. 28.1C**).

Uses of Headgear

- Restrains the forward and downward growth of the maxilla and redirects maxillary growth
- Molar distalisation
- Reinforce anchorage
- Maintain arch length
- Maintain or correction of molar rotation.

Limitations of Headgear Therapy

- Dental changes inevitable
- Patient non-compliance.

Face Mask

- Headgear which causes a forward pull on the maxilla is called reverse pull headgear
- A face mask works on the principle of pulling the maxillary sutures forward with the help of anchorage from the chin or forehead of usually both
- A forward maxillary pull is applied with the help of "heavy elastics" that are attached to the hooks on the rigid framework.

Indications

- Retrusive maxilla—Class I, Class II
- Correction of post-surgical relapses after osteotomies
- Selective rearrangement of palatal shelves in cleft patients.

Parts

- Metal framework
- Chin cup/pad
- Forehead cap
- Intra-oral appliance
- Heavy elastics.

Types

- Hickam
- Delaire
- Turbinger
- Petit.

Chin Cup

- Class III malocclusion due to protrusive mandible but a relatively normal maxilla **(Figs. 28.3A and B)**
- Chin cup therapy attempts to retard or redirect the growth of the mandible in order to obtain a better antero-posterior relation between the two jaws.

Question 2

What are headgears? Explain in detail?

Answer

Classification of Headgears

According to the area of attachment, headgears are classified into:

- Cervical area of the neck (cervical strap)
- Occipital area of the head (occipital strap)
- Combination of cervical and occipital [straight pull or combination (combee)]
- Chin (chin cup)
- Reverse pull
- High pull (parietal).

According to the purpose of usage:

- Growth Modulators
- Protractors
  - Reverse pull
  - Space regaining
  - Molar distalisation
  - Intrusion of maxilla.
- Retractors
  - High pull
  - Straight pull
  - Cervical pull
  - Combination.
- Control vertical excess.
  - Chin cup.

Uses of Headgears

- Anchorage reinforcement
- Distalisation of upper molars
- Space maintenance
- Canine retraction using J hooks
- Overjet reduction
- Intrusion of molars and incisors
- Growth redirection: When used as an orthopaedic appliance, headgears can redirect the maxillary growth and allow normal growth to be expressed clinically by removing dento-alveolar compensations
- Expansion or contraction of the arch
- Uprighting of molars
- Space closure
- Torquing roots
- Correction of molar rotation
- Restriction of mesial drift of teeth, associated with age
- Restricting the eruption of teeth into the inter-maxillary growth space.

Headgear Selection

It depends on the location of anchorage in a headgear:

- **High pull headgear**: Intrusive and distal force to the maxilla and the maxillary dentition
- **Cervical pull**: Extrusive and distalising force on the maxilla
- **Combination headgear**: No moment is produced and a distalising force is applied to the maxilla.

Age

- The ideal age is around 8 years (because in some cases, juvenile acceleration of jaw growth occurs at the age of 7–8 year just before pubertal growth spurt)
- According to Proffitt, Growth modification should be done early in girls, since girls undergo pubertal changes by an average of 2 years before boys
- Age is 8–9 year in girls
- 10–11 year in boys, depending on the developmental status.

Selection Based on Mandibular Plane Angle (MPA)

According to Alexander:

- A low angle or normal growing [Sella-Nasion to mandibular plane (SNMP) less than 37°] case is suitable for cervical headgear
- If SNMP is between 37° and 41°, a combination headgear is used
- If SNMP more than 41°, then a high pull headgear (HG) is used.

Based on occlusal plane requirements **(Table 28.1)**:

Table 28.1: Headgear according to occlusal plane requirements

Action desired	Headgear type
Extrusion and steepening	Cervical HG; outer bow even or low
Extrusion and flattening	Cervical HG; outer bow very high
Intrusion and steepening	High pull HG; outer bow posterior to Cres
Intrusion and flattening	High pull HG; outer bow anterior to Cres
Distal force and flattening	Combination; outer bow above Cres
Distal force and steepening	Combination; outer bow below Cres
Distal force and no moment	Combination; outer bow at Cres

Indications

Patients with Maxillary Excess

- Skeletal Class II malocclusion with a component of excessive horizontal or vertical growth of the maxilla
- Some protrusion of maxillary teeth
- Reasonably good mandibular dental and skeletal morphology as this is minimally affected by extra-oral forces
- Potential for continued mandibular growth.

Patients with Horizontal Maxillary Deficiency

- Using the reverse pull headgear
- Causes reciprocal downward and backward rotation of the mandible
  - Ideal patients should have:
  - Normally positioned or slightly retrusive but not protrusive maxillary teeth
  - Normal or short but not long anterior facial height
  - Ideal age of 8 years.

Patients with Vertical Maxillary Excess

In these patients, restriction of vertical maxillary growth is needed.

- High pull headgear for upper molars is given
- Interocclusal bite blocks can also aid in prevention of eruption of posterior teeth, e.g., high pull head gear with functional appliances.

Components of Headgear

The principal components of headgear are **(Fig. 28.4)**:

- **Force delivering unit:** Usually a face bow or a J-hook that delivers force to the intra-oral location.
- **Force generating unit**: This is the active unit—usually springs of elastic bands.
- **Anchor unit:** Its location depends on the direction of the force applied and is usually from the neck or the head.

Force is transmitted to the dental arch by:

- **Face bow:** The force is delivered to the first molar by the face bow which is engaged in the buccal tube
- It can be attached to removable appliances'
- The face bow has an inner bow and an outer bow
- The inner bow is available in either 0.045–0.051 inch, dependent on the size of the headgear tubes on the first molars
- The outer bow is usually 0.072 inch.

The different methods of making the inner bow stop mesial to the first molar buccal tube are:

- **U-loop**: Advantage is that the length of the arm can be altered by adjusting the loop
- **Bayonet bend**: Horizontal inset bend that keeps the anterior segment of the bow away from the brackets
- **Friction stops**: Stops can be fixed at the desirable location by crimping it
- **Stop screws:** The position of these screws can be changed and can be reused.

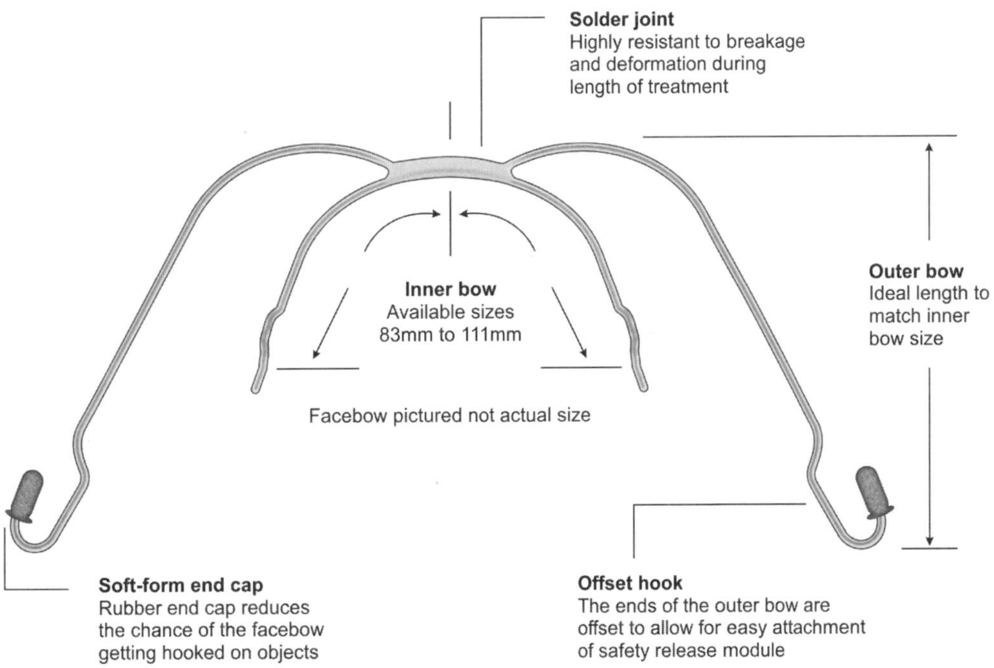

Fig. 28.4: Components of headgear

Outer bow is attached to the anchor unit and can be of different types depending on its length:

- **Short**: Outer bow shorter than the inner bow
- **Medium**: Outer bow almost the same length as that of the inner bow
- **Long**: Outer bow is longer than the inner bow.

Adjustments to the inner bow can be made in:

- **Bucco-lingual**: Constrict the inner bow—expansive force on the molars
- **Superoinferiorly**: Passive position—patient closes his mouth and relaxes his lips—the anterior junction of the inner and outer bows should not be pushing either lip in a vertical direction
- **Anteroinferiorly**: The inner and outer bow junction is just anterior to the point where the lips seal.

Types of headgears are as follows:

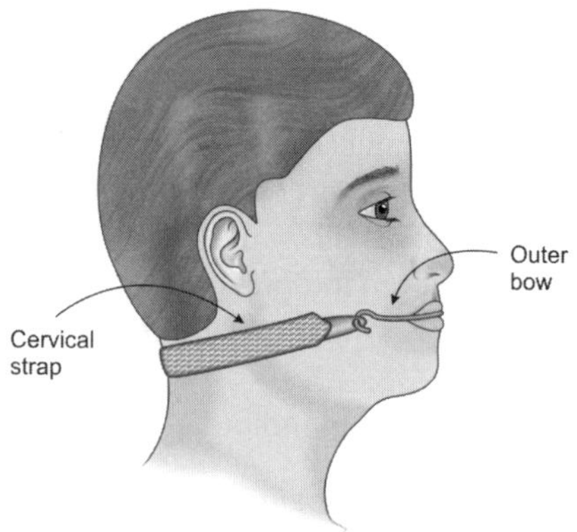

Fig. 28.5: Cervical headgear

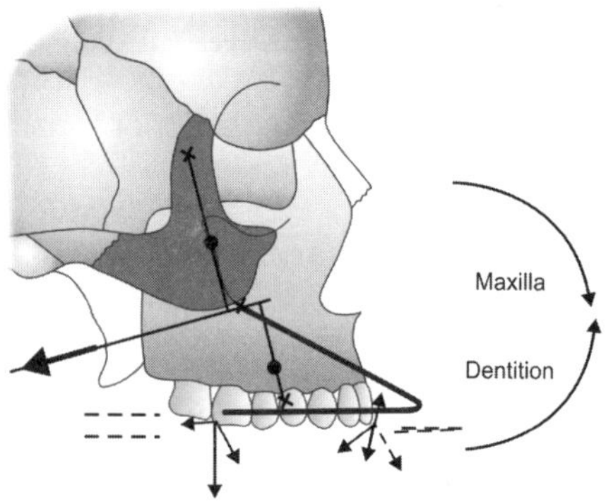

Fig. 28.6: Cervical pull of headgear

Cervical Headgear

- First described by Silas Kloehn in 1947
- Growing patients with decreased vertical dimension
- Purpose of the face bow is to restrict the forward growth of the maxilla
- The vector of force is below the occlusal plane producing both extrusive and distalising effects.

Component parts of headgear:

- Molar tubes with headgear tubes
- Inner and outer bow soldered together in the centre
- A neck strap that is placed around the back of the neck to provide traction to the dentition.
  - Effects of cervical headgear (**Figs. 28.5 and 28.6**):
    - Extrusion of the entire upper jaw
    - Tends to move the upper jaw distally
    - Steepens the occlusal plane
    - Expansion of the upper arch.

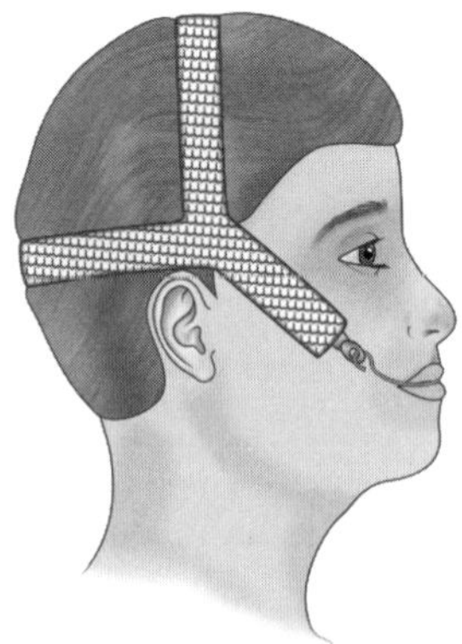

Fig. 28.7: Occipital headgear

Occipital Headgear

- Anchorage: Occiput of the head (**Fig. 28.7**)
- Forces generated are distalising and intrusive forces since the force is exerted above the occlusal plane
- Such forces are used in conditions where vertical control of the molars is important.

Indications

- Steep mandibular plane
- Certain open bite cases caused due to excessive eruption of buccal teeth
- As growth guiding appliance
- To decrease the vertical development of the maxilla
- Allowing for autorotation of the mandible
- Maximising the horizontal expression of mandibular growth.

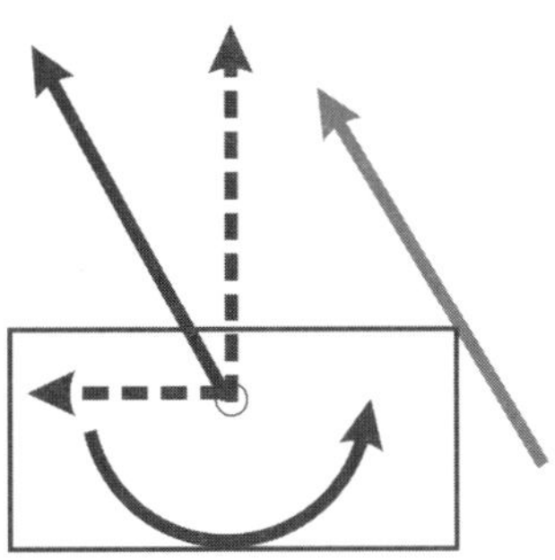

Fig. 28.8: Occipital pull with short outer bow

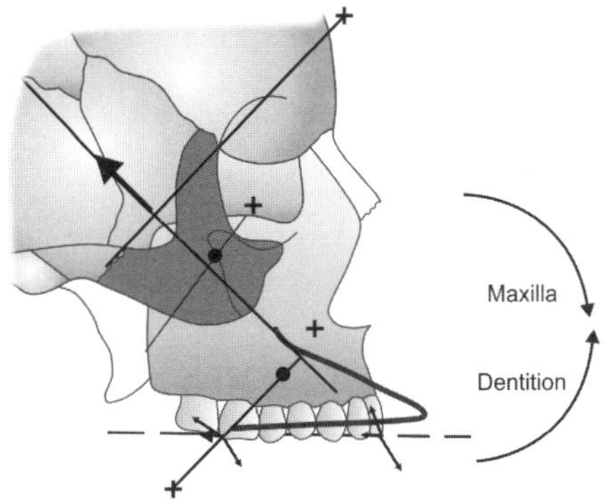

Fig. 28.9: Occipital pull with force passing through Cres

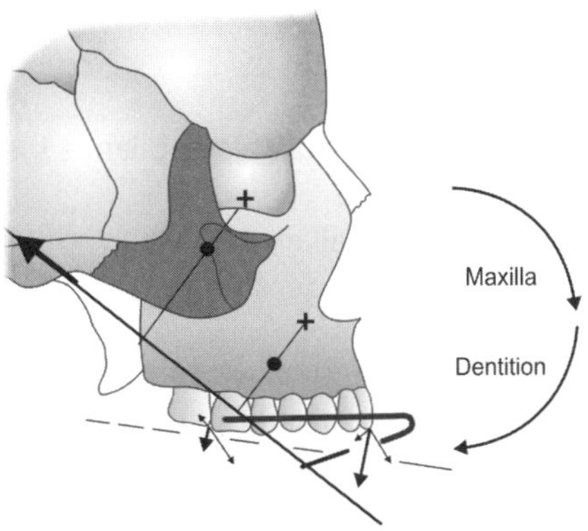

Fig. 28.10: Occipital pull with long outer bow

Occipital pull with short outer bow [force anterior to Cres (**Fig. 28.8**)]

- This results in a force system at the unit's Cres with a moment that tends to flatten the occlusal plane
- Creates distalising and intrusive components.

Occipital pull with force passing through Cres (**Fig. 28.9**):

- No moment that is created and hence there is no change in the cant of the occlusal plane
- Intrusive and distal components of force are produced.

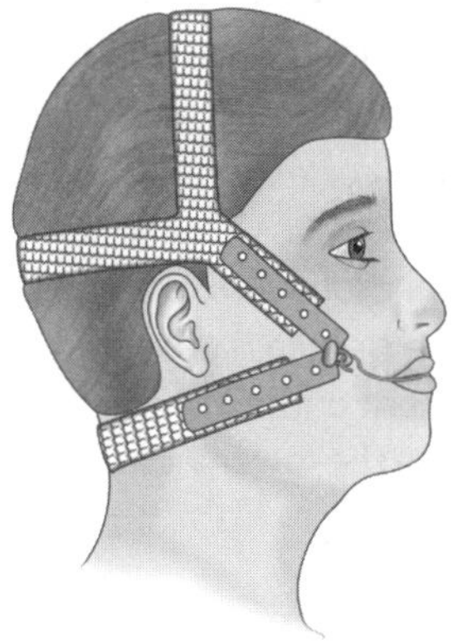

Fig. 28.11: Both occipital and cervical traction springs

Occipital pull with long outer bow [force posterior to Cres (**Fig. 28.10**)]:

- The force system at the unit's Cres has a moment that tends to steepen the occlusal plane
- Intrusive and distalising forces are produced
- Indicated in Class II open bite patients.

Combination Headgear

- Combination headgears have both occipital and cervical traction springs
- The most versatile type because the pull can be readily controlled by selecting the force level of the springs and by controlling the length of the outer bow
- For distal translation of the upper posteriors, a distal traction is needed that passes through the Cres (**Fig. 28.11**).

Question 3

What is face mask?

Answer

Face Mask

- With conventional extra-oral anchorage at cranial or cervical locations, the principal action in the direction of force delivery with headgear is posterior.
- The application of extra-oral anchorage combined with the clinical need at times for anteriorly directed active force has led to the development of reverse-pull headgear
- Orthopaedic facial mask is appliance of choice for most Class III patients in early mixed dentition or late deciduous dentition
- It has the widest application and produces the most dramatic results in the shortest period of time.

Face mask, especially when combined with a maxillary anchorage unit can produce following treatment effects:

- Correction of CO-CR (centric occlusion- centric relation) discrepancy: This correction is immediate and usually observed in pseudo-Class III patients
- Maxillary skeletal protrusion: Usually 1–2 mm of forward movement of the maxilla is observed
- Forward movement of the maxillary dentitions
- Lingual tipping of the lower incisors.

Classification

- Face mask
  - Old type (Petit facial mask)
  - New type (Delaire face mask).
- Reverse pull headgear
- Chin cup
  - Occipital pull
  - Vertical pull.

Components of Facial Mask

- Facial mask **(Fig. 28.12)**
- Bonded maxillary expansion splint
- Heavy elastics.

The Facial Mask (Jean Delaire)

- Delaire's approach involves applying traction to the maxillary sutures while reciprocally pushing on the mandible and the forehead through the anchorage provided by the facial mask
- This approach provides a repositioning of the bones of the craniofacial complex to a greater extent than that could be carried out by traditional orthodontic methods.

Petit Facial Mask

- The Petit facial mask originally was constructed on a patient by patient basis, using 0.25" round lengths of stainless steel, to which pads for the forehead and chin were attached **(Fig. 28.13)**
- The design was later simplified and made available commercially
- The positions of the pads are adjustable through the loosening and tightening of a set screw. The midline framework also can be bent to conform better to the outline of the face of the individual patient
- In the centre of the midline framework is a crossbar made from 0.075" stainless steel that is secured to the main framework by a set screw, thus, allowing the position of the crossbar to be adjusted vertically.

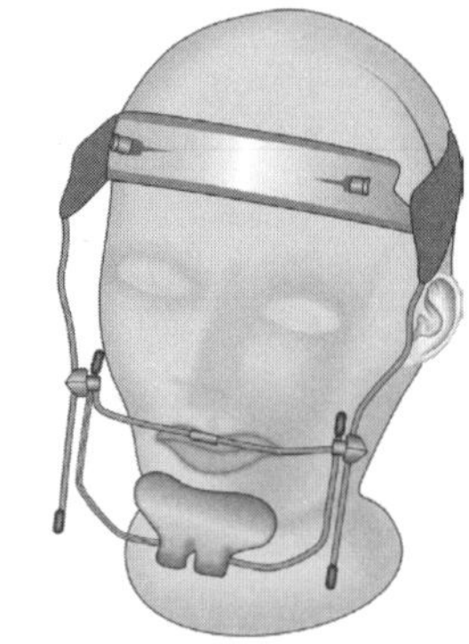

Fig. 28.12: Components of facial mask

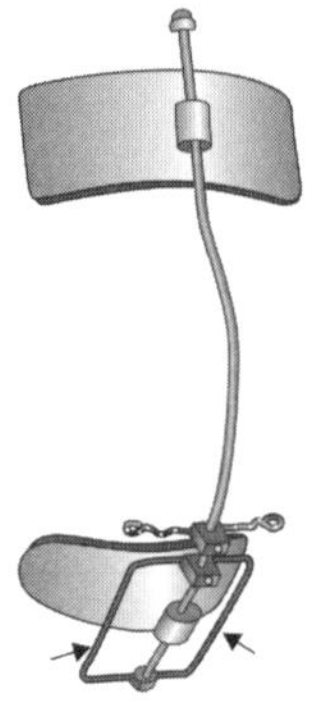

Fig. 28.13: Petit facial mask using 0.25" round lengths of stainless steel

Bonded Maxillary Splint

- The second component of this appliance system is the maxillary splint
- An acrylic and wire maxillary expansion appliance that is bonded to the posterior dentition.

Activation of the Splint

The patient is instructed to turn the midline expansion screw of the appliance once per day, generally before bedtime. In the majority of Class III individuals for whom the use of an orthopaedic facial mask is indicated, some maxillary expansion is beneficial.

Elastic Traction

- The facial mask is secured to the face by stretching elastics from the hooks on the maxillary splint to the crossbow of the facial mask
- Heavy forces are generated usually through the use of a sequence of elastics ultimately resulting in 14 oz force being generated by 5/16" elastics
- Lighter forces may be used during the break-in period but forces should be increased as the patient adjusts to the appliance.

SHORT ESSAYS

Question 1

What is chin cup/chin cap?

Answer

Chin Cup / Chin Cap

- It is an extra-oral orthopaedic appliance which has a device that covers the chin and is attached to the head gear **(Fig. 28.14)**
- It restricts downward and forward growth of mandible.

Types

- The occipital chin cup is used in cases of mandibular prognathism
- The vertical pull chin cup is used in cases of steep mandibular plane angle and excessive anterior facial height.

Occipital Pull Chin Cup

Indications

- Mild to moderate mandibular prognathism
- Success is greatest in those patients who can bring their incisors close to an edge-to-edge position, when in centric relation
- This treatment is particularly useful in patients who begin treatment with a short lower anterior facial height, as this type of treatment can lead to an increase in lower anterior facial height
- The occipital chin cup also is indicated in patients who have normally positioned or slightly protrusive lower incisors
- Since, the chin cup generates some force against the soft tissue in the chin region, some backward tipping of the lower incisors often is observed

Vertical Pull Chin Caps

- This appliance derives anchorage from the parietal region
- It is indicated in patients with steep mandibular plane
- It has seen in patients with excessive lower anterior facial height
- It has seen in patients with anterior open bite.

Question 2

What is the basis of orthopaedic appliances?

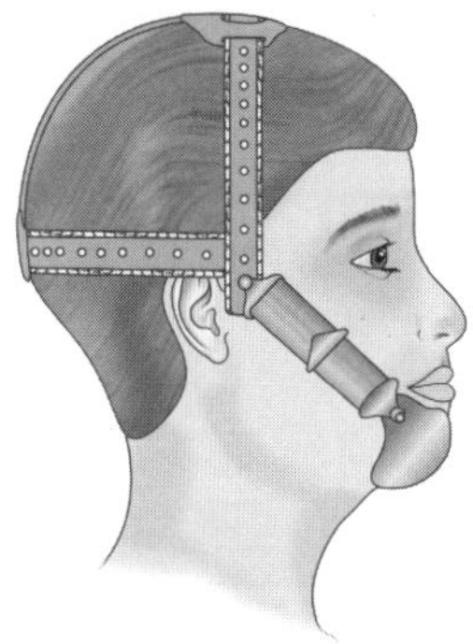

Fig. 28.14: Occipital pull chin cup

Answer

Orthopaedic appliances apply force on teeth through which force is transmitted to the underlying skeletal structures and bring about a change.

Orthopaedic therapy depends upon:

- Amount of force
- Duration of force
- Direction of force
- Age of patient.

Amount of Force

Force magnitude should be high:

- 400–600 g/side
- Maximum of 2–3 lb
- Bring about undermining resorption.

Duration of Force

- Intermittent forces: Skeletal changes
- Continuous forces: Dental changes
- 12–14 hour wear
- Increased wear: dental changes.

Direction of Force

Should be such as to maximize skeletal effect.

Age of Patient

- Most effective during pre-pubertal growth spurt
- But treatment should be maintained till growth is complete as these appliances change only the expression of growth and not the underlying growth pattern, which may latter reassert.

CHAPTER 29 Treatment Planning

LONG ESSAYS

Question 1

What are the steps of orthodontics treatment planning?

Answer

Steps of orthodontic treatment planning are as follows:

- Setting up treatment goals
  - Improvement in aesthetics
  - Improvement in function
  - Achieving treatment stability.
- Setting up of problem list
  - Skeletal
    - Prognathic maxilla
    - Prognathic mandible
    - Retrognathic maxilla
    - Retrognathic mandible
    - Protrusive chin
    - Recessive chin.
  - Dental
    - Class II molar relationship
    - Class III molar relationship
    - Increased overjet
    - Increased overbite
    - Open bite (anterior or posterior)
    - Cross bite (anterior or posterior)
    - Crowding
    - Spacing
    - Rotations
    - Deep bite
    - Impacted tooth/teeth
    - Proclination
    - Retroclination
    - Midline diastemas.
  - Soft tissue
  - Incompetent lips
  - Short upper lip
  - Hyperactive muscle activity
  - Lip trap
  - Habits.
    - Thumb sucking
    - Tongue thrusting
    - Mouth breathing.
- Treatment objective
  - It consist of formulating a list of problem that can be treated, considering the chief complaint of the patient and the willingness of the patient to undergo the required treatment procedures.
- Assessing the growth potential of the patient
  - The orthodontist has to carefully assist the growth potential of the patient in case of skeletal defect to decide. For example, skeletal Class II malocclusion and skeletal Class III malocclusion.
- Space analysis: In this, the space requirement is calculated to carry out the orthodontic treatment.
  - Correction of crowding: For correcting every millimetre of crowding, equal space is required in the arch
  - Rotations: Derotation of Anterior rotated teeth require space for corrections while rotated posterior teeth provide space
  - Curve of Spee: Flat curve of Spee occupies more space in the arch as compared to increased curve of space thus, space is required to flatten the curve of Spee
  - Correction of proclination: Retraction of proclined teeth requires space
    - For 1 mm of retraction, double the amount of space is required.
  - Molar correction: Protraction of molars requires space, while distalisation of molar gives spaces.

Considering the above factors, the orthodontist calculates how much space is required and then carries out the required method for gaining space like extractions, proximal shipping or distalisation.

- Planning extraction
  - Depending on the malocclusion, arch length and tooth material discrepancy, the extraction of teeth is planned
  - In Class I bidental proclination cases, the upper and lower 1st or 2nd premolar extraction are carried out, depending on the space requirement.
- Planning anchorage (Please refer chapter on Anchorage)
- Selection of appliances
  - In growth modification cases like skeletal Class II or Class III malocclusion, the functional appliances selection is carried out depending on the malocclusion and treatment goals
    For example, activator, twin block, frankel, chin cap, etc.
  - For fixed appliance cases, preadjusted edgewise appliance is commonly used
  - Habits: For elimination of habits, the appliances are given to the patient, e.g., tongue crib, oral screen, etc.
- Planning pretention protocols
  - Retention appliances like Hawley's retainer, begg retainer, fixed retainers, etc. are given
    - In mid-line diastema cases with high frenum attachment, frenectomy is carried out
    - Pericision is carried out in teeth, where large rotations are corrected
    - Growth modification cases require lengthy retention protocols
- Follow up: Regular follow-up of the cases should be carried-out post orthodontic treatment.

CHAPTER 30 Management of Some Common Malocclusions

LONG ESSAYS

Question 1

What is midline diastema? What are its causes? What are the diagnostic aspect and how can midline diastema be managed?

Answer

Midline diastema is referred to an anterior midline spacing between the two maxillary incisors.

Causes

- Transient malocclusions
- Tooth material - Arch length discrepancy
- Abnormal frenal attachment
- Pressure habits
- Midline pathology
- Iatrogenic
- Racial predisposition.

Diagnostic Aspects

- A proper history and clinical examination should be done
- Blanch test should be done to identify a high frenum attachment
- Presence of a notching in the interdental alveolar bone as seen on a radiograph is also diagnostic of a thick and fleshy frenum
- Midline radiographs are a valuable aid in diagnosing midline pathology that causes spacing
- Tooth material arch length discrepancies can be determined using model analysis.

Treatment

It can be done in three phases:

1. Removal of the cause
2. Active treatment
3. Retention.

- **Removal of the cause**: Habits should be removed by using fixed or removable habit breakers
  - Unerupted mesiodens should be extracted
  - Frenectomy.
- **Active treatment**: It can be done by using removable appliance or fixed appliance.
  - Removable appliances: Finger spring or a split labial bow can be used to close the midline spacing **(Fig. 30.1)**
  - Fixed appliance: Fixed appliances incorporating elastics or spring bring about the most rapid correction of midline diastema **(Fig. 30.2)**.
- **Retention**: In this, retaining of the treated malocclusion is done. It can be achieved by using retainers
  - Lingual-bonded retainers can be used since, prolonged retention is indicated
  - Other retainers are bonded retainers, Hawley's retainers, etc.

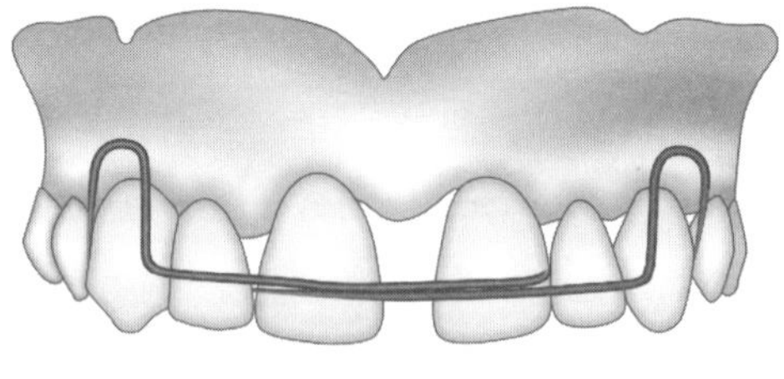

Fig. 30.1: Removable appliance

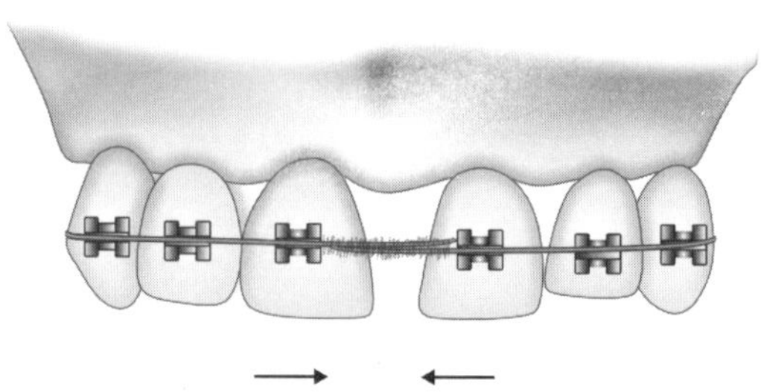

Fig. 30.2: Fixed appliance

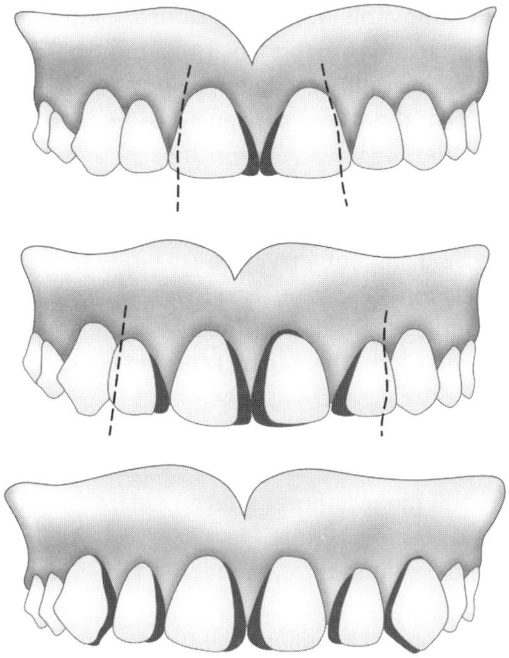

Fig. 30.3: Cosmetic Restoration

- **Cosmetic restoration**: Aesthetic composite resins can be used for midline diastema correction by gradual composite build up **(Fig. 30.3)**
- Prosthesis/Crown

Question 2

What is the aetiology, diagnosis and treatment of spacing?

Answer

Spacing between teeth is one of the commonly seen manifestations of Class I malocclusion.

Aetiology

- Disproportion between arch length and tooth material. For example, in cases of oligodontia and microdontia
- Because of alteration in tooth morphology. For example, in case of peg-shaped laterals
- Habits such as thumb sucking and tongue thrusting
- Because of abnormally large tongue, i.e., macroglossia
- Premature loss of permanent teeth
- Unerupted supernumerary teeth or other pathology and cystic lesions between the teeth.

Diagnosis

- Model analysis
- Radiographic examination.

Treatment

- **Removal of aetiology**: Spacing due to habits can be treated by using habit breakers
  - Bony pathology or cystic lesions should be removed.
- **Use of removable and fixed appliance**: Active removable appliance incorporating labial bow can be used, and fixed appliances along with elastic chains or elastic threads can be used
- **Crowns and prosthesis**: Spacing due to microdontia can be treated using crown
  - For example, in cases of peg-shaped maximally lateral incisors, spacing is commonly seen
  - This can be treated using a removable appliance incorporating finger spring or fixed appliances incorporating an open coil spring.

Question 3

What is the aetiology of crowding? Discuss diagnosis and treatment plan?

Answer

Aetiology of crowding is as follows:

- Arch length: Tooth material discrepancy because of decreased arch length or an increased tooth material
- Presence of supernumerary or extra teeth
- Retained deciduous teeth
- Premature loss of a deciduous tooth results in drifting of adjacent teeth
- Abnormalities in size and shape of teeth can also lead to crowding.

Diagnosis

- Clinical examination
- Model analysis.

Treatment

- **Gaining space**: There are various methods of gaining space. For example, proximal stripping, expansion, extraction, molar distalisation, derotation and uprighting of posterior teeth and proclination of anteriors
- **Use of removable appliance**: Removable appliance can be used, which incorporate coil springs, canine retractors, lateral bow, etc
- **Use of fixed appliances**: Fixed appliances that make use of multi-looped arch wires or resilient nickel-titanium wires are very effective is corrections of crowding.

Question 4

What are rotations? Discuss the treatment of rotation?

Answer

Rotations are tooth movements that occur around their long axis.

There are two types of rotations:

1. Mesio-lingual or disto-buccal rotations
2. Disto-lingual or mesio-buccal rotation.

- Anterior teeth that are rotated require additional space for their derotation
- Posterior teeth occupy more space when they are rotated, therefore space is gained when posterior teeth are derotated.

Treatment

- **Space management**: Treatment of anterior tooth rotation requires space
  - Therefore provision should be made in the treatment plan for obtaining required space.
- **Use of removable appliance**: Double cantilever spring, i.e., Z spring along with a labial bow can be used
- **Use of fixed appliance**: When multiple rotations of teeth are present then fixed appliance can be used. There are various methods of derotation, they are as follows:
  - Rotations wedges can be used which can be wedged between the arch wire and the tooth
  - By using resilient arch wires like nickel titanium
  - Elastic threads can be used to rotate the teeth
  - A couple of force is also effective in the treatment of a rotated tooth. This can be achieved by elastic threads both buccally and lingually.
- **Retention of rotation**: There is a high risk of relapse because of the stretching of the supra-alveolar and transeptal gingival fibres which readapt very slowly to the new position.
  - Therefore, long-term retention is required to achieve stability of treatment
  - Pericision or circumferential supracrestal fibrotomy is an adjunctive surgical procedure where the gingival fibres are incised to prevent relapse.

CHAPTER 31 Management of Class II Malocclusion

LONG ESSAYS

Question 1

What is class II malocclusion? What are its forms? Discuss its clinical features, aetiology and treatment of both the forms of class II malocclusions?

Answer

Class II malocclusion is the malocclusion where the disto-buccal cusp of the upper first permanent molar occlude in the buccal groove of the lower first permanent molar.

It has two main forms:

1. Class II, Division 1 (**Fig. 31.1**)
2. Class II, Division 2 (**Fig. 31.2**).

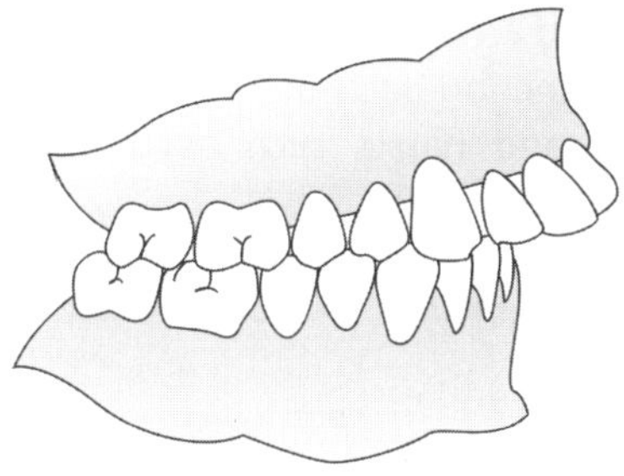

Fig. 31.1: Class II, Division I

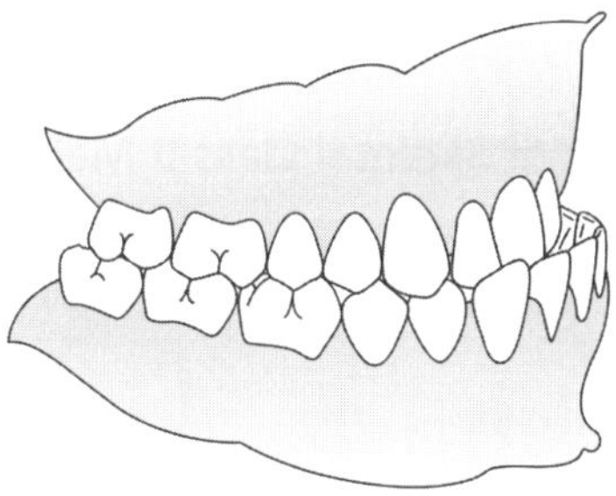

Fig. 31.2: Class II, Division II

Skeletal Features

Abnormal skeletal features are as follows (**Fig. 31.3**):

- Maxillary protrusion
- Mandibular retrusion
- Maxillary protrusion and mandibular retrusion.

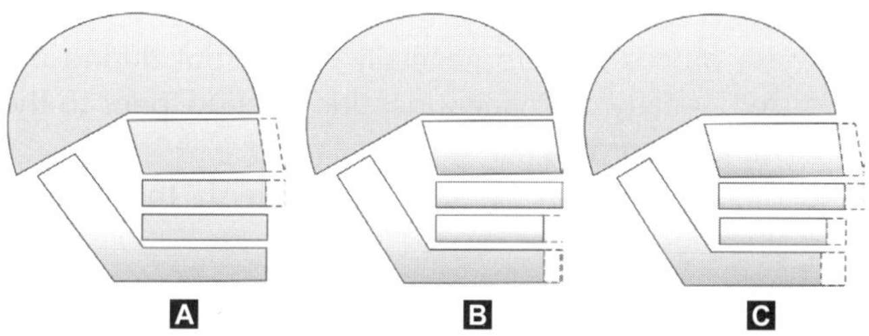

Fig. 31.3: Skeletal features. (A) Maxillary protrusion; (B) Mandibular retrusion; (C) Maxillary protrusion and mandibular retrusion

Aetiology

It can be classified as:

- Pre-natal factor
- Natal factor
- Post-natal factors.

Pre-natal Factor

- **Hereditary**: Size, position and relationship of the jaws is dependent upon the familial factors
  - Thus, presence of prognathic maxilla or a retrognathic mandible may be because of hereditary causes.
- **Teratogenesis**: Certain drugs at the time of pregnancy can lead to abnormal development. Such drugs are known as teratogens
- **Irradiation**: Exposure to radiation in a pregnant female can lead to abnormal development
- **Intra-uterine foetal posture**: Abnormal posture like hands across the face can affect the mandibular growth.

Natal Factor

- Sometimes trauma can be induced by improper forceps application during delivery
- This can lead to injury to the condylar region
- The temporomandibular joint (TMJ) in such cases can get ankylosed or fibrosed leading to under development of the mandible.

Post-natal Factors

- Traumatic injury to TMJ or mandible
- Long-term irradiation therapy of the skeletal craniofacial region
- Mandibular growth can be affected by conditions such as rheumatoid arthritis
- Abnormal function such as oral respiration, abnormal swallowing and habits such as thumb sucking can prevent muscle activity.

Treatment Objectives

- Reduction in overbite
- Reduction in overjet
- Correction of unstable molar relationship
- Correction of crowding and local irregularities
- Normalising the musculature
- Correction of posterior crossbites, if any.

Management of Skeletal Class II Malocclusion

There are three basic approaches to the treatment. They are:

- Growth modification
- Camouflage
- Surgical correction.

Growth Modification

- Functional and orthopaedic appliances can be used for growth modifications
- These procedures are generally carried out during the mixed or early permanent dentition period, prior to the cessation of growth
- Cephalograms can be used to establish the skeletal malrelationship.

Corrections of Mandibular Deficiency

- It can be done during the mixed dentition period by use of myofunctional appliances like activator, twin block, bionator, functional regulator
- If the patient is at the end of the growth period, then fixed functional appliances such as Herbst appliance or Jasper jumper is indicated.

Correction of Maxillary Prognathism

- Face bow with headgear can be used to restrict further maxillary growth
- If in a patient, there is maxillary prognathism as well as mandibular deficiency, then in such patient appliance such as activator with headgear is used to restrict maxillary growth and promote mandibular growth.

Camouflage

- If the patient is beyond growth, it is not possible to undertake growth modification procedure
- Therefore, orthodontic tooth movement can be done to camouflage the underlying skeletal discrepancy
- This can be achieved by extracting certain teeth and shifting the rest of the teeth into the space created.

Ideal Requirements for Camouflage

- Patient too old for successful growth modification using myofunctional appliances
- Reasonably well-aligned teeth so that extraction space is available for retraction, and not for correction of crowding
- Mild to moderate skeletal class II malocclusion
- Good vertical facial proportions with neither deep bite nor open bite
  - Space is required in the upper arch for reducing the overjet, overbite and to correct minor irregularities of teeth
  - To correct the unstable molar relations, corrections of crowding, deep bite and minor irregularities in the arch, extraction may be necessary
  - First premolar are the teeth that are most frequently extracted
  - Second premolars are extracted in those cases, where the space requirement is not much
  - Distal driving of maxillary molars can also be done in cases of mild class II malocclusion prior to eruption of second molar.

Surgical Correction

- Surgery may be ideal treatment in patients with existing severe skeletal malrelationships
- Depending upon the skeletal pattern either a maxillary set back or a mandibular advancement or both can be performed after the completion of growth.

Correction of Deep Bite and Crossbite

Anterior deep bite can be seen in cases of class II malocclusions. It can be corrected in following ways:

- By using removable anterior bite planes to encourage vertical development of the posterior dento-alveolar segments
- By using fixed appliances to intrude the upper and lower anteriors
- Cross bite can also be seen in cases of class II malocclusions. It can be treated in following ways:
  - Using appliance incorporating screws or springs that expand the maxillary arch.

Class II. Division 2 Malocclusion

In this condition, there is a class II molar relationship with retroclined upper central incisors that are overlapped by the lateral incisors.

Features of Class II Division 2

Features of class II division 2 are as following:

- Molars are in distal occlusion
- Retroclined central incisors
- Deep overbite
- Pleasing straight profile
- Broad square face
- Backward path of closure
- Deep mentolabial sulcus
- Absence of abnormal muscle activity.

Treatment Objectives

- Relief of gingival trauma
- Correction of incisor relationship
- Relief of crowding and local irregularities
- Correction of buccal segment relationship.

The increased anterior overbite and retroclination which are characteristics of division 2 malocclusion, can be treated by:

- Reduction in incisal overbite
- Alteration of incisal inclination
  - Anterior bite planes or fixed appliances incoroporating anchor bends or reverse curve of Spee can be used to reduce the deep overbite
  - Torquing springs can be used to treat incisor inclinations and to move the upper incisor roots lingually and the crowns labially
  - Functional appliance can also be used to correct class II division 2 into class II division 1 and further class II division 1 can be treated as described earlier.

CHAPTER 32 Management of Class III Malocclusion

LONG ESSAYS

Question 1

Discuss the clinical features and skeletal features of class III malocclusion. What is the aetiology, diagnosis and treatment plan for class III malocclusion?

Answer

Features of class III malocclusion are as follows:

- Patient has a class III molar relationship
- There may be an edge-to-edge relationship or an anterior cross-bites, seen in incisors
- Frequently the upper arch may be narrow or short, while the lower arch is broad
- Therefore, posterior cross-bites are a common features of class III malocclusion
- Because of presence of prominent chin, the patient has a concave profile
- Anterior open bite may be present in vertical growers, exhibiting an increased inter-maxillary height
- Since the arch is narrow and short, it is common for the upper teeth to be crowded, while the mandibular arch is often spaced
- Pseudo class III malocclusion is characterised by the presence of occlusal prematurities resulting in a habitual forward positioning of the mandible
- These patients might have a forward path of closure.

Skeletal Features of Class III Malocclusion

Skeletal features of class III malocclusion are as follows:

- Normal maxilla and prognathic mandible
- Maxillary retrognathia and normal mandible
- Maxillary retrognathia and mandible prognathic

Aetiology

- Usually inherited
- They have a very strong genetic basis
- Other reasons could be habitual forward positioning of the mandible because of occlusal prematurities or enlarged adenoids.

Diagnosis

- Diagnosis should determine whether the malocclusion is dental, skeletal, true or pseudo. Clinical examination should include observation of path of closure
- Study models and radiographs should also be taken
- A lateral cephalogram can be taken to understand the skeletal nature of the malocclusion.

Treatment

- Class III malocclusions should be recognized early in life and treated early because of following reasons:
  - Identifying the malocclusions at an early age makes it possible to intercept the abnormal skeletal pattern so as to reduce the severity of the developing malocclusion
  - Continued forward growth of the mandible is encouraged when the occlusal forces on the mandibular incisors are exerted by the maxillary incisors, further worsening the prenormalcy.

Interception During Growth

- Class III relation needs an early treatment to intercept the developing skeletal malocclusion
- Certain growth modulation procedures that can be carried out are as following:
  - Frankel III, a myofunctional appliance which can be used during growth to intercept a class III
  - Chin cup with a high pull headgear can be used to intercept class III malocclusion because of mandibular prognathism
  - Reverse activator. Severe class III malocclusions that are a result of maxillary retrusion can be treated by a reverse headgear or a face mask to protract the maxilla.

Treatment of Anterior Cross-bite

- Lower anterior inclined planes can be used for treatment of mild anterior cross-bite
- Removable appliances incorporating screws can be used for anterior expansion.

Treatment of Posterior Cross-bite

Rapid maxillary expansion can be done for treating posterior cross-bite.

Role of Extractions

- Class III malocclusions having lower arch length deficiency and anterior cross-bite can be treated by extracting the lower first premolar followed by fixed mechanotherapy
- To retract the lower anterior, class III intermaxillary elastics should be used **(Fig. 32.1)**
- In cases of arch length deficiency involving both the arches, the first premolars should be extracted in both the upper and lower arches.

Treatment of Severe Class III after Growth

- It can be treated by surgical and corrective procedures
- Class III because of maxillary deficiency can be treated by maxillary advancement procedures like Le Fort I osteotomy

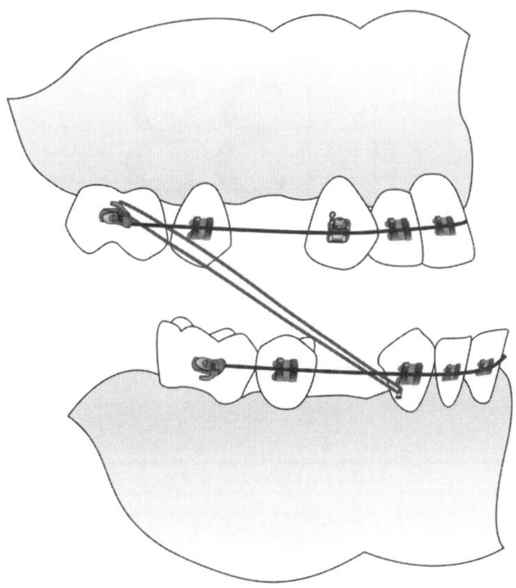

Fig. 32.1: Fixed mechanotherapy

- Class III malocclusions that are a result of mandibular prognathism are treated by mandibular set back procedures.

Treatment of Pseudo Class III

By removal of the cause pseudo class III can be corrected. E.g. by correcting the occlusal prematurity.W

CHAPTER 33

Management of Open Bite

LONG ESSAYS

Question 1

What is open bite, define and classify it? Explain the various methods of treatment of open bite?

Answer

Open bite is a malocclusion that occurs in the vertical plane, characterized by lack of vertical overlap between the maxillary and mandibular dentition.

Open bite is defined as a condition where a space exists between the occlusal or incisal surfaces of the maxillary and mandibular teeth in the buccal or anterior segments when the mandible is brought into a habitual or centric occlusion (Graber).

According to Moyers, there are two definitions of open bite:

1. The first defines open bite as the absence of vertical incisal overlap
2. The second defines open bite as the absence of an occlusal stop.

Open bite is the failure of a tooth or teeth to meet antagonists in the opposite arch or the occlusal planes.

Classification

According to location open bite is divided into:

- Anterior open bite
- Posterior open bite.

According to Moyers

- **Simple open bite**: When the cephalometric analysis reveals no abnormal measures and the sole problem is the failure of some teeth to meet the line of occlusion
- **Complex or skeletal open bite**: When the cephalometric analysis reveals disharmonies in the skeletal components of the anterior face height.

Etiology of Open Bite

Anterior Open Bite

- Disturbances in the eruption of teeth and alveolar growth, e.g., ankylosed primary molars
- Mechanical interference with eruption and alveolar growth, e.g., finger sucking, foreign body in mouth (pins, pencil)
- Vertical skeletal dysplasia which may be genetically determined
- **Mouth breathing**: Can cause different head, jaw and tongue position which would affect the jaw growth and tooth positions
- Different postures seen in mouth breathing:
    - Lowering the mandible
    - Positioning the tongue downward and forward
    - Tipping back of the head.
- The type of open bite associated with mouth breathing is called "skeletal open bite or adenoid facies".
    - Excessive eruption of posterior teeth
    - Tendency towards maxillary constriction
    - Excessive overjet
    - Anterior open bite.
- Thumb sucking can cause:
    - Flared and spaced maxillary incisors
    - Anterior open bite
    - A narrow upper arch.
- Lip sucking and lip biting
- Foreign bodies: Pipes, pen, pencil
- Trauma or pathology of condyle.

Features of Skeletal Open Bite

Extraoral Features

- Long face due to increased lower anterior facial height
- Incompetent lips

- An increased mandibular plane angle
- An increased gonial angle
- Marked antegonial notch
- A short mandible is a possibility
- Maxillary base may be more inferiorly placed.

Intraoral Features

- Mild crowding
- Gingival hypertrophy
- Maxillary occlusal and palatal plate tilt upwards
- Mandibular occlusal plane canted downwards.

Features of Dental Anterior Open Bite

- Proclined upper incisors
- Vertical space between maxillary and mandibular anteriors
- Narrow maxillary arch.

Posterior Open Bite

Causes

1. Mechanical interference with eruption:
   Before tooth emerges from alveolar bone, mechanical interference may be:
   Ankylosis of tooth to the alveolar bone (trauma), e.g., trauma, supernumerary teeth, non-resorbing deciduous roots.
   After the tooth emerges from the alveolar bone:
   - Pressure from the soft tissues (cheek, finger, tongue) can be obstacle to eruption.
2. Failure of the eruptive mechanism of tooth so that expected amount of eruption does not occur.

Treatment

In Deciduous Dentition Stage

Interception of habit (**Table 33.1**):

- Another level of intervention is reminder therapy.
  - Bitter medicine may be placed on adhesive , which is wrapped around the thumb
  - Reward system can be implemented. Reward for not engaging into the habit
  - Elastic bandage loosely wrapped around the elbow prevents the arm from flexing and fingers being sucked.
- Treatment of open bite in the mixed and early permanent dentition:
  - Headgear
  - Functional appliance with bite blocks
    - Activator
    - FR4
    - Bionator.

Table 33.1: Interception of habit

Etiology	Age of the patient	Appliance used for correction
Tongue thrust	Pre-adolescent	Fixed tongue crib/rake
Tongue thrust	Adolescent or adult	Fixed or removable tongue cirb/take
Digit sucking	Pre-adolescent	Motivation and/or medicaments. Acrylic digit caps. Fixed tongue crib/rake
Digit sucking	Adolescent (Rarely seen)	Fixed tongue crib/rake
Mouth breathing	Pre-adolscents	ENT check-up followed by Breathing exercises mouth shield
Mouth breathing	Adolescents and adults	ENT check-up followed by Breathing exercises Orthodonitc trainers

- Treatment of open bite in the mixed and early permanent dentition:
  - Headgear
  - Functional appliance with bite blocks.
- Treatment in permanent dentition:
  - Fixed appliance therapy with screening appliance
  - Box elastics
  - Repelling magnets placed in the posterior bite plates
  - Anterior attractive and posterior repelling mode to achieve normal over bite
  - Palatal bars and lingual arches: Reduce the vertical eruption of molars
  - Posterior bite planes on the upper or lower posterior teeth
  - High pull face bow and chin caps: Limit the vertical eruption of molars.

Surgical Correction

Maxilla

- This allows mandible to rotate around the condyle, thereby reducing the mandibular plane angle and shortening the face
- Le fort 1 down fracture of the maxilla with superior reposition of the maxilla after removal of the bone from the lateral walls of the nose, sinus and nasal septum
- Results are quite stable.

Mandible

Inferior border osteotomy of the mandible to reduce vertical height of the chin.

CHAPTER 34

Management of Cross Bite

LONG ESSAYS

Question 1

What is cross-bite? Classify cross-bite. What is the aetiology of cross-bite? Discuss in detail the management of cross-bite?

Answer

Cross-bite is an abnormal occlusion in the transverse plane.

According to Graber, cross-bite is a condition where one or more teeth may be abnormally malposed bucally or lingually or labially with reference to the opposing tooth or teeth.

Classification of Cross-bite

Cross-bite can be classified according to location:

- Anterior cross-bite
  - Single tooth
  - Segmental.
- Posterior cross-bite
  - Unilateral
  - Bilateral.

Based on the nature of the cross-bite as:

- Skeletal cross-bite
- Dental cross-bite
- Functional cross-bite.

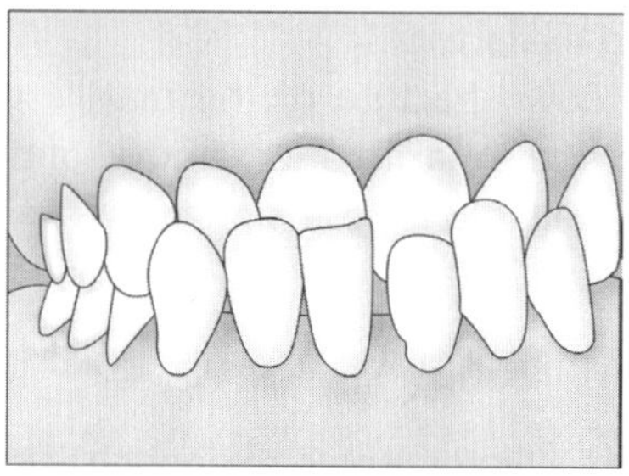

Fig. 34.1: Anterior crossbite

Anterior Cross-bite

It can be defined as a malocclusion resulting from the lingual position of the maxillary anterior teeth in relationship with the mandibular anterior teeth (**Fig. 34.1**).

Posterior Cross-bite

- It is an abnormal relationship between the upper and lower posterior teeth
- In this condition, the mandibular buccal cusps occlude buccal to the maxillary buccal cusps (**Fig. 34.2**).
- Posterior cross-bite can be unilateral or bilateral.

Buccal non-occlusion: It is a form of posterior cross-bite where the maxillary posterior occludes entirely on the buccal aspect of the mandibular posterior. It is also referred to as scissors bite (**Fig. 34.3**).

Lingual non-occlusion: It is a form of posterior cross-bite where the maxillary posterior occludes entirely on the lingual aspect of the mandibular posteriors (**Fig. 34.4**).

Skeletal Cross-bite

- It is associated with a discrepancy in the size of the maxilla and the mandible
- This kind of cross-bite is usually inherited or may result from defective embroyological development

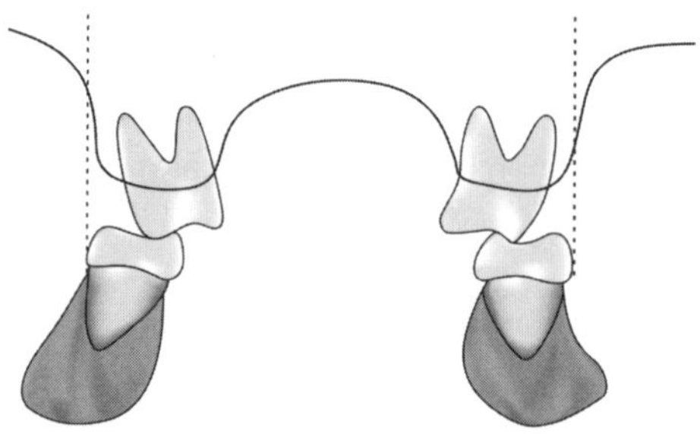

Fig. 34.2: Posterior crossbite

- They may present either in the anterior or the posterior region
- Skeletal anterior cross-bites are usually as a result of retarded maxillary growth or a maxilla that is backwardly positioned **(Fig. 34.5A)**
- It can also occur as a result of excessive mandibular growth **(Fig. 34.5B)**
- Narrow upper arch is seen in skeletal posterior cross-bite.

Dental Cross-bite

These are generally localised and is characterised when single or a group of teeth of mandibular arch are in abnormal relationship to the maxillary teeth.

Causes

- Lingual eruption of maxillary tooth/teeth
- Buccal eruption of mandibular tooth/teeth
- Arch length—tooth material discrepancy in mandibular arch causing crowding with teeth being displaced labially/buccally.

Functional Cross-bite

- Presence of occlusal interferences result in deviation of mandible during jaw closure leading to the development of unilateral cross-bite
- Habitual forward positioning of the mandible leads to anterior cross-bite.

Management

- Management of dental cross-bite
- Management of skeletal cross-bite
- Management of dental cross-bite in:
  - Primary dentition
  - Early mixed dentition
  - Late mixed dentition
  - Permanent dentition.

Primary Dentition

- **Anterior cross-bite**: Removing the interferences by occlusal grinding or extracting the primary incisor.
- **Posterior cross-bite**: If the inter-molar width is satisfactory, grinding primary canines to eliminate defective contact. If both molar and canine width are narrow, expansion of the upper arch is indicated.

Early Mixed Dentition Period

- **Anterior cross-bite**: Lingually trapped incisors can be corrected by extracting the adjacent canines, if sufficient space is not available.

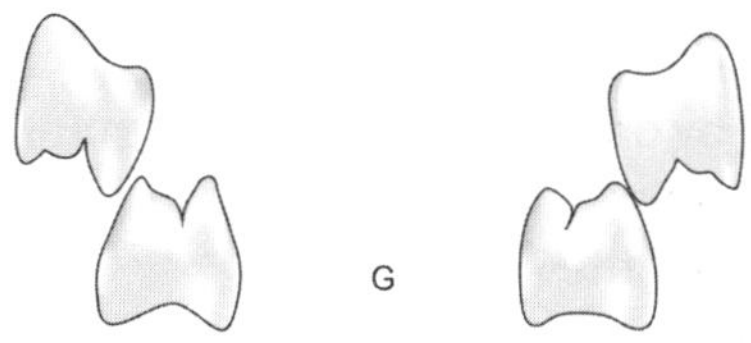

Fig. 34.3: Buccal crossbite, bilateral

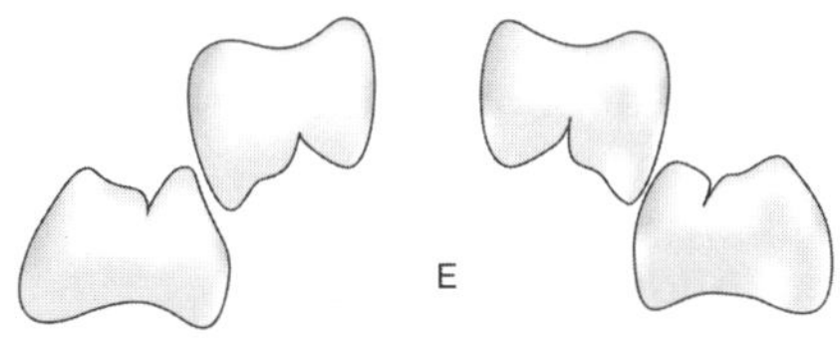

Fig. 34.4: Complete lingual, bilateral

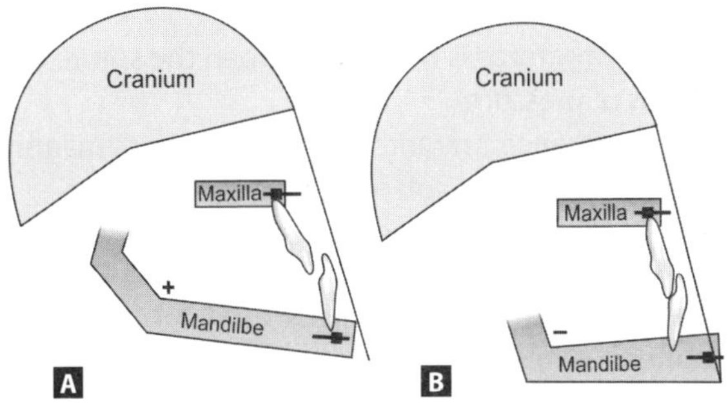

Figs. 34.5A and B: Skeletal crossbite

If sufficient space is available, a maxillary removable appliance is usually the best mechanism to correct a simple anterior cross-bite that requires tipping movement.
- **Posterior cross-bite**: Both removable and fixed appliances are used. The maxillary arch should be overexpanded and then held passively in this overexpanded position for approximately 3 months before it is removed.

Three basic approaches to the treatment of posterior cross-bite in children are:

1. Equilibration to eliminate mandibular shift
2. Expansion of the constricted maxillary arch
3. Repositioning of individual teeth to deal with intra-arch asymmetries.

Late Mixed Dentition Period

- **Anterior cross-bite**: Best method for tipping maxillary and mandibular teeth out of cross-bite is by using finger spring, double helical cantilever, Z spring along with an anterior bite plate to prevent any hindrance to tooth movement
- Fixed appliances are also used for the correction. For example, maxillary lingual arch with finger springs. Use of posterior bands and anterior bonded attachments with a round arch wire is done.

Pre-Adolescent Children

- Corrected by opening the mid palatal suture
- Growth at this suture continues in most children until late teens and then ceases
- Less force is required to open the suture in primary and early mixed dentition period
- W-arch, Quad Helix and Jack screw appliances are used. They deliver less than 2 pounds of force
- A fixed banded or bonded jack screw appliance can be used.

Adolescent Children

- As age increases, the sutures becomes more and more tightly interdigitated and opening it becomes eventually difficult
- A very heavy force is required to open the suture (10–20 pounds of pressure).
- A fixed appliance is required because the force magnitude is large enough to displace removable appliance.

Question 2

What are the different appliances used for correction of cross-bite?

Answer

Various Appliances for Correction of Cross-bite

Coffin Spring

- Made of 1.25 mm stainless-steel wire **(Fig. 34.6)**
- Differential expansion in molar and premolar region
- Disadvantages: Unstable, lack control in molars, frequent activation needed and force applied varies.

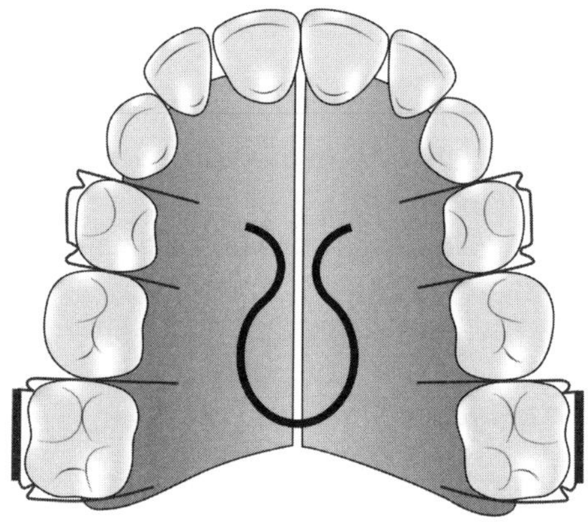

Fig. 34.6: Coffin spring

W-arch

- Moves both primary and permanent teeth and accelerate the rate of normal expansion of the mid palatal suture
- Activated by simply opening the apices of W **(Fig. 34.7)**
- Expansion should continue at the rate of 2 mm per month.

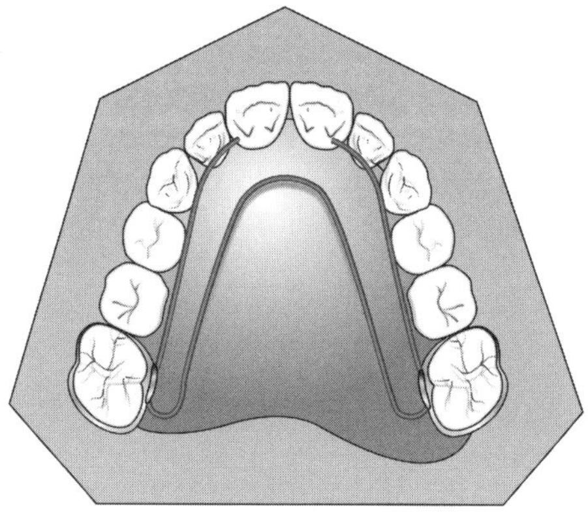

Fig. 34.7: W-arch

Quad Helix

- Helices in the anterior plate helps in stopping sucking habit **(Fig. 34.8)**
- Indicated for the correction of cross-bite and finger sucking habit
- Forces are produced when the appliance is widened by 3–8 mm
- 3 months of retention is recommended.

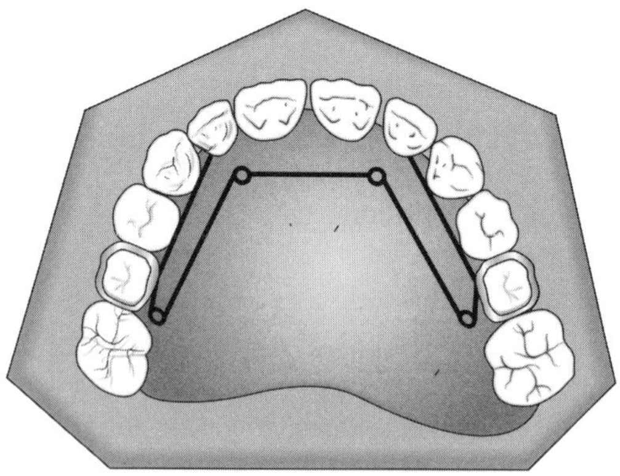

Fig. 34.8: Quad helix

Indications

- Cross-bites in which upper arch need to be widened
- Thumb sucking or tongue thrusting cases
- Cleft palate conditions either unilateral or bilateral
- Cases of class II and class III conditions in which the upper arch needs to be widened.

Disadvantages

- Excessive tipping of teeth buccally
- Movements are not long enough and hence, not retained long enough
- Restriction of tongue space so, tongue function is hampered
- Intermittent forces
- Frequent activations are required
- Uncomfortable for patient.

Cross Elastics

- Typically run from lingual of upper molar to buccal of lower molar
- For scissors bite, opposite is followed **(Fig. 34.9)**
- Indicated for a short period to correct simple cross-bite
- Effective in correction of unilateral cross-bites.

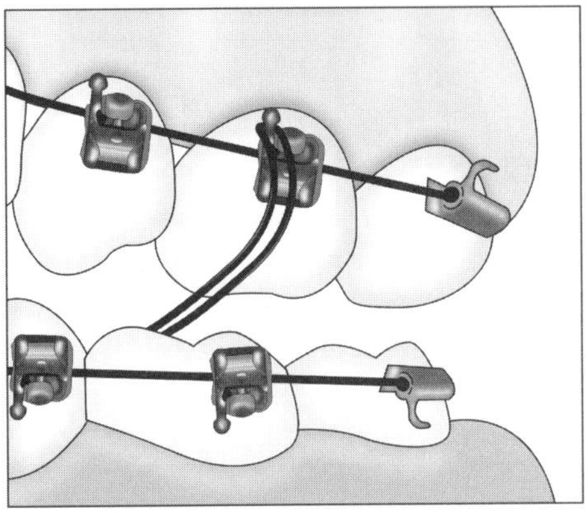

Fig. 34.9: Cross elastic

NiTi Palatal Expander

- It is a temperature-activated palatal expander **(Fig. 34.10)**
- Apply light continuous pressure on the mid-palatal suture
- Self-activated
- Action is due to NiTi's shape memory and transition temperature effects.

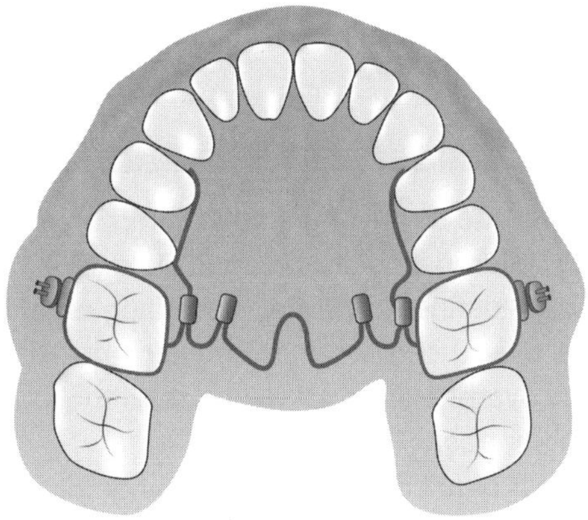

Fig. 34.10: NITI palatal expander

Advantages

- Little clinical manipulation
- Absence of lab work
- Reduced treatment time
- Exerts light continuous forces
- Requires no adjustments
- Comfortable and minimal patient co-operation
- It has a safety system and helps the patient to mitigate the pressure response.

ELSAA

- Expansion and Labial Segment Alignment Appliance
- Used for the purpose of expansion and labial segment alignment prior to treatment by functional appliance
- Until 4–6 month into the functional treatment, the previous ELSAA must be worn whenever the functional appliance is out of mouth.

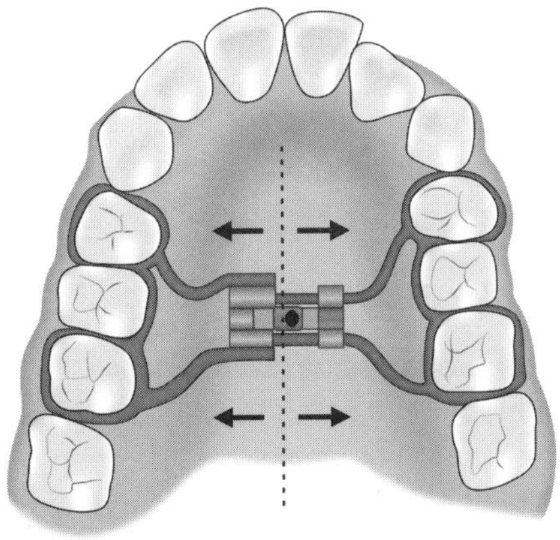

Fig. 34.11: Rapid palatal expander (HYRAX)

Rapid Palatal Expander (HYRAX)

- It involves appliance activation of at least 0.5 mm daily **(Fig. 34.11)**
- The force is transmitted immediately to the teeth and then to the suture
- 1-–20 pounds of pressure is applied
- The expansion occurs faster and to a greater extent in the anterior portion of the palate because of the buttressing effect of the other maxillary structures in the posterior region.

CHAPTER 35 Management of Deep Bite

LONG ESSAYS

Question 1

Define and Classify Deep-bite. Explain different methods for treatment of deep-bite?

Answer

- Deep overbite is one of the most common malocclusion seen in children as well as in adults **(Fig. 35.1)**
- Strang has defined overbite as overlapping of the upper incisors over the lower in a vertical plane. He described average overbite as equal to one third the length of the maxillary incisor
- Graber has defined deep-bite as a condition of excessive overbite, where the vertical measurement between the maxillary and mandibular incisal margins is excess when the mandible is brought into habitual or centric occlusion.

Classification

- Dento alveolar deep-bite
- Skeletal deep-bite.

Dentoalveolar Deep-bite

- Dental deep-bite occurs due to:
  - Over eruption of anteriors (true deep-bite)
  - Infra occlusion of molars (pseudo deep-bite).
- Deep-bite due to over eruption of anteriors:
  - Dental deep-bite associated with over eruption of lower incisors are usually seen in class II malocclusions.
- Deep-bite due to infra occlusion of molars:
  - Deep-bites can occur due to infra occlusion of the molars
  - The presence of a lateral tongue posture or lateral tongue thrust may prevent the molars from erupting to their normal occlusion level

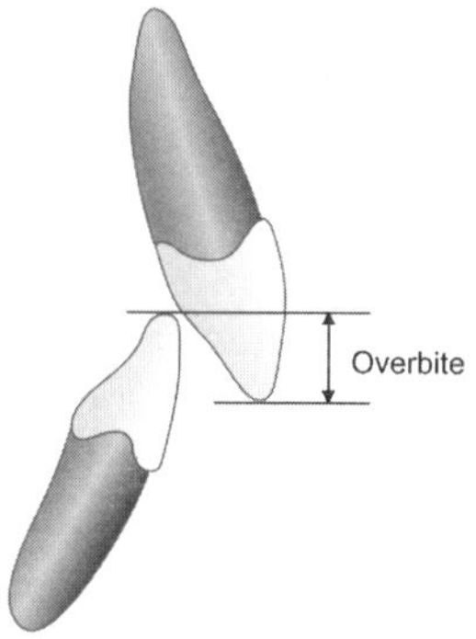

Fig. 35.1: Overbite

  - It can also occur due to premature loss of posterior teeth
  - Deep-bite caused by infra occlusion of molars are characterized by the presence of partially erupted molars (i.e., Reduced crown height) and large inter-occlusal clearance.

Skeletal Deep-bite

- The mandible in skeletal deep-bite shows certain distinct features:
  - The ramus is broad anteroposteriorly with a big coronoid
  - Flaring of the gonial process laterally is seen indicating a strong masseter action, with the absence of the ante gonial notch
  - The ramus and corpus lengths are almost equal
  - The mandibular symphysis is broad antero posteriorly but short vertically.
- Methods of correcting deep-bite:
  - Extrusion of the posterior teeth
  - Intrusion of the anterior teeth
    - Absolute Intrusion
    - Relative intrusion
    - Pseudo intrusion.

- Combination of both
- Uprighting the posterior teeth
- Increasing the inclination of the anterior teeth.

Anterior Bite Plane

Bonded biteplanes achieve **(Fig. 35.2)**:

- Intrusion of maxillary anterior teeth
- Intrusion of mandibular anterior teeth
- Extrusion of maxillary posterior teeth
- Extrusion of mandibular posterior teeth.

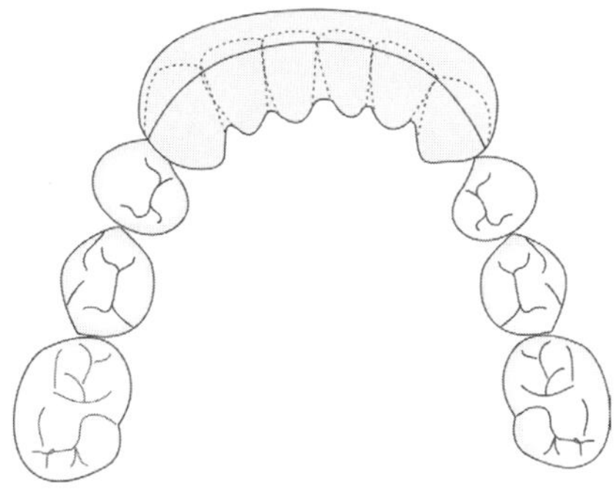

Fig. 35.2: Anterior bite plane

Intrusion of Anterior Teeth

In vertical growth pattern bite opening should be achieved by the of intrusion of incisors.

Indications

- Large interlabial gap
- Large incisor stomion-distance
- Short upper lip
- High gingival smile line
- Large lower facial height.

Intrusion

- True or absolute intrusion is achieved by moving the root apices of the anteriors closer to the bony base
- Relative intrusion is achieved by keeping lower anteriors where they are, while the mandible grows and the posterior teeth erupt
- Apparent intrusion is achieved by extrusion of the posterior teeth
- According to Proffit the optimum force for intrusion is 15-25 gm
- Values depend in part on the size of the tooth
- Smaller values appropriate for incisors
- Higher values are for multirooted posterior teeth.

According to Burstone the average force values for intrusions are given in **Table 35.1**.

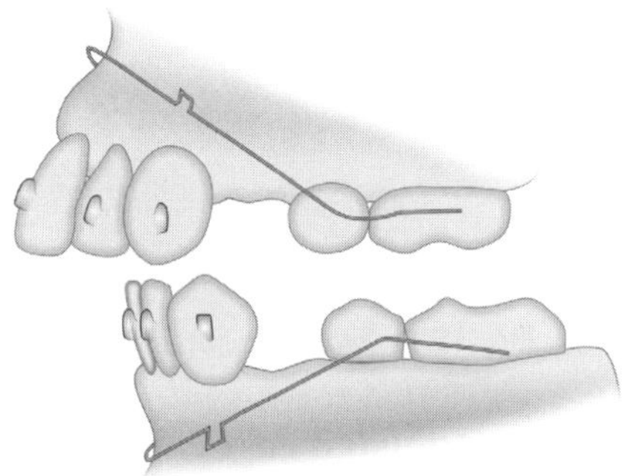

Fig. 35.3: Anchor bends with Begg's appliance

Table 35.1: Burstone's average force values for intrusions

Teeth	*Force / Side*	*Total force in midline*	*Moment/ side (gm-mm)*
Upper			
Central incisors	25	50	750
Central and lateral incisors	50	100	1,500
Central and lateral incisors and canine	100	200	3,000
Lower			
Central and lateral incisors	20	40	600
Central and lateral incisors and canines	80	160	2,400

Bite Opening with Begg's Appliance

Anchor Bends

Anchor bend is placed 3 mm mesial to the molar tube in such a way that there is an intrusive force acting on the anterior segment **(Fig. 35.3)**.

Gable Bend

- Gable bends placed distal to the canines, normally made in the third stage archwire to maintain bite opening attained in the earlier stages
- This has a more intrusive effect on central and lateral incisors **(Fig. 35.4)**.

Swain's Modification

Swain advocates giving a mild gingival curve in the anterior region which starts from mesial side of one canine to the mesial side of the other canine for the better intrusion of the anteriors **(Fig. 35.5)**.

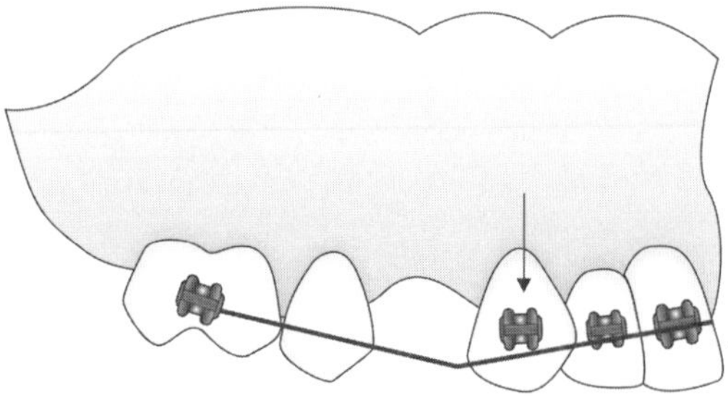

Fig. 35.4: Gable bend

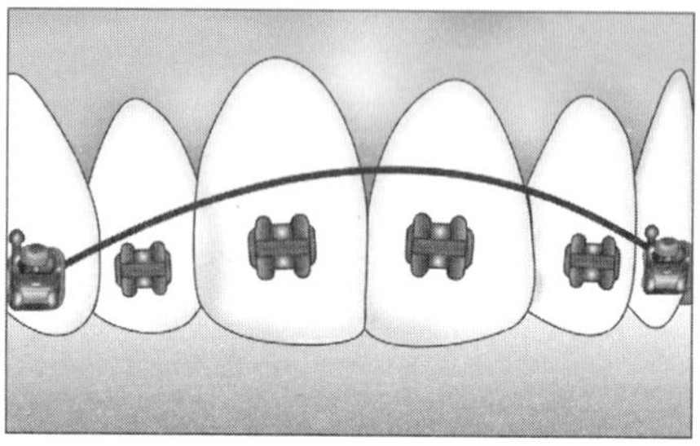

Fig. 35.5: Swain's modification

Intrusion In Pre-adjusted Edgewise Appliance

Burstone Intrusion Arch

Intrusive arch normally consists of an 0.018/0.025 SS or TMA wire with a 3 mm helix wound 2½ times placed mesial to the auxiliary tube **(Figs. 35.6A to C)**.

Intrusion Utility Arch

This appliance consists of a continuous wire that extends across both buccal segments but engages only the first permanent molars and four incisors therefore also called 2 × 4 appliance **(Figs. 35.7 and 35.8)**.

- Molar segment
- Posterior vertical segment
- Vestibular segment
- Anterior vertical segment
- Incisal segment
- Fabricated from 0.016 × 0.016 Blue Elgiloy wire
- Utility arch mechanics used in the intrusion of lower incisors require forces of 15 to 20 gram per lower incisor or 60 to 80 gram for all four lower incisor teeth and approximately 160 gram or 40 gram per each tooth for upper incisors.

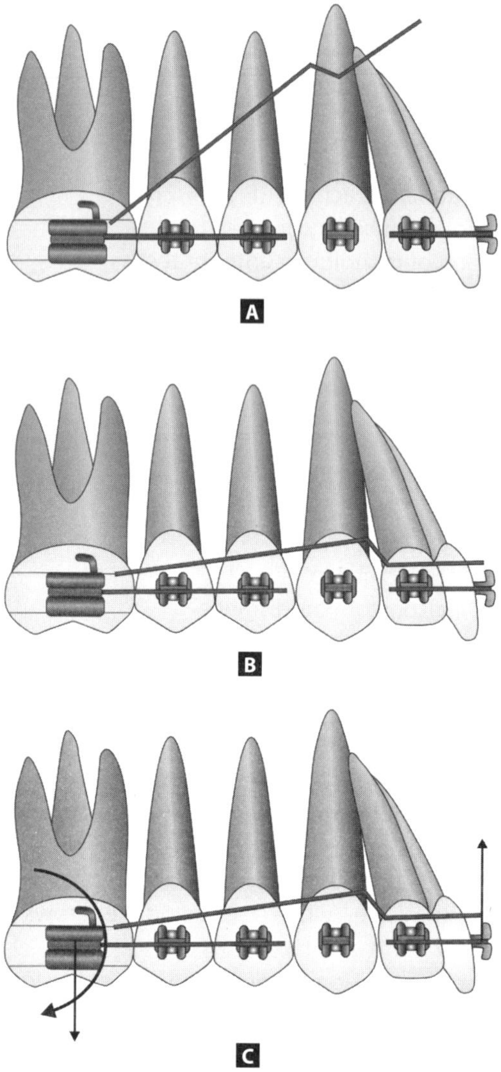

Figs. 35.6A to C: Burstone's intrusion arch: (A) Arch placed mesial to the auxiliary tube; (B) Curvature is placed in the ntrusive arch; (C) Arch is tied to the level of the incisors

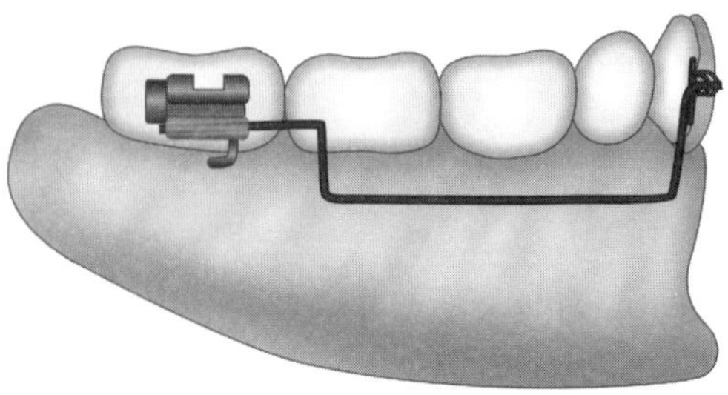

Fig. 35.7: Intrusion utility arch

The Connecticut Intrusion Arch

- Fabricated from a nickel titanium alloy **(Fig. 35.9)**
- Two wire size are available 0.016″ × 0.022″ and 0.17″ × 0.25″
- The maxillary and mandibular versions have anterior dimensions of 34mm and 28mm, respectively
- In most cases, the wire is not directly ligated into the bracket slots, the anterior wire dimension is adequate to allow for it

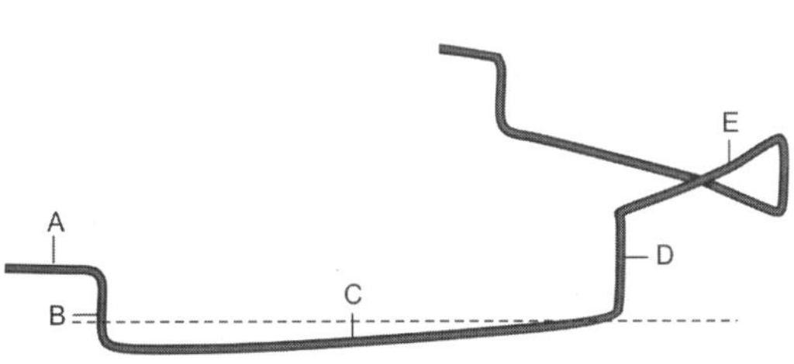

Fig. 35.8: Utility arch: 2 × 4 appliance (A) Molar segment; (B) Posterior vertical segment; (C) Vestibular segment; (D) Anterior vertical segment; (E) Incisal segment

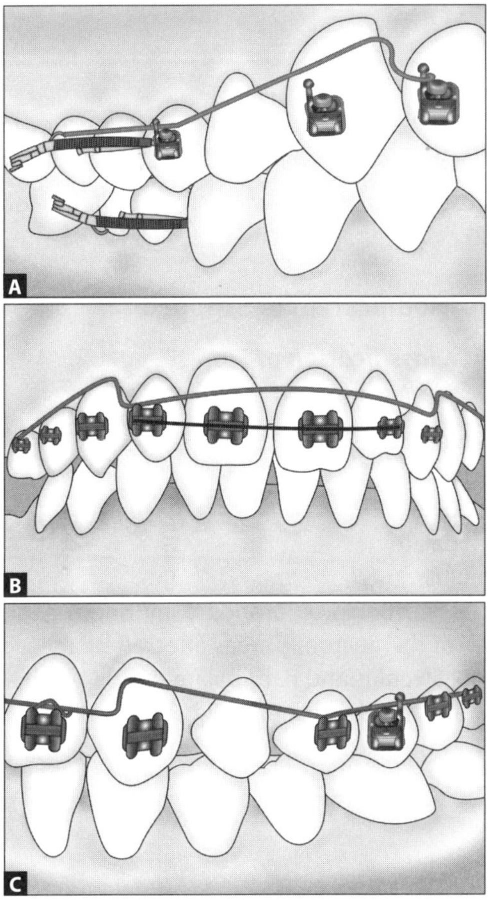

Fig. 35.9: The Connecticut intrusion arch

- The bypass, located distal to the lateral incisors, is available in two different lengths to accommodate for extraction, nonextraction, and mixed dentition cases.

Three Piece Intrusion Arches

- Three piece intrusion arches can achieve deep overbite correction and close extraction spaces simultaneously

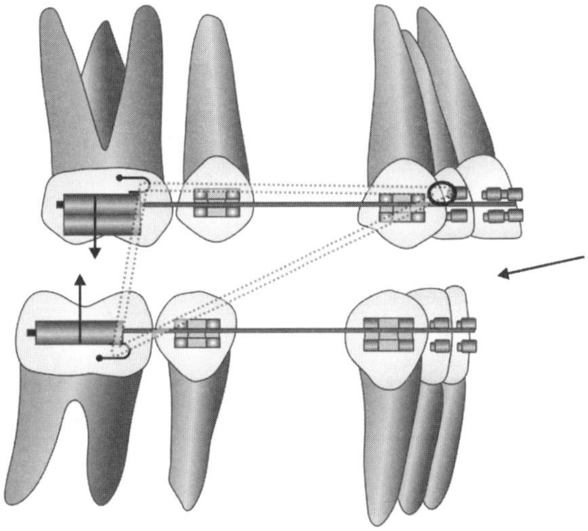

Fig. 35.10: Intermaxillary elastics

- This appliance was introduced by Burstone, modified by Shroff, Lindhauer
- 0.017 × 0.025 TMA wire is used to fabricate the appliance.

Intrusion with Micro-Implants

- Micro implants can be used to bring about intrusion of incisors or all anterior teeth in both maxilla and mandible
- Micro implants can be placed between the roots of central and lateral incisor to bring about intrusion of incisors
- They can also be placed between premolar and molar roots to bring about intrusion and distal movement of whole anterior segment.

Inclusion of Second Molars

Inclusion of second molar in fixed orthodontic therapy bring about their extrusion thus leading to early closure of mandible resulting in downward and backward rotation of mandible leading to reduction in over bite.

Intermaxillary Elastics

- The action of the elastics is to reduce deep-bite by obtaining extrusion of the molars **(Fig. 35.10)**
- Class II elastics can be used in a triangular configuration with the elastic extended form the lower molar to the upper molar to encourage extrusion of the posterior teeth.

CHAPTER 36 Cleft Lip and Palate

LONG ESSAYS

Question 1

What is cleft lip and palate, classify cleft lip and palate?

Answer

Davis and Ritchie's Classification of Clefts (1922)

Davis and Ritchie's classified cleft into three categories are:

- **Group I**: Pre-alveolar cleft. These are Lip clefts only. Can be further divided into unilateral, median, bilateral
- **Group II**: Post-alveolar cleft. There is different degree of involvement of hard palate and soft palate
- **Group III**: Alveolar clefts. They are complete clefts of palate, alveolar ridge and lip. These can be further divided into unilateral, median and bilateral.

Veau's Classification of Clefts (1931)

Veau classified clefts into four groups, which are:

- **Group I**: Cleft of the soft palate only
- **Group II**: Cleft of the hard and soft palate up to the incisive foramen
- **Group III**: Complete unilateral cleft of the soft palate, hard palate and the lip and alveolar ridge
- **Group IV**: Complete bilateral cleft of the soft palate, hard palate, and the lip and alveolar ridge.

Schuchardt and Pfeiffer's Classification (Graphic)

- Chart made up of a vertical block of three pairs of rectangles
- Inverted triangle represents the soft palate.
  - Areas affected by clefts are shaded (**Fig. 36.1**).

Kernahan's Stripped "Y" Classification

- Block 1 and 4—Lip
- Block 2 and 5—Alveolus
- Block 3 and 6—Hard palate anterior to incisive foramen
- Block 7 and 8—Hard palate posterior to the incisive foramen
- Block 9—Soft palate.

The boxes are shaded where the cleft has occurred (**Fig. 36.2**).

Millard's Modification of Stripped "Y"

LAHSHAL Classification of Lip

- L: Lip
- A: Alveolus
- H: Hard palate
- S: Soft palate
- H: Hard palate
- A: Alveolus

This classification was proposed by Kriens. Lashal is a paraphase of the anatomic areas affected by the cleft. The clefts of lip, alveolus and hard palate can be bilateral while clefts of soft palate is unilateral (**Fig. 36.3**).

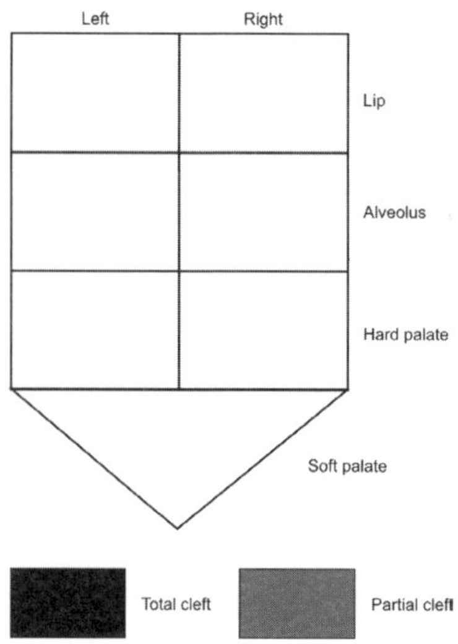

Fig. 36.1: Schuchardt and Pfeiffer's classification

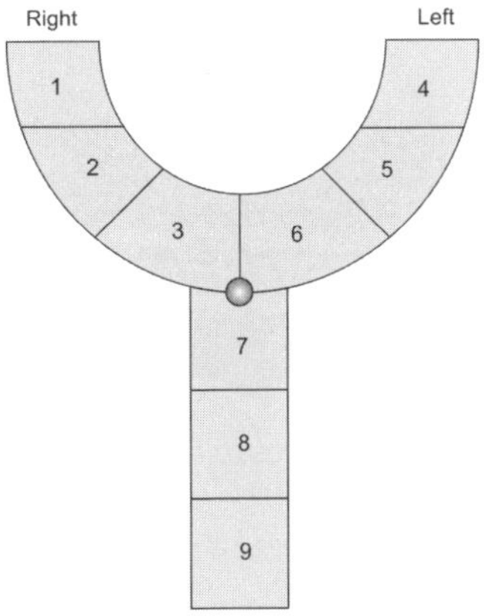

Fig. 36.2: Kernahan's stripped "Y" classification

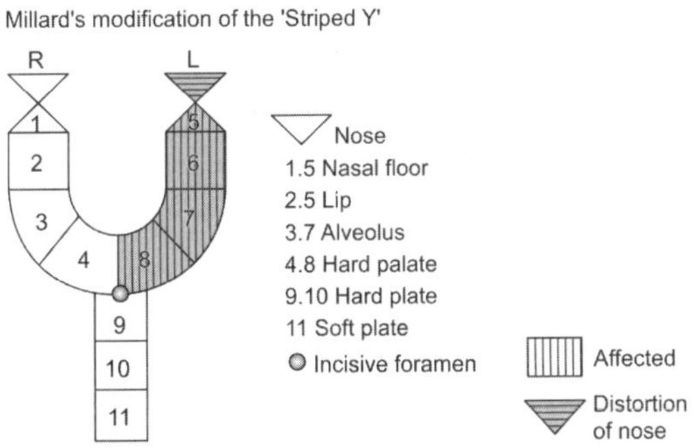

Fig. 36.3: Millard's modification of stripped "Y"

For example, L_ _S_ _ _: This denotes involvement of right lip and soft palate.
_A _ S_ A L: This denotes bilateral involvement of alveolus while unilateral left lip and soft palate involvement.

Question 2

What are the problems associated with cleft lip and palate?

Answer

Cleft lip and palate affects the growth of the face in all the three dimensions and also on the contiguous structures and functions.

The problems associated with clefts are:

- Psychosocial
- Airway and feeding
- Hearing
- Effects on associated facial structures
- Functional.

Psychosocial

- **Parental attitudes**: Birth of cleft child places the parents under stress of being unable to carry out the usual social rituals associated with the birth of a new baby
- **Intelligence**: Mean intelligence quotient (IQ) tend to be somewhat lower than the non-cleft population.

Airway and Feeding

- **Airway**: Clefts if associated with Pierre Robin syndrome can cause airway and breathing problems
- **Feeding**: Nasal regurgitation is the most common problem associated with clefts. Despite problems in maintaining suckling pressures, swallowing mechanisms are normal.

Hearing

Many studies have reported that the cleft palate patients suffer from conductive hearing loss and associated middle ear disease.

Associated Facial Structures

Nose

- In patients with clefts of lip and palate, asymmetries of the nostrils are almost always present
- In patients with unilateral clefts, the size of the nasal cavity is narrower on the affected side
- This impairs nasal respiration and also influences nasal resonance causing hyponasality.

Upper Lip

Short upper lip, impaired motility and abnormal lip function.

Upper Jaw

Cleft in upper jaw can affect the:

- Dentition
- Impaired growth of midface
- Oro-nasal fistulas.

Hard Palate

- Hard palate separates the oral and nasal cavity
- Clefts of the palate affects speech by preventing the building up of adequate intra-oral air pressure necessary for articulation of the high pressure consonants.

Speech

- During swallowing, speech and other activities like whistling, the oropharynx must be separated from the nasopharynx
- This is done by the velopharyngeal muscles
- Its main component is the elevation of the soft palate to meet the posterior pharyngeal wall
- In cleft patients, the development of speech and language may be impaired because of this defect and is termed as velopharyngeal incompetence.

Question 3

Describe the management of cleft lip and palate?

Answer

The clinical care of the child with a cleft lip/palate require a team of specialists who will coordinate their diagnosis and treatment.

The specialists involved include:
- Obstetrics
- Paediatrics
- Plastic surgery
- Dentistry
- Orthodontics
- Geneticist
- Social worker
- Otorhinolaryngology (ENT)
- Audiology and speech therapist.

General Management Overview

It is proposed by Centre for Craniofacial Anomalies, University of California, San Francisco.
- **Immediately after birth**: Paediatric consultation, evaluation by geneticist
- **Within first few week**: Team evaluation
- **10–12 weeks**: Surgical repair of cleft lip
- **Before 1 year**: Surgical repair of cleft palate
- **3 months after palate repair**: Team evaluation, speech and language assessment
- **Between 2 years and 5 years**: Medical and behavioural intervention, if needed
- **At 5–6 years**: Lip and nose revision, if necessary
- **At 7 years**: Start orthopaedic/orthodontics (phase I)
- **Between 9 years and 11 years**: Bone grafting of alveolar bony defects
- **At 12 years or later**: Phase II orthodontics
- **At the end of orthodontic treatment**: Replacement of missing teeth
- **When most growth is completed**: Orthognathic surgical procedures.

Orthodontic treatment is performed at different stages of development:
- Neonatal maxillary orthopaedics as an infant
- Orthodontic-orthopaedics in deciduous dentition
- Orthodontics in the mixed dentition
- Orthodontics alone or in conjunction with maxillofacial surgery (with or without distraction osteogenesis) in the permanent dentition
- Pre-surgical obturator plates, moulding plates, and feeding plates (**Figs. 36.4 and 36.5**).

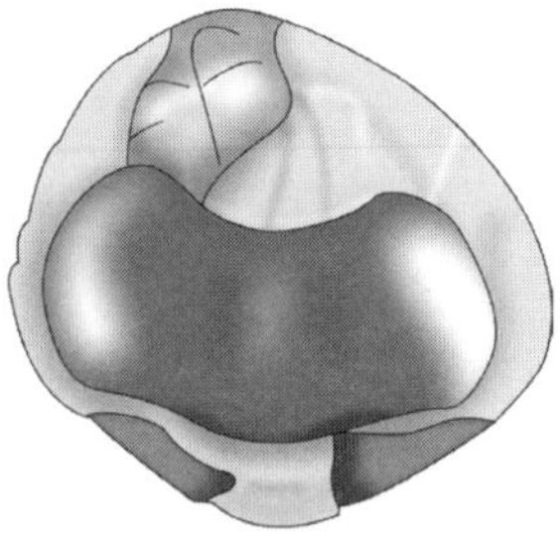

Fig. 36.4: Feeding plates to assist in early feeding

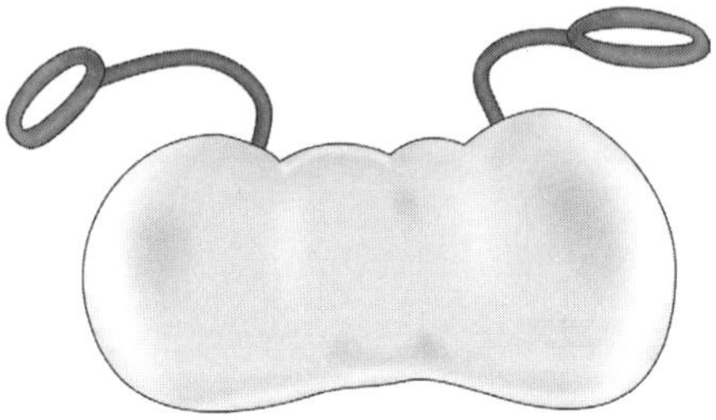

Fig. 36.5: Obturator plate

Surgical Management

- Surgical correction of cleft lip and palate
- Alveolar bone grafting
- Oronasal fistulas.

Surgical Correction of Lip

It is technically possible to correct the lip during the first day or two.

The criteria followed are the "Rule of 10" for the patient to be eligible for surgery:
- 10 weeks of age
- 10 pounds of weight (4.5 Kg)
- 10 g/dL of haemoglobin
- 10,000 WBC count.

Surgical Techniques for Lip

- The Rose and Thomson operation
- Triangular flap operation
- The rotation advancement operation by Millard
- The Skoog technique.

Surgical Correction of Cleft Palate

- The aim in cleft palate surgery is to restore a functioning, anatomical structure that will improve speech, oronasal physiology and aesthetics
- There is no consensus as to the timing of palatal surgeries
- But most surgeons do it during 18–24 month of age, which is prior to the development of speech habits.

Surgical Techniques for Cleft Palate

- The Langenbeck operation
- The three flap Wardill-Kilner pushback operation
- The four flap modification of Wardill-Kilner.

Alveolar Bone Grafting

Goals of alveolar bone grafting:

- Closing of oronasal fistulae
- Continuity between cleft segments
- Proper alveolar contour
- Supporting tooth eruption and orthodontic tooth movement
- Periodontal health of the teeth.

Orthodontic Treatment in Mixed Dentition

- A tentative decision on extraction of supernumerary teeth and over-retained teeth
- Correction of crossbites by jack screw, rapid maxillary expansion (RME), quad helix, NiTi expanders
- Maintain space for proper eruption of teeth
- Expand the collapsed segment to improve surgical access to the graft site
- Traumatic occlusion is eliminated in preparation of alveolar graft (by aligning the offending tooth)
- Correction of jaw relationship by face mask therapy.

Orthodontic Treatment in Permanent Dentition

The objectives of an orthodontic treatment should be "to produce optimum alignment and relationship of the dental arches for speech, mastication, oral health and function.

Treatment procedures include:

- Expansion of maxilla
- Extraction of hopeless teeth
- Orthodontic alignment
- If skeletal disparity is severe, orthognathic surgery at a later date.
- Clinical Feature of this Stage Medial displacement of the maxillary segment causing buccal crossbite
- Relative maxillary retrognathism leading to reversed incisal overjet
- Deficiency of vertical growth of the upper jaw leads to reduced facial height
- Rotation, malposition and hypodontia of teeth
- Supernumerary teeth
- Accentuated curve of spee in maxilla
- Collapsed arch forms
- Poor oral hygiene and caries

Alignment of Incisor Teeth

Incisors are usually rotated and in crossbite. Corrected by means of fixed orthodontic appliance.

Correction of Lateral Dimension

By expansion appliance. Patients with cleft lip and palate have Class III malocclusion because of maxillary deficiency [anteroposterior (AP) and vertical], coupled with mandibular overclosure. In such cases, use of Class III elastics after levelling and aligning results in upper molar extrusion and favourable downward and backward rotation of mandible.

Orthognathic Surgery Combined with Orthodontics

Due to severe skeletal discrepancy, there is deterioration of aesthetics and occlusion, psychological implications leading to low self-esteem, defective speech, and oronasal fistulas. Such cases require a combined orthodontic and orthognathic approach.

To correct the transverse problem multiple segment Le Fort I osteotomies may be required. For a bilateral cleft lip and cleft palate three-piece maxillary surgery (allows rotation of segments also) is required while for unilateral cleft lip and cleft palate a two piece is sufficient.

Decompensation

- Usually requires 12 months
- Multiple segment maxillary osteotomies require segmental treatment
- The bracket positions are altered for teeth adjacent to the osteotomy site
- Dental compensations in the lower arch also should be addressed, i.e., alleviation of crowding and proclination
- Gaps present in the arches due to the missing teeth must be closed
- In cases with an overjet of more than 8 mm, mandibular surgery [bilateral sagittal split osteotomy (BSSO)] also must be considered

Post-surgical orthodontics:

- Involves detailing of occlusion, closure of residual spaces and maintenance of transverse dimension (overlay arches)
- It lasts for 4-6 months

Retention: After removal of appliance, retainers should be placed immediately.

CHAPTER 37 Surgical Orthodontics

LONG ESSAYS

Question 1

Explain different surgical procedures during orthodontic treatment?

Answer

Surgical procedures in orthodontics can be broadly classified into:

Minor Surgeries

- Extractions
  - Therapeutic extractions
  - Serial Extractions
  - Extraction of grossly carious tooth
  - Extractions of malformed teeth
  - Extractions of supernumerary teeth
  - Extraction of unfavourably impacted teeth.
- Surgical uncovering of impacted/submerged teeth
- Frenectomy
- Pericision
- Corticotomy.

Major Surgeries

- Orthognathic surgeries
- Cosmetic surgeries
- Surgeries in cleft lip and palate patients
- SARPE (Surgically Assissted Rapid Palatal Expansion).

Extractions

Therapeutic Extractions

- Therapeutic extractions are commonly done during fixed orthodontic treatment to gain space
- They are generally done in cases of arch length–tooth material discrepancy cases like crowding and proclination
- These extraction should be atraumatic with special emphasis on the preservation of integrity of buccal and lingual cortical plates
- Pre-operative radiographs act as a valuable aid in planning and execution of the procedure.

Serial Extraction

- Serial extraction is a commom procedure employed during mixed dentition stage to intercept potential malocclusion
- Clinician should carefully plan the treatment before carrying out serial extraction procedure.

Extraction of Grossly Carious Tooth/Supernumerary/Unfavourly Impacted/Ankylosed Tooth

- These extractions are carried out in order to remove the cause of malocclusion and to gain space
- Extraction of grossly carious tooth is preferred over a healthy tooth for gaining space
- During removal of these teeth, care should be taken to prevent any damage to adjacent tooth/root or any other neighbouring structures.

Surgical Uncovering of Impacted Tooth

- Impacted tooth are a common cause of malocclusion as they lead to arch length- tooth material discrepancies
- Most common impacted tooth encountered during fixed orthodontic treatment is maxillary permanent canine
- These canine if favourably placed can be guided into their anatomic position with the help of fixed orthodontic appliance
- Steps undertaken to manage impacted canine are:
  - **Location of tooth**: the exact location of the impacted tooth is determined i.e., buccal or lingual placement
    - Upon Clinical examination a bulge may be seen on the palatal or buccal side in the mucosa
    - Radiographically Clark's tube shift technique is used to locate the exact positioning of tooth.

- **Evaluation of favourability**: The orientation of the impacted tooth is evaluated and seen whether the tooth can be successfully brought into its anatomic position orthodontically without damaging adjacent tooth and other structures.
- **Evaluation of space**: the treatment is planned according to the space requirement for bringing the tooth into the dental arch.
  - Adequate space is created prior to disimpaction for bringing the tooth into the arch.
- **Surgical exposure**: the flap is raised and the bone is removed to gain access to the crown of the impacted canine.
  - The bone should be removed upto the maximum height of the contour.
- **Fixing orthodontic attachment**: Post crown exposure, an orthodontic attachement like button, bracket, eyelet, etc are bonded onto the surface of the crown.
  - Ligature wire is wound over the attachment which is exposed outside after flap closure on which the traction force is applied.
- **Flap closure**: Post the bonding of attachment the gingival flap is closed.
  - Care should be taken to keep the ligature wire exposed while closing the flap.

Frenectomy

- Frenectomy is a surgical procedure involving excision of the frenum and the deeply embedded fibrous tissue.
- It is most commonly done in cases of Midline Diastema.

Timing of the procedure: Some authors advise frenectomy prior to fixed orthodontic treatment while some authors prescribe is post orthodontic treatment as that reduces chances of scar tissue formation.

Corticotomy

- Corticotomy is a surgical procedure involving giving shallow vertical cuts in the labial and lingual cortical plates to hasten fixed orthodontic treatment.
- The philosophy behind this procedure is "due to trauma induced by surgical cuts, inflammation occurs which brings about influx of chemical mediators. This influx of chemical mediators bring out rapid orthodontic tooth movement."

Pericison

- Also called as circumferential supra- crestal fibrotomy
- This procedure is carried out to prevent relapse due to uncoiling of the stretched trans- septal and alveolar crestal group of fibres
- This is indicated in cases where large derotation movements have been carried out
- This involves surgical sectioning of the above mentioned gingival fibres by a sharp scalpel passed through gingival sulcus around the tooth to a depth of 2 mm apical to alveolar crest.

Orthognathic Surgeries

- The term orthognathic orginates from the greek words 'ortho' meaning straight and gnathos meaning jaw
- These surgeries are procedure by which dentofacial deformities and malocclusions are corrected with both orthodontic alongwith the surgical modification of the facial morphology and various soft tissue structures
- Once growth has ceased, surgery becomes the only means of correcting a severe jaw discrepancy.

Indications

- Skeletal open bite
- Skeletal deep bite
- Skeletal class-II
  - Prognathic maxilla, normal mandible.
  - Normal maxilla, retrognathic mandible
  - Prognathic maxilla, retrognathic mandible.
- Skeletal Class III
  - Normal maxilla, Prognathic mandible
  - Retrognathic maxilla, normal mandible
  - Retrognathic maxilla, Prognathic mandible.
- Vertical maxillary excess
- Facial asymmetry
- Deficient chin/prominent chin
- Decreased or increased anterior facial height
- Cleft lip and palate
- Constricted maxilla/mandible.

Diagnosis and Treatment Planning

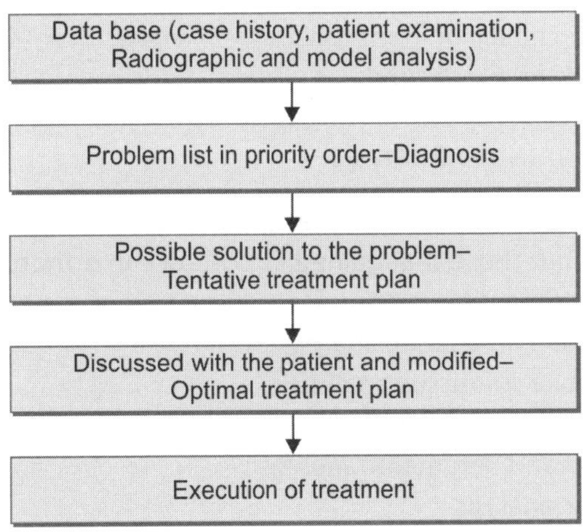

Execution of Treatment

Pre Operative Evaluation

- Medical history
  - Patient's medical information must aim to obtain information regarding medical conditions like history of medication, allergies to drug, bleeding disorder, Respiratory problem, cardiac problem, asthma, diabetics, anemia, rheumatic fever etc that may complicate correction of a skeletal deformities
  - Additional lab investigations and consultation with the patients physician should be completed whenever compromised medical situation exist.
- Socio psychological evaluation
  - Psychologic makeup of the patient is important because, despite an objectively favorable treatment result, certain patients will express dissatisfaction with their results due to unrealistic patient expectations regarding the result of the treatment
  - Unrealistic expectations are most likely to occur in two types of patients, patients with acquired deformities and those with external motivations
  - Treatment of such patients must be executed only after careful consideration and psychologic consultation
  - Frequently it is best not to treat the patients since they are generally unhappy with the results achieved
  - These kind of patients can be distinguished by a deliberate social psychologic evaluation.

Radiographic Examination

- Basic radiographs required will include Lateral cephalogram, orthopantomogram specialized views like IOPA, occlusal view
- PA cehalogram in the case of facial asymmetry
- Trans cranial or trans pharyngeal views for TMJ are requested if indicated.

Cephalomatric Analysis

Various cephalometic analyses are put forward by various authors but those that gained importance in orthognathic surgery are:

- Burstone hard tissue analysis
- Burstone soft tissue analysis
- Grummon's analysis
- Arnett and Bergmann analysis
- Tomac analysis.

Pre-Surgical Orthodontics

Selection of the Appliance

- Stability
- Esthetics
- Slot Size
- Bonding vs Banding

Stability

- Stabilize the teeth against stresses encountered at surgery and during inter maxillary fixation (IMF)
- Pre-adjusted edgewise appliance is preferred.

Esthetics

- Lingual appliance has to be removed and labial appliance fixed just before the surgery and continued till end of treatment
- Metal brackets are preferred over ceramic brackets in surgical cases.

Slot Size

- In 0.018 slot, the surgery should be done on 0.017 x 0.025" stainless steel wire
- In 0.022 slot, the surgery should be done on 0.021 x 0.025" stainless steel wire.

Bonding vs Banding

- Anteriors should be bonded while posteriors banded
  - 2nd molars should be banded
- Procedures that need to be done before surgery include:
  - Alignment of teeth
  - Leveling – by intrusion
  - Arch compatibility.
- Procedures that can be done before and/or after surgery:
  - Post crossbite correction
  - Leveling by extrusion.
- Procedures necessary after surgery:
  - Settling and leveling by extrusion
  - Root paralleling at osteotomy sites
  - Detailed tooth positioning.

Alignment of the Arch

- This stage is similar to any orthodontic patient
- Principles of alignment remain the same
- Initial tipping of the teeth into their correct position, using undersized, round and resilient wires
- This permits free sliding, freedom to tip mesio distally and labio lingually, and light continuous forces, with longer range of action.

Leveling of the Arch

- When the mandible is moved forward or back surgically, the final vertical height of the face is determined by the position of the lower incisors
- If it is desired to increase the face height, the lower incisors should not be intruded, and leveling of the arch should be done post-surgically, by extrusion
- In patients with normal or excessive face height, the lower incisors must be intruded pre-surgically
- If segmental procedures are to be done, the teeth should be leveled within the segments, and the final leveling among the segments will be done post-surgically
- Mechanics to be employed for leveling:
  - Intrusion : Segmented mechanics
  - Extrusion : Continuous wire mechanics.

Antero-posterior Positioning of the Incisors

- Antero-posterior postion of the teeth affect the amount the jaws can be moved sagitally
- In any malocclusion, some amount of dental compensation occurs to partially correct the malocclusion
- During presurgical orthodontic phase, dental compensations must be removed
- Hence tooth movement is often in the direction opposite to what they would be moved for camouflage treatment
- This has an effect to seemingly worsening the malocclusion, either increasing the overjet, or creating a reverse jet
- For the same reason extraction patterns used in presurgical orthodontics are opposite to those used for camouflage treatment.

Arch Compatibility

- The final step is to assure that the maxillary and mandibular archforms are compatible to each other, so that the teeth fit into each other after surgery
- This includes shape and width
- Usually, one of the arches has a U shape and the other has a V shape
- The narrower regions need to be expanded
- This can be done by using co-ordinated arch wires from the beginning, and slowly proceeding to heavier archwires
- Sometimes exaggerated arch wire forms may be needed to correct the archform
- After archform correction, the roots will have to be torqued, so as to prevent cuspal interferences
- At the end of the pre-surgical phase, the patient should be in a full sized rectangular steel wire which will help stabilize the teeth during surgery.

Stabilization of the Arches during Surgery

As discussed earlier, the stabilizing archwire should have the following characteristics:

- Full dimension, filling the slot—17 × 25 SS for 18 slot, and 21 × 25 SS or TMA for 22 slot. A 19 × 25 wire in a 0.022 slot is acceptable, but it is prefered to place at least a 21 × 25 TMA wire
- Attachments for IMF—the surgeon will require to at least tie the arches together into the splint towards the end of the surgery. Thus hooks are soldered on arch wire
- The stabilizing wire must be passive—so that no tooth movement occurs after model surgery.

Final Surgical Planning and Preparation

After the patient is ready for surgery the following set of records are taken, usually about 2 weeks before surgery, after the final rectangular wires have been in place for 3 weeks or more so that they are passive:

- OPG
- Lat. Ceph
- Casts
  - Photos—intra and extra-oral
  - PA ceph—if there is facial asymmetry
  - IOPAs and occlusal view if needed
  - Face bow transfer onto an articulator if needed.
- OPG is used to verify that root positions will not interfere in osteotomy cuts. The roots should be slightly divergent or parallel, but not converging
- The Ceph. is to be used for cephalometric predictions, to guide the model surgery
- Casts are to be used for the model surgery itself.

Model Surgery

- Soon after the completion of pre-surgical orthodontic treatment, mock surgery is performed on the upper and lower models
- Upper and lower models are recorded
- Facebow transfer is done
- Models are mounted on the articulator
- Cut the model exactly similar to surgery
- Avoid apices or root surfaces of teeth during cutting
- Detect the problem areas-proximity of roots, bony interferences, etc.
- Observe and note the movement of dento-osseous segments-rotations and expansion
- Consider best aesthetics, functional requirement, axial inclination, vertical relationship, and maximum interdigitation

- Consider difference in movements of bony segments of one side to the other side as in the case of facial asymmetry cases in superior positioning of maxilla
- With the final positioning achieved, occlusal splints are fabricated.

Orthognathic Surgery

- Treatment of skeletal Class II malocclusion **(Fig. 37.1)**
- Treatment of maxillary protrusion **(Fig. 37.2)**
- Treatment of Class III skeletal pattern due to mandibular prognathism **(Fig. 37.3)**
- Treatment of Class III skeletal pattern due to maxillary retursion **(Fig. 37.4)**
- Treatment of Class III skeletal pattern due to mandibular protrusion and maxillary retrusion **(Fig. 37.5)**

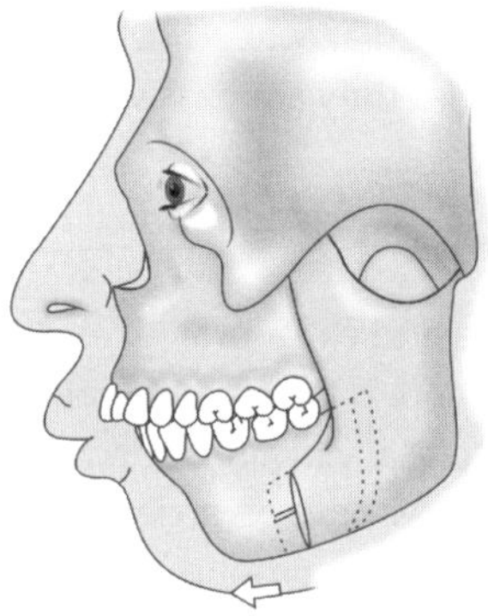

Fig. 37.1: Skeletal Class II malocclusion due to mandibular retrognathism treated by sagittal split osteotomy with mandibular advancement

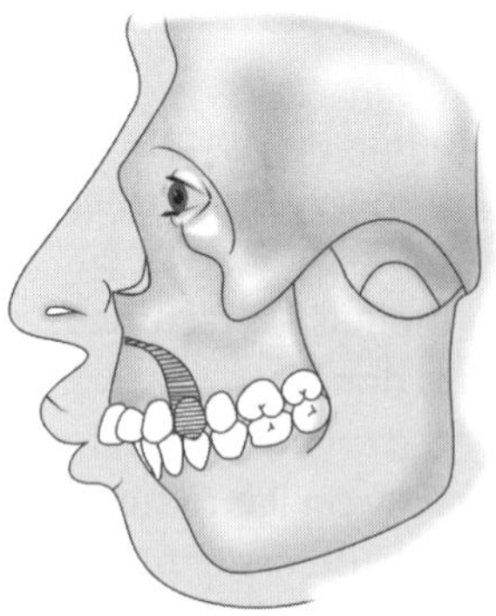

Fig. 37.2: Maxillary protrusion treated by maxillary segmental (anterior) set back

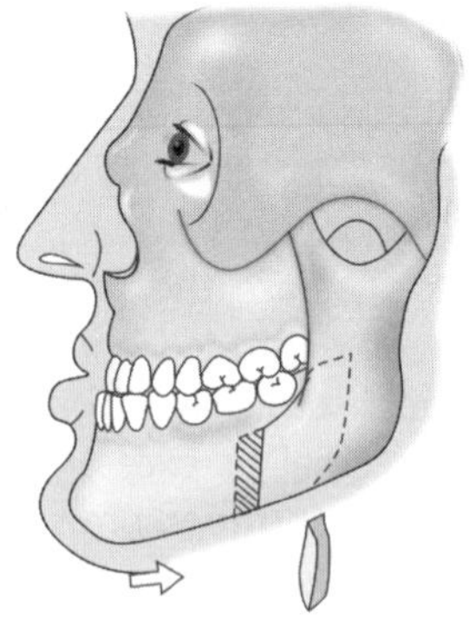

Fig. 37.3: Class III skeletal pattern due to mandibular prognathism treated by sagittal split osteotomy with mandibular set back

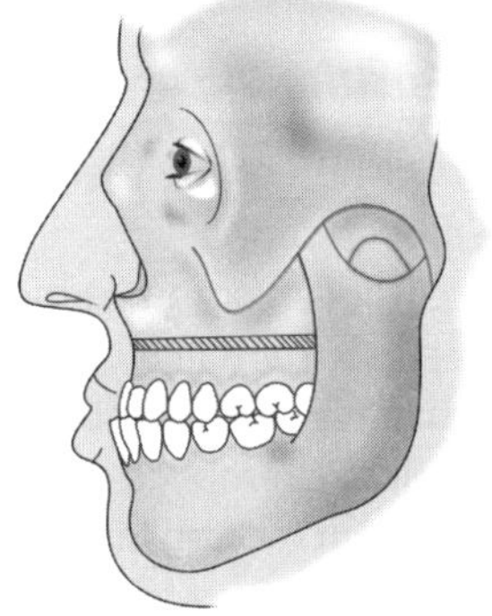

Fig. 37.4: Class III skeletal pattern due to maxillary retrusion of hypoplasia treated by le Fort I osteotomy with maxillary advancement

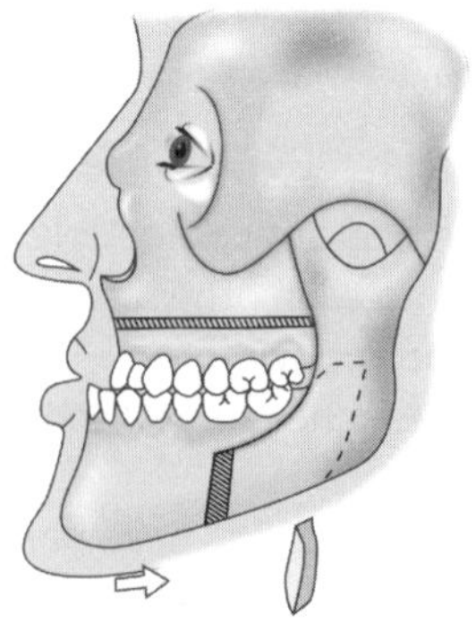

Fig. 37.5: Class III skeletal pattern due to maxillary retrusion or hypoplasia and mandibular prognathism treated by le Fort I osteotomy with maxillary advancement and sagittal split osteotomy with mandibular set back

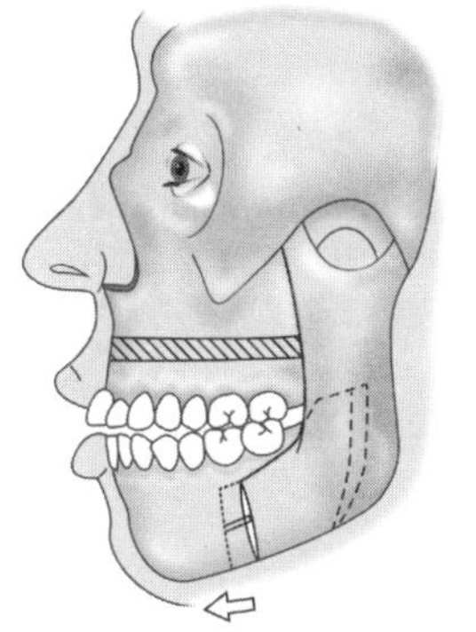

Fig. 37.6: Skeletal open bites along with Class II skeletal pattern require le Fort 1 with maxillary impaction with sagittal split osteotomy for mandibular advancement

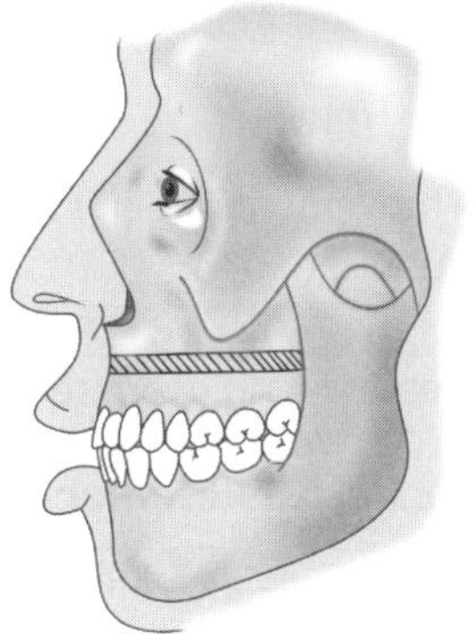

Fig. 37.7: Long face is usually associated with vertical maxillary excess. They are treated by le Fort 1 with maxillary impaction

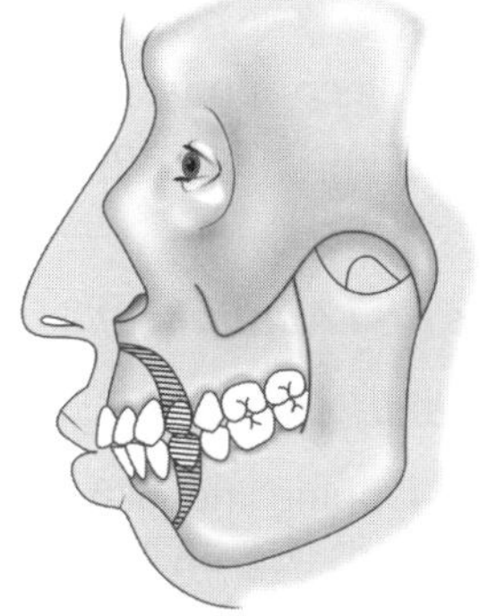

Fig. 37.8: Bimaxillary protrusion require maxillary and mandibular segmental osteotomy for set back of anterior maxilla and mandible

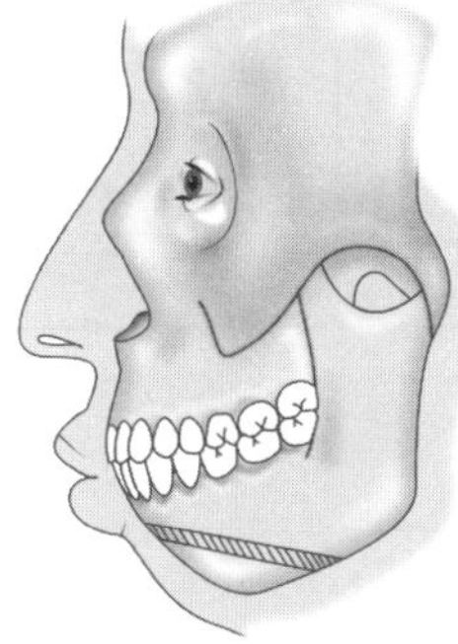

Fig. 37.9: Horizontal chin deficiency often require genioplasty.

- Treatment of skeletal open bite along with Class II skeletal pattern **(Fig. 37.6)**
- Treatment of long face associated with vertical maxillary excess **(Fig. 37.7)**
- Treatment of bimaxillary protrusion **(Fig. 37.8)**
- Treatment of horizontal chin deficiency **(Fig. 37.9)**

Post Surgical Orthodontics

- The first step is to remove the splint and the stabilizing arch wires
- Any repairs to the appliance can then be made
- Then the working orthodontic wires can be placed
- The splint and stabilizing wires must be removed at the same time
- The purpose of the stabilizing archwire is to prevent the movement of teeth.
- Torque control of anterior teeth is achieved
- Vertical elastics are given (green or blue).

Elastics serve 2 purposes:

1. The help in settling of the teeth, bringing them into a good, solid occlusion
2. Override the patient's proprioceptive drive towards positioning the mandible in maximum intercuspation.

Goals of post surgical orthodontics can be summed up as follows:

- Establishment of final occlusion, including final alignment, interdigitation, torque, artistic positioning
- Establishment of correct root parallelism, especially at osteotomy sites, where roots of adjacent teeth may have been left divergent.

CHAPTER 38 Retention and Relapse

LONG ESSAYS

Question 1

What are different types of retainers?

Answer

Retainers are classified into:

- Removable retainers
- Fixed retainers
- Aesthetic retainers.

Removable Retainers

The ideal removable retainers should be:

- Able to allow functional occlusion
- Sturdy enough to withstand long-term use
- Convenient for the orthodontist to provide and maintain
- Patient friendly, in comfort and routine wear.

Hawley Retainers

Hawley retainer is the most commonly used retainer, designed in 1920.

Standard Appliance

- Consists of labial bow with loops from canine to canine
- Adams clasps on molars
- Acrylic palatal coverage in upper arch.

Modifications of Hawley's Appliance

Many modifications were performed for various purposes:

- Hawleys with bite plate (to control bite depth)
- Hawleys with labial bow soldered to clasps on molars (to prevent reopening of extraction space)
- Hawleys with labial bow wrap around entire arch with C clasps on second molars (to prevent reopening of extraction space).

Removable Wrap Around Retainer

This is the second most commonly used removable retainer.

Disadvantages Over Hawley's

- Individual tooth movements are not allowed to stimulate periodontal reorganisation
- Less comfortable
- Not effective in maintaining overbite correction.

Removable Plastic Herbst Retainer

It has property of both single arch and dual arch retainers.

Components

Upper and lower plastic splints connected on each side by the telescoping Herbst mechanism. It can also be used as:

- Finishing appliance
- Re-treatment appliance
- Post-surgical retainer
- Aid for obstructive sleep apnoea
- Anterior repositioning splint for temporomandibular joint (TMJ) disorders.

Crozat Appliance (4-4 Appliance)

Components of Labial Bow

- Recurved double-lapping lingual finger springs
- Cribs on first bicuspids **(Fig. 38.1)**.

Advantages

- Firm retention, flexibility, good labio-lingual control
- Aesthetics and good oral hygiene.

Disadvantages

Expensive, require quality laboratory, breakable.

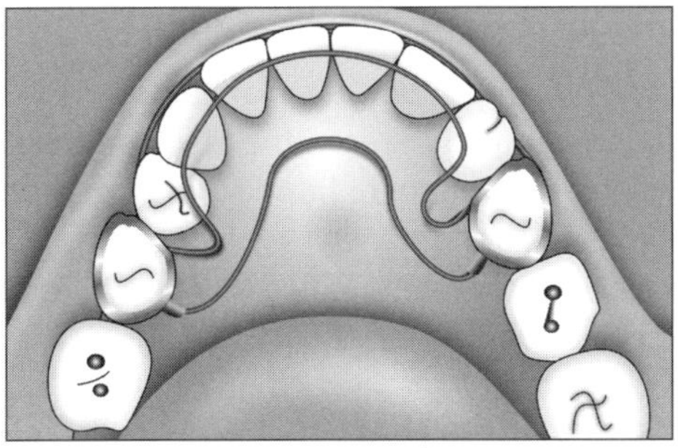

Fig. 38.1: Crozat Appliance

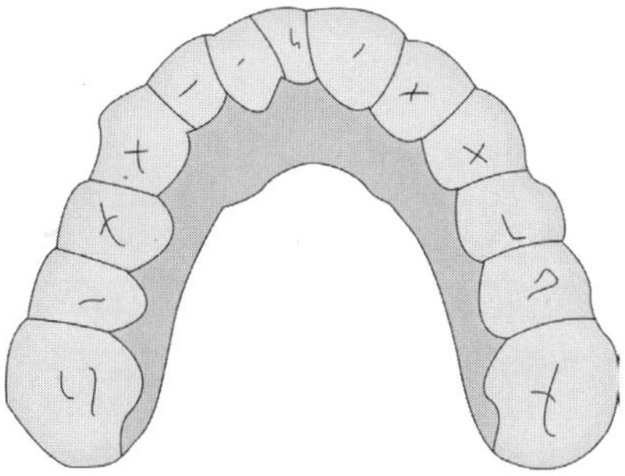

Fig. 38.2: Tooth positioners

Tooth Positioners as Retainers

- Tooth positioners can be used as removable retainers
- They should be worn at least 4 hours day time and full night time wear (**Fig. 38.2**).

Problems

- Difficulty in wearing the appliance due to its bulkiness
- Difficulty in retaining incisor irregularities and rotations and overbite corrections due to poor patient cooperation.

Advantages

It can be effective in maintaining occlusal relationships and intra-arch tooth positions.

Fabrication

- It is necessary to separate the teeth by 2–4 mm.
- Articulator mounting to record patient's hinge axis
- Positioner made with incorrect hinge axis leads to separation of posterior teeth when incisors are in contact.

Fixed Retainers (Bonded)

The various forms of fixed bonded retainers allow more differential retention than before.

Advantages of Bonded Retainers

- Completely invisible from front
- Reduced risk of caries under loose bands
- Reduced need for long-term patient cooperation
- Prolonged semi-permanent and even permanent retention when conventional retainers do not provide the same degree of stability.

Various types of retainers and splints are available. The most commonly used bonded retainers are:

- Mandibular canine-to-canine (3-3) retainers
- Flexible spiral wire retainers.

Mandibular Canine-to-Canine Retainers

In differential philosophy the purpose of a bonded 3-3 retainer is:

- To prevent incisor re-crowding
- To achieve lower incisor position in space
- To keep the rotation centre in incisor area when mandibular anterior growth rotation tendency is present.

These are classified into three groups:

1. First generation retainers
2. Second generation retainers
3. Third generation retainers.

First Generation Canine-to-Canine Retainers

The retainer is made of plain 0.032–0.036" Blue Elgiloy wire with loop at each terminal end adapted to lingual surface of anterior teeth and bonded to canines (**Fig. 38.3**).

Second Generation Canine-to-Canine Retainers

The plain Elgiloy was replaced with twisted three stranded 0.032 inch wire (**Fig. 38.4**).

Difficulties encountered were:

- Distortion due to lack of rigidity
- Difficult to bend to optimal fit.

Third Generation Canine-to-Canine Retainers

It is made of round 0.032 inch stainless steel wire or 0.030 inch gold coated wire with ends sandblasted for mechanical retention (**Fig. 38.5**).

Flexible Spiral Wire Retainers

Indications

- Prevention of space reopening
  - Median diastemas
  - Spaced anterior teeth

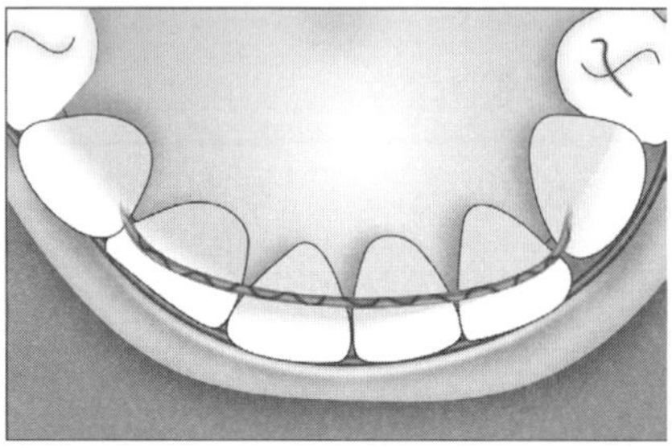

Fig. 38.3: First generation 3-3 retainers

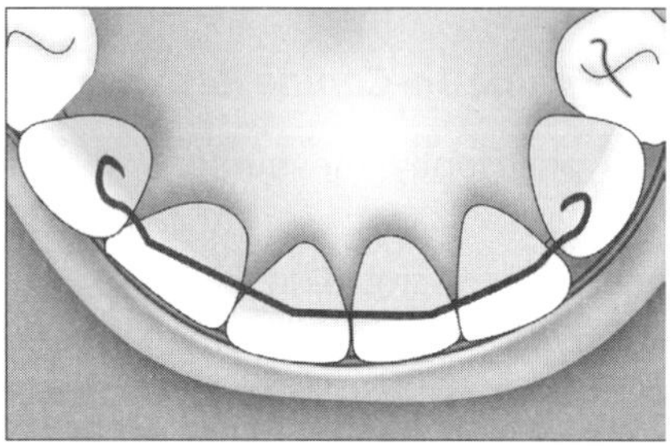

Fig. 38.4: Second generation 3-3 retainers

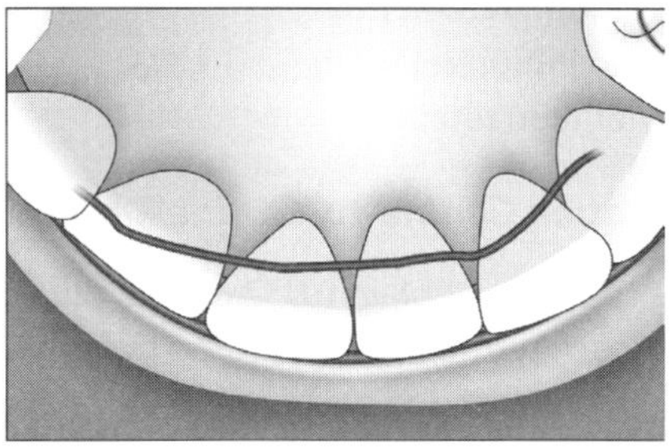

Fig. 38.5: Third generation 3-3 retainers

  - Adult periodontal conditions with potential for post-orthodontic tooth migration
  - Mandibular incisor extractions.
- Holding the individual teeth
  - Severely rotated maxillary incisors
  - Palatally impacted canines.

Advantages

- They may allow safe retention of treatment results when proper retention is difficult or even impossible with traditional retainers
- They allow slight movement of all bonded teeth and segment of teeth
- They are invisible
- They are neat and clean
- They can be placed without occlusal interference
- They can be used alone or in combination with removable retainers.

Disadvantages

- Good oral hygiene should be maintained
- Daily flossing should be recommended gingival to the wire
- Undesirable movement of bonded teeth may occur if the wire is too thin or not passive while bonding
- Not indicated in deep bite cases where wire cannot be placed out of occlusion.

Aesthetic Retainers (Essix)

These are thermoplastic co-polyester vacuum formed retainers.

Advantages

- Aesthetic and absolute stability of anterior teeth
- Less expensive, good durability, easy oral hygiene maintenance
- Less bulk and thickness (0.015 inch).

Drawbacks

- Cannot be used for expanded arches
- Prolonged use can cause anterior open bite
- Less durable when compared to Hawley retainer.

Surgical Procedures Aiding in Retention

Most common surgical procedures employed to aid in retention are:

- Frenectomy procedure (to remove abnormal frenum preventing diastema closure)
- Circumferential supracrestal fiberotomy (to prevent rotational relapse).

Question 2

What are the Raleigh Williams keys to eliminate lower anterior teeth retention?

Answer

Raleigh Williams put forward six keys to eliminate need for lower retention in anterior teeth and achieve lower arch stability post-orthodontic treatment.

1. The incisal edge of lower incisor should be placed on the patient Pt. A to Pogonion (AP) line or 1 mm in front of it **(Fig. 38.6)**. This creates optimum balance of soft tissue in lower third of face.
2. The lower incisor apices should be spread distally to the crowns more than is generally considered appropriate, and the apices of the lower lateral incisors must be spread more than those of the central incisors **(Fig. 38.7)**.

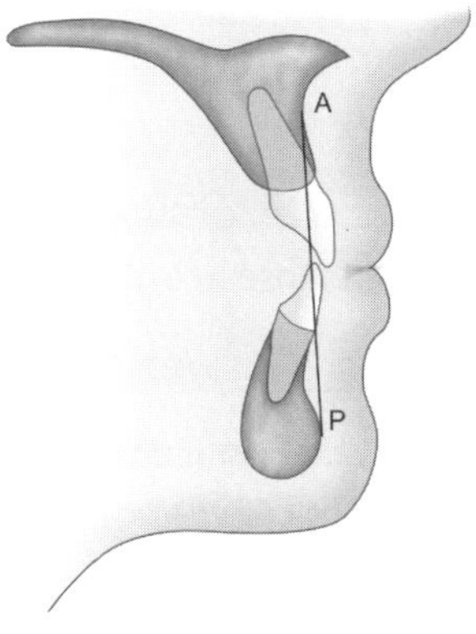

Fig. 38.6: Antero-posterior line in lower incisor

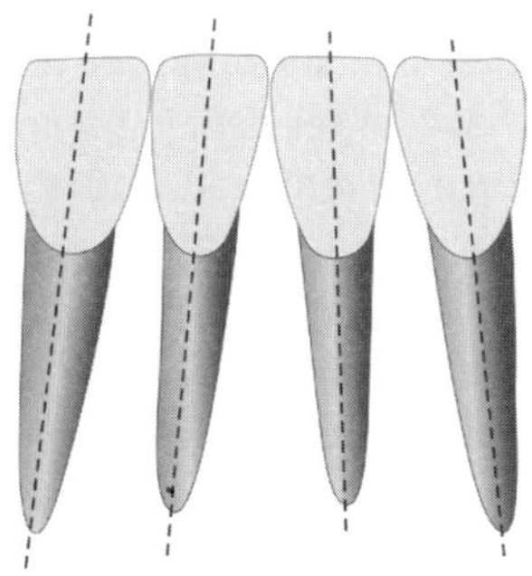

Fig. 38.7: Lower incisor apices spread distally

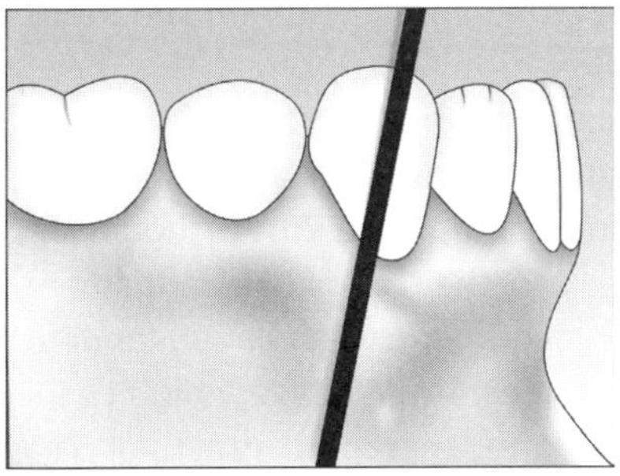

Fig. 38.8: Apex of the lower cuspid

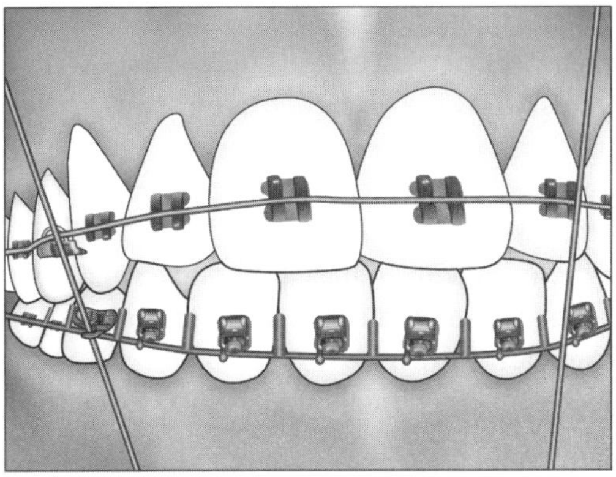

Fig. 38.9: The lower cuspid root apex

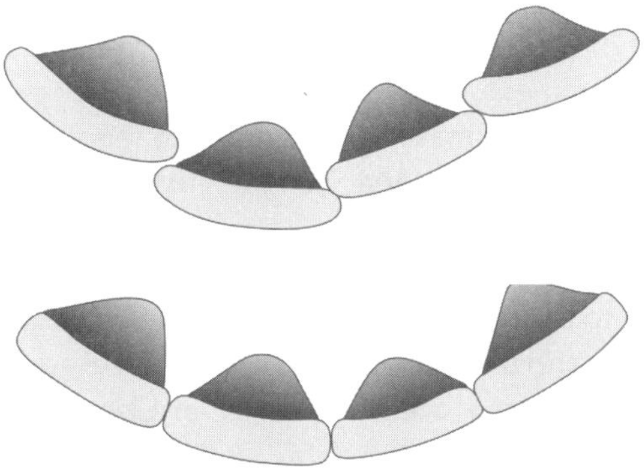

Fig. 38.10: Sixth key: slenderise the lower incisors to resolve minor crowding

3. **Third key**: The apex of the lower cuspid should be positioned distal to the crown **(Fig. 38.8)**. The occlusal plane should be used as a positioning guide.
4. **Fourth key**: All four lower incisor apices must be in the same labio-lingual plane **(Fig. 38.9)**
5. **Fifth key**: The lower cuspid root apex must be positioned slightly buccal to the crown apex
6. **Sixth key**: The lower incisors should be slenderised as needed after treatment **(Fig. 38.10)**.

SHORT ESSAYS

Question 1

What are the different kinds of retention protocols?

Answer

There are three kinds of retention:

1. Natural or no retention.
2. Limited or short-term retention.
3. Permanent retention.

Natural or No Retention

Correction of certain malocclusions does not require any retention like:

- Corrected crossbites:
  - Anterior crossbite when adequate overbite has been established
  - Posterior crossbite where axial inclinations of posterior teeth remain reasonable after corrective procedures have been completed.

- Dentitions treated by serial extraction.
- High cuspid eruption cases
  - Occasionally the extraction of one or more teeth (as in subdivision types of malocclusion).
- Corrections achieved by retarding maxillary growth whether skeletal or dental
- Dentitions in which maxillary and mandibular teeth have been separated to allow for eruption of previously blocked out teeth, usually
- Partially impacted mandibular second bicuspids and maxillary canines.

Limited Retention

Most typical orthodontic cases probably fall into this category:

- Class I non-extraction cases characterized by protrusion and spacing of maxillary incisors, they require retention until normal lip and tongue function has been achieved
- Class I and Class II extraction cases probably require that teeth to be held in contact, particularly in maxillary arch until lip and tongue functions can be achieved
- Corrected deep overbites, either in Class I or Class II malocclusions
- Early correction of rotated teeth to their normal position, perhaps before root formation has been completed
- Cases involving ectopic eruption of teeth or the presence of supernumerary teeth
- Class II division 2 type of corrected malocclusion generally require extended periods of retention to allow the adaptation of musculature
- These cases allow for some increase in mandibular inter-canine width, which is maintained out of retention.

Permanent or Semi-permanent Retention

- Cases in which expansion has been choice of treatment (particularly in the mandibular arch) may require permanent retention or semi-permanent retention to maintain normal contact alignment
- Cases of considerable or generalised spacing may require permanent retention after space closure has been completed
- Instances of severe rotations (particularly in adults) and severe labio-lingual malposition sometimes require permanent retention
- Spacing between maxillary central incisors in otherwise normal occlusions sometimes requires permanent retention.

Question 2

Discuss the causes of relapse in orthodontics?

Answer

Relapse is defined as "the loss of any correction achieved by orthodontic treatment".

Causes of Relapse

- **Periodontal ligament traction**: During orthodontic tooth movement, the periodontal principle fibres and the gingival fibres that surround the teeth are stretched. These fibres have a tendency to contract once the orthodontic force is removed and thus, are a potent cause for relapse
  - Studies have shown that the principle fibres reorganise themselves to newer positions in about 25–30 days while supra-alveolar gingival fibres can take almost up to 8–10 months for adapting to newer positions.
- **Relapse due to growth changes**: Patients with skeletal malocclusions like Class II, Class III, deep bite and open bite may show relapse due to the continuation of abnormal growth pattern after orthodontic therapy
- **Bone adaptation**: The bony trabeculae are normally perpendicular to the long axis of the tooth, but during orthodontic therapy, they align themselves parallel to the direction of the host. Post-orthodontic therapy, they revert back to their original arrangement. During this phase of realignment, teeth have a tendency to relapse
- **Muscular forces**: There are very high chances of relapse post-orthodontic therapy, if structural balance between the muscular forces of orofacial apparatus is not achieved Removal of the aetiology of malocclusion is necessary to prevent relapse
- **Role of third molars**: Third molars generally erupt around the age of 21 years. If the patient has completed orthodontic therapy prior to this age, they might develop late anterior crowding due to lack of space availability for the eruption of third molars
- **Role of occlusion**: To prevent relapse, the centric relation and centric occlusion (CR-CO) should coincide or their discrepancy should not be greater than 2 mm.

SHORT NOTES

Question 1

What are theories of retention?

Answer

According to Riedel:

- **Theorem 1**: Teeth that have been moved tend to return to their former positions
- **Theorem 2**: Elimination of the cause of malocclusion will prevent relapse
- **Theorem 3**: Malocclusions should be overcorrected as a safety factor
- **Theorem 4**: Proper occlusion is a potent factor in holding teeth in their corrected positions
- **Theorem 5**: Bone and adjacent tissues must be allowed time to reorganize around newly positioned teeth
- **Theorem 6**: If the lower incisors are placed upright over the basal bone, they are more likely to remain in good alignment
- **Theorem 7**: Corrections carried out during periods of growth are less likely to relapse
- **Theorem 8**: The farther the teeth have been removed, the lesser is the risk of relapse
- **Theorem 9**: Arch form, especially in the mandibular arch cannot be permanently altered by appliance therapy

According to Moyers:

- **Theorem 10**: Many malocclusions require permanent retention.

Question 2

What are the different school of thoughts for basis of retention?

Answer

The different school of thoughts for basis of retention are:

- The Occlusion School 1880 by Kingsley stated that the occlusion of teeth is the most potent factor in determining the stability of the new position
- The apical base school 1920 by Alex Lundstrom suggested that apical base is the most important factor in the correction of malocclusion and maintenance of correct occlusion.
- The mandibular incisor school by Grieves and Tweed in 1952 suggested that the mandibular incisors must be kept upright and over the basal bone.
- The musculature school 1922 suggested that the proper functional muscle balance was necessary for maintenance of stability.

CHAPTER 39 Lab Procedures

LONG ESSAYS

Question 1

What is soldering? What are dental solder? Explain ideal requirements, types of soldering and steps in soldering?

Answer

Soldering is defined as a process of joining metal by the use of a filler metal which has a substantially lower fusion temperature than that of the metals being joined.

- Dental solder are the alloys which are used for joining two or more metallic parts in the form of an intermediary or a filler metal.
- Ideal requirement of a dental solder are as follows:
  - Fusion temperature of the dental solder must be less than that of the parts being joined, approximately it should be 50–100°C less than the parts which are to be joined
  - Dental solder should have sufficient tarnish and corrosion resistance
  - It should aid in achieving excellent adhesion by free-flowing and by wetting the metal parts it joins
  - Dental solder should have strength equivalent to metal parts being joined
  - Dental solder should be of the colour similar to the parts being soldered.
- Copper, nickel, gold, silver, zinc and tin are main constituents of the dental solder. Copper gives a yellow colour to the solder, while nickel gives whitish appearance to the solder.

Types of soldering are as follows:

- Investment soldering
- Free hand soldering.

Investment soldering: It is done in those cases where precision is required while joining the metals and also when the contact areas between the metallic parts being joined are large.

In this procedure, the metallic parts are embedded in an investment. A gap of about 0.13 mm is left in between the metals.

Free hand soldering: This is the most commonly used soldering method.

In this process, two metallic parts are soldered together after adequate stabilization, without the use of investment.

Steps in soldering are as follows:

- Surfaces, which are to be joined, should be cleaned properly
- Parts to be joined together are assembled
- Right solder and flux should be selected
- Proper joint between the metal being joined should be selected
- Application of flux
- Heating and introduction of solder
- Quenching.

There are few factors which should be considered during soldering which are as follows:

- Reducing flame of the soldering torch should be used
- To limit the spread of heat, wet cotton and asbestos should be used
- Polishing should not be done of the soldered joint as it causes weakening of the joint
- To prevent excessive spread of solder, antiflux should be used.

Application of soldering in orthodontics are as follows:

- To join the parts of orthodontic appliances
- To fasten the attachment to bands.

Question 2

What is welding? What is the principle of spot welding? Discuss its procedure and applications of it in orthodontics?

Answer

Welding is the process of joining of two or more metal pieces directly under pressure without the involvement of an intermediary material.

Two Types of Welding

1. **Cold welding**: It is done by hammering, e.g., Gold foil filling
2. **Hot welding**: It is done by the use of heat of sufficient intensity to melt the metals being joined.

- Spot welding is the welding which is used to join the orthodontic components
- High amperage electricity is generally the heat source.

Principles of Spot Welding

- There are two basic principles involved in spot welding, i.e., heat and pressure
- In a step down transformer, an electric current is made to pass through it, because of which low voltage and high amperage current is generated
- This current is conducted on either side of the metals being joined, through two copper electrode
- Resistance is offered by stainless steel to current of high amperage, which produces very high temperature at the electrodes
- Therefore, the area of metal under the electrodes becomes plastic
- The metals are squeezed into each other as the copper electrodes apply pressure on the metals.

In a welding process, the copper electrodes serve the following functions:

- They help in transmitting the current to the metals which are to be joined in order to increase the temperature
- The electrodes help in holding the two metal together
- Electrodes put pressure on the metals, which help in squeezing the metal into each other
- To preserve the properties of stainless steel around the weld spot, the electrodes help in conducting the heat produced away from the area.
  - Current should be of very short duration, i.e., not more than 1/10 of a second
  - If the time extends for a longer duration, it can lead to weld decay because of precipitation of carbides from the metal.

Spot-welding Procedure

- An appropriate electrode should be attached with the desired shape and thickness of the material
- Any kind of carbide precipitates should be removed
- Surface of every electrode should be smooth, flat and perpendicular to its long axis
- Electrode should be in contact totally when they are together
- The metal are placed between the two electrodes, which are to be joined and the switch is turned on
- The presence of the electrodes can be maintained for a few seconds to help obtain a good joint.

Application of Welding in Orthodontics

Application of welding in orthodontics is as follows:

- To join metal strips during banding
- To fix attachment like brackets and molar tubes onto the bands.

Question 3

Define orthodontic study models. What is its importance? What are its ideal requirement; discuss about steps involved in construction of a study model?

Answer

Study Models

These are the accurate plaster reproduction of the teeth and their surrounding soft tissues.

Importance of study models is as follows:

- Help in studying occlusion from all aspects
- Help in making accurate measurement in a dental arch
- They help in assessment of treatment progress
- Help in describing the treatment plan to the patient
- Help in motivating the patient
- Help in assessing the nature and severity of malocclusion
- Help in transferring the records in case the patient is to be treated by some other clinician.

Ideal Requirements of a Study Model

- Models should produce accurate teeth and surrounding soft tissues without any destruction
- Models should be symmetrical
- They should accurately reproduce occlusion
- Models should have clean, smooth and nodule free surface
- Models should depict teeth as well as alveolar process as possible.

Parts of Study Models

They have two parts:

1. **Anatomic portion**: It is the actual impression of the dental arch and its surrounding structures

2. **Artistic portion:** It contains a plastic base which supports the anatomic portion.

Steps of Constructing a Study Model

- **Impression making**: A good impression is made by recording the details of both soft and hard tissues of the dento-alveolar regions
  - Special emphasis should be given on recording the vestibular sulcus and lingual sulcus up to its complete depth
  - High flange impression trays are recommended to record orthodontic impression.
- **Disinfecting the impression**: Impression should be washed in water and then a disinfecting solution is used
  - After disinfecting, the impression is again rinsed with water.
- **Casting the impression**: The air bubbles are eliminated with the help of a vibrator
- **Basing and trimming**: Once the models are poured and set, the basing of the cast is done.
  - After pouring of base, it is trimmed.
- **Finishing and polishing**: The base of the model is sand papered to give it a smooth finish and is then polished with the help of soap water, which after drying the cast is buffed to obtain a smooth and shiny appearance.

Question 4

What is flux and antiflux?

Answer

Flux

It is basically a Latin word which means flow.

Flux basically helps in:

- Removing the oxide layer from the metallic surfaces in order to increase the flow of the molten solder
- Flux also helps in dissolving any surface impurity
- It prevent oxidation of the metals
- It also reduces the melting point of the dental solder.

Composition of Flux

- Borax glass—55%
- Boric acid—35%
- Silica—10%.

Antiflux

- It helps in confining the flow of the molten solder over the metal being joined
- Antifluxes can be graphite lines, lead pencil marking and iron rouge.

CHAPTER 40 Genetics Factors in Orthodontics

SHORT ESSAYS

Question 1

Discuss genetics in orthodontics?

Answer

Genetics like in other branches also plays an important role in orthodontics.

- Its importance was described in 1836 by Frederick G Kussel. He said that malocclusion both skeletal and dental can be transmitted from one generations to another
- Dentofacial disturbances of genetic origin are as follows:
  - Micrognathia
  - Macrognathia
  - Cleft lip and palate
  - Down syndrome (trisomy of chromosome 21)
  - Gardner's syndrome
  - Marfan's syndrome
  - Cherubism
  - Cleidocranial dysplasia
  - Mandibulofacial dysostosis
  - Osteogenesis imperfecta
  - Bimaxillary atresia
  - Bimaxillary protrusion
  - Hypodontia, anodontia and oligodontia
  - Retarded eruption of teeth
  - Abnormal overjet and overbite
  - Open bite
  - Abnormal number and arrangement of teeth
  - Deep palatal vault.
- Research in the genetic influence of dento-facial complex has thrown light on new vistas of thought and at the same time disapproval from of the misconceptions within the subject.
- For example: Earlier racial crossing between humans was considered to be one of the factors of malocclusion
- Later on, this was disproved by studies stating that human racial crossing presented very little risk to dental occlusion
- In the same way, another study on relapse of treated cases showed that relapse can be caused by hereditary tendencies that come into play and upset the results after treatment gets over
- Occlusal positions, jaw positioning and abnormal pressure habits which impart untoward forces that tend to move the orthodontically treated teeth back into malocclusion can also be of genetic origin.

Question 2

What are the various methods of studying role of genes?

Answer

- Various methods of studying role of genes are as follows:
  - Twin studies
  - Pedigree studies
  - Inbreeding.
- Twin studies: These studies are carried out to check the influences of genes in malocclusions.
  - These studies are done by analysing monozygotic and dizygotic twins, which are as follows:
    - Monozygotic twins: These twins develop from single fertilised ovum and possess an identical genetic makeup to each other
    - Dizygotic twins: These twins develop from two separate ova that are ovulated and fertilised at the same time.
  - As they develop from two different embryos, they have a different genetic make up from each other.
  - Twin studies, in case of monozygotic twins are carried out by altering the environmental factors and conditions for each twin

  - Thus, the influences of environmental factors can be analysed in the two individuals having similar genetic makeup
  - In cases of dizygotic twin, the environmental factor for both the twin are kept similar
- The influence of genetic factors is then checked in both the twin.
- **Pedigree studies**: In these kind of studies, single trait of a person is studied along his whole family tree, and a correlation of any hereditary influences is checked, e.g. bimaxillary protrusion, missing teeth, deep vault palate, etc.
- **Inbreeding**: This kind of study is used to study dominated and recessive characteristic in communities in which polygamy and marriages within the families are seen.

SECTION 2

RECENTLY ASKED QUESTIONS

CHAPTER 41 Recently Asked Questions

INTRODUCTION TO ORTHODONTICS

Long Essays

1. What is orthodontia? Describe the various sequelae of malocclusion of teeth. [MUHS]
2. What is orthodontia? Describe the various sequelae of malocclusion of teeth. [MUHS]
3. Describe briefly about the aims, objectives, scope and limitations of orthodontic treatment. [MUHS]
4. Define orthodontics. Describe about aims and science of orthodontics. [NTR ORA]

Short Essay

1. Objectives of orthodontics. [MUHS]

Short Notes

1. Define orthodontics. [NTRUHS]
2. Definition and scope of orthodontics. [NTR-NR]
3. Adult orthodontics. [RGUHS]
4. Contributions of EH Angle to orthodontics. [MUHS]
5. Aims and scope of orthodontics. [NTRUHS]
6. Describe Andrew Jackson's triad. [MUHS]
7. Jackson's triad. [NTR-OR; TN; RGUHS; MUHS; NTRUHS]
8. Aims of orthodontics. [NTR-OR; RGUHS]
9. Aims and objectives of orthodontics. [NTR-NR; TN]
10. Aims of orthodontic treatment. [RGUHS (OS); NTR]
11. Unfavourable sequelae of malocclusion. [RGUHS]

GENERAL PRINCIPLES AND CONCEPTS OF GROWTH

Long Essays

1. Enumerate theories of bone growth. [MUHS]
2. Enumerate various theories of growth. Describe functional matrix theory of Moss. [RGUHSA]
3. Describe the methods of studying growth. Discuss postnatal growth of mandible. [RGUHS]
4. Describe the prenatal and postnatal growth of mandible. [TN]
5. What are growth spurts? What according to you is of a good use for orthodontic treatment and why? [MUHS]
6. What are growth studies? What is the importance of studying growth in orthodontics? [MUHS]
7. Enumerate the various theories of growth. Explain in detail about the functional matrix theory. [RGUHS]
8. Enumerate the various methods of measuring growth. Discuss in detail about the clinical implications of growth and development in orthodontics. [TN]
9. How and why will you analyse growth in orthodontics? [MUHS]
10. Describe growth and development of jaws, theories of growth and how disturbances cause malocclusion. [RGUHS]
11. Describe the growth and development of mandible and its clinical importance in orthodontics. [NTRUHS]
12. What are growth trends? Give their significance in diagnosis, treatment planning and retention. [MUHS]
13. Define growth and development. Mention various theories of growth and write in detail about functional matrix hypothesis. [NTR-OR, RGUHS]
14. Discuss briefly about clinical application of knowledge of growth and development in orthodontics. [RGUHS; BUHS]
15. Define growth and development. Describe various methods of studying bone growth. [MUHS]

Short Essays

1. Neurotrophism. [RGUHS]
2. Growth trends. [RGUHS]
3. Scammon's curve. [RGUHS]
4. Safety valve mechanism. [RGUHS]
5. Methods of gathering growth data. [RGUHS]
6. Trajectories of facial skeleton. [RGUHS]
7. Y-axis. [RGUHS; TN]
8. Growth site versus growth centre. [RGUHS]
9. Pubertal growth spurts. [RGUHS]
10. Explain differential growth and Scammon's growth curve. [RGUHS]
11. Functional matrix theory of growth and development. [RGUHS]
12. Sutural growth. [MUHS]
13. Growth spurts. [RGUHS; MUHS]
14. Functional matrix theory. [RGUHS, TN; NTRUHS]
15. Methods of studying growth. [RGUHS]
16. Growth spurts and their two clinical importance. [RGUHS]
17. Endochondral and intramembranous bone formation. [NTR]
18. Cephalocaudal gradient of growth. [RGUHS]
19. Expanding 'V' principle. [NTRUHS]
20. Pressure-tension theory. [RGUHS]
21. Trajectories of forces. [RGUHS]

Short Notes

1. Growth trends. [RGUHS]
2. Differential growth. [RGUHS]
3. Scammon's curve. [RGUHS; TN]
4. Fontanelles. [RGUHS]
5. Genetic counselling. [RGUHS]
6. Prepubertal growth spurt. [NTR-NR]
7. Prepubertal growth periods. [NTR-OR]
8. Functional matrix theory. [NTR-OR; MUHS; RGUHA; TN]
9. Scammon's growth curves. [MUHS; RGUHS; NTRUHS]
10. Growth spurts. [NTR-OR; MUHS; TN; NTRUHS]
11. Growth sites. [NTR-NR; RGUHS]
12. Growth curve. [NTR-OR]
13. Methods of studying growth. [RGUHS]
14. Growth spurts and their two clinical importance. [RGUHS]
15. Twin studies. [NTR-NR]
16. Neurotrophism. [RGUHS]
17. Piezoelectric screws. [RGUHS]
18. Spheno-occipital synchondrosis. [TN]
19. Moss's functional matrix theory. [TN]
20. Types of bone growth movements. [RGUHS]
21. Wolff's law of bone transformation. [NTRUHS]
22. Safety valve mechanism. [RGUHS]
23. Methods of gathering growth data. [RGUHS]
24. Give at least four definitions of growth and at least four applications of it in orthodontics. [MUHS]
25. Enumerate the various tissues for which Scammon's growth curves are plotted. [MUHS]
26. Define and distinguish between growth centre and growth site, giving examples. [MUHS]
27. Enumerate the periods of postnatal growth. [MUHS]
28. Enumerate various theories of growth. [MUHS]
29. Adenoid facies. [RGUHS]
30. Growth centres. [RGUHS]
31. Wolff's law. [RGUHS]
32. Cortical drift. [RGUHS]
33. Trajectories of forces. [RGUHS]

GROWTH AND DEVELOPMENT OF CRANIAL AND FACIAL STRUCTURES

Long Essays

1. Describe growth and development of mandible. [RGUHS]
2. Describe in detail about prenatal and postnatal growth of mandible. [NTR-OR]
3. Explain in detail about prenatal and postnatal growth and development of maxilla. [NTR-OR]
4. What are growth sites? Explain how maxilla increases in width, length and height? [RGUHS]
5. Discuss in detail about the clinical application of growth and development in orthodontics. [TN]
6. What are the clinical implications of growth and development? [TN]
7. Enumerate the various theories of growth. Explain in detail about the functional matrix theory. [TN]
8. Describe the aetiology, diagnosis and treatment of Angle's class III malocclusion patients. [TN]
9. Describe postnatal growth of maxilla. [RGUHS]
10. Describe growth and development of mandible. [BUHS]
11. Define growth. Write in detail about the prenatal and postnatal growth of mandible. [TN]
12. What are growth sites? Explain how maxilla increases in width, length and height? [RGUHS]

13. What are the different theories of growth? Explain the functional matrix hypothesis in detail. [TN]
14. Define growth and development. How will you differentiate between growth and development? Describe mandibular postnatal growth and its application in orthodontics. [MUHS]
15. Define growth and development. Discuss postnatal growth of maxilla. [TN; MUHS]
16. What are the various definitions related to growth? Discuss in detail about the postnatal growth of maxilla with diagrams. [TN]
17. Define growth and development. Discuss in detail about the postnatal growth of the mandible. [TN]
18. Mention the theories of growth. Describe in detail about postnatal growth of mandible. [TN]
19. Describe the prenatal and postnatal development of mandible and its clinical implications. [RGUHS]
20. Discuss prenatal and postnatal growth of mandible and its clinical application in orthodontics. [NTR-NR]
21. Discuss prenatal and postnatal growth of mandible and its clinical implications in orthodontics. [NTR-NR]
22. Define growth and development. What are the theories of growth? How growth disturbances can cause malocclusion? [NTR-NR]
23. Describe in detail about prenatal and postnatal development of mandible. Development of mandible. [RGUHS]
24. Write in detail about the development of maxilla. Elaborate on aetiology and treatment of cleft palate. [RGUHS]
25. Discuss in detail about the clinical applications of growth and development in orthodontics. [NTRUHS]
26. Define growth. Mention the various theories of growth and discuss in detail about the functional matrix hypothesis. [NTRUHS]

Short Essays

1. Trajectories of forces. [NTRUHS]
2. Describe the role of mandibular growth in orthodontics. [MUHS]
3. Cephalocaudal gradient of growth. [RGUHS]
4. Skeletal age. [MUHS]
5. Growth spurts. [RGUHS; NTR]
6. Functional matrix theory. [RGUHS]
7. Define growth and development. Explain the postnatal growth of mandible. [RGUHS]
8. Clinical application of growth and development. [NTR]
9. Wolff's theory of bone transformation. [NTRUHS]
10. Postnatal growth and development of the mandible. [NTRUHS]
11. Spheno-occipital synchondrosis. [NTRUHS]
12. Define growth and development. Describe in detail about the postnatal development of maxilla. [MUHS]
13. How is 'form' related to 'function'? Explain the above statement in relation to growth of mandible. [MUHS]

Short Notes

1. Growth charts. [TN]
2. Nasal septal cartilage. [TN]
3. Palatally impacted canine. [TN]
4. Differential growth. [NTRUHS]
5. Compare drift versus displacement, with examples. [RGUHS]
6. Capsular matrix. [NTR-OR]
7. Cranial base synchondrosis. [RGUHS]
8. Pressure-tension hypothesis. [TN]
9. Growth rotations. [TN]
10. Growth spurts. [TN, RGUHS; NTRUHS]
11. Synchondrosis. [NTR-OR; RGUHS]
12. Wolff's law and trajectories of forces. [TN]
13. Examples of functional matrix theory. [TN]
14. Safety changes following orthodontic tooth movement. [TN]
15. Envelope of discrepancy. [TN]
16. Down's syndrome. [TN]
17. Meckel's cartilage. [RGUHS-BUHS; NTRUHS]
18. Spheno-occipital synchondrosis. [NTR-NR; RGUHS; TN; NTRUHS]
19. Mechanism of bone growth. [NTR-NR]
20. Functional matrix theory. [TN]
21. Endochondral bone formation. [TN]
22. Expanding 'V' principle. [TN]
23. Cephalocaudal gradient of growth. [TN]
24. Twin studies. [TN]
25. Methods of studying growth. [TN]
26. Sutural growth. [NTR-NR]
27. Wolff's law. [RGUHS]
28. Define synchondrosis. [MUHS]
29. Neurotrophic theory of craniofacial growth. [NRUHS]
30. Development of palate. [TN]
31. Congenital defects. [TN]
32. Piezoelectric theory. [NTRUHS]
33. Y-axis. [RGUHS]
34. Scammon's curve. [RGUHS]

DEVELOPMENT OF DENTITION AND OCCLUSION

Long Essays

1. Describe briefly about development of occlusion and its clinical significance. [RGUHS]
2. Discuss the development of dentition between 6 and 12 years of age. [TN]
3. Write briefly about leeway space. [NTR]
4. Discuss ill-effects of early loss of deciduous teeth on developing dentition. [MUHS]
5. Describe briefly about development of occlusion and its clinical significance. [BUHS]
6. Discuss ill-effects of early loss of deciduous teeth on developing dentition and write in detail about various space regainers. [MUHS]
7. Describe gum pad occlusion in a newborn. What are the factors enhancing the development of normal occlusion? [MUHS]
8. Define optimum orthodontic force. Discuss the various theories of tooth movement. [NTRUHS]
9. Discuss the role of lip and tongue in relation to normal occlusion. [NTR-OR]
10. Describe the development of dentition and intra-arch tooth relationships from 6th to 12th year of a child's life? [RGUHS]
11. Describe various factors for development of normal occlusion. [MUHS]
12. Define normal occlusion. Describe normal occlusion in deciduous dentition and its further development till the age of 12 years. [MUHS]
13. Describe the development of normal occlusion. [NTR-OR; RGUHS-BUHS]
14. Discuss the various stages of development of occlusion from birth to adolescence. [NTR-NR]

Short Essays

1. Syndrome and malocclusion. [RGUHS]
2. Physiologic spaces. [RGUHS]
3. Leeway space. [MUHS]
4. Premature loss of second deciduous molars. [MUHS]
5. Andrews' keys to normal occlusion. [RGUHS]
6. Ugly duckling stage. [RGUHS; NTR]
7. Curve of Spee. [RGUHS]
8. Safety valve mechanism. [RGUHS]
9. Anthropoid spaces. [MUHS]
10. Discuss the role of TMJ in orthodontics. [RGUHS]
11. Space of Nance. [RGUHS]
12. Incisal liability. [RGUHS]

Short Notes

1. Explain Scammon's curves. [MUHS]
2. What is ugly duckling stage? [MUHS]
3. Enumerate self-correcting malocclusions. [MUHS]
4. Describe ugly duckling stage. [MUHS]
5. Centric relation. [RGUHS]
6. Leeway space of Nance. [NTR-OR; TN; RGUHS-BUHS]
7. Distal flush terminal plane. [NTR-OR]
8. Flush terminal plane. [NTR-OR; RGUHS; NTR]
9. Theories of eruption. [NTR-NR]
10. Gum pads. [NTR-OR; RGUHS; NTRUHS]
11. Primate spaces. [NTR-NR; TN; RGUHS; MUHS]
12. Incisor liability. [NTR-NR; RGUHS; TN, MUHS]
13. Ugly duckling stage. [NTR-OR; RGUHS; TN, MUHS]
14. Freeway space. [NTR-OR; RGUHS]
15. Premature loss of second deciduous teeth. [RGUHS]
16. Premature loss of deciduous teeth,. [RGUHS]
17. Transitional period. [NTRUHS]
18. Andrews' six keys to normal occlusion. [NTRUHS]
19. Gum pads. [NTRUHS; RGUHS]
20. Leeway space. [NTR-OR; MUHS; RGUHS]
21. Sequence of eruption of permanent teeth. [NTR-OR]
22. Transient malocclusion. [RGUHS; TN; MUHS]
23. Dental age. [RGUHS]
24. Growth spurts. [TN]
25. Early loss of deciduous teeth. [TN]
26. Physiologic spaces. [TN]
27. Abnormal eruptive path. [TN]
28. Space of Nance. [BUHS]
29. Stages of eruption of permanent teeth. [NTR-NR]
30. Ugly duckling stage of dentition. [MUHS]
31. Ectopic upper canines. [TN]
32. Dental formula at the age of 9. [RGUHS]

FUNCTIONAL DEVELOPMENT

Long Essays

1. Discuss in detail about various functions of stomatognathic system. [MUHS]

Short Essays

1. Anterior crossbite. [RGUHS]
2. Trajectories of force. [RGUHS; TN]
3. Buccinator mechanism. [RGUHS; RGUHS; NTRUHS]
4. Deglutition. [MUHS]

Short Notes

1. Trajectories of forces. [RGUHS; TN]
2. Trajectories of facial skeleton. [RGUHS; NTR-NR]
3. Trajectories of occlusal forces. [NTR-NR]
4. Trajectories of forces in mandible. [NTR-OR]
5. Wolff's law of transformation of bone. [NTR-OR; TN]
6. Infantile swallow. [RGUHS]
7. Infantile swallow. [BUHS]
8. Pterygoid response. [RGUHS]
9. Buccinator mechanism. [TN; RGUHS]
10. Buccinator mechanism. [RGUHS]
11. Discuss about Wolff's law of transformation of bone. [NTR-NR; TN]
12. Centric relation and centric occlusion. [RGUHS]

OCCLUSION—BASIC CONCEPTS

Long Essays

1. What are the forces of occlusion? Give the factors that determine and maintain position of tooth and dental arches. [MUHS]
2. What are the six keys of normal occlusion? State how Ack-erman-Proffit system is an improvement over Angle's classification. [NTR-OR]

Short Essays

1. Andrews' six keys to normal occlusion. [NTRUHS]
2. Muscles of mastication. [NTR]
3. Describe six keys to normal occlusion. [RGUHS]
4. Dewey's modification of Angles' classification. [RGUHS]
5. Flush terminal plane. [NTRUHS]
6. Occlusal plane. [NTRUHS]
7. Incisal liability. [NTRUHS]
8. Six keys to normal occlusion. [RGUHS]
9. Terminal planes. [NTRUHS]
10. Trajectories of occlusal forces. [NTRUHS]
11. Supernumerary teeth. [NTRUHS]

Short Notes

1. Incisal liability. [NTRUHS]
2. Supernumerary teeth. [RGUHS]
3. Overjet and overbite. [NTR-OR]
4. Occlusion and malocclusion. [NTR-OR]
5. Enlist Andrews' six keys to normal occlusion. [MUHS]
6. Six keys to normal occlusion. [RGUHS; TN]
7. Features of normal occlusion. [RGUHS]
8. Andrews' six keys to normal occlusion. [TN; RGUHS; NTRUHS]
9. Centric relation and centric occlusion. [NTRUHS]
10. Normal occlusion concept. [NTR-OR]
11. Enumerate Andrews' six keys to normal occlusion. [MUHS]
12. Curve of Spee. [NTR-OR, RGUHS]
13. Late incisor crowding. [TN]
14. Simon's law of cuspid. [NTRUHS]
15. Overjet. [RGUHS]
16. Six keys to normal occlusion. [RGUHS]
17. Describe six keys to normal occlusion. [RGUHS]

CLASSIFICATION OF MALOCCLUSION

Long Essays

1. Describe the various classifications of malocclusion. Enumerate the merits and demerits of Angle's classification. [RGUHS; TN, BUHS]
2. Discuss in brief about Angle's classification of malocclusion along with its merits, demerits and modifications. [RGUHS-BUHS]
3. Describe Angle's and Simon's classifications of malocclusion, and their merits and demerits. [RGUHS-BUHS]
4. What is classification? Discuss the different classifications on malocclusion. What is the latest classification on malocclusion? [NTR-NR]
5. Define various classifications of malocclusion and explain in detail about Angle's classification and its validity? [NTR-OR]
6. Describe Angle's classification of malocclusion and mention its limitations. [NTR-OR]
7. Classify class III malocclusion. Discuss in brief about the management of class III malocclusion. [TN]
8. Define Angle's class I crowding. State its clinical and occlusal features. Give step by step description of the treatment planning of typical class I crowding. [TN]
9. What is the purpose behind classifying malocclusion? Enumerate the three basic types of malocclusion. What are the demerits of Angle's classification system? Describe Dewey-Anderson's modification of Angle's classification in detail. [TN]
10. Describe the shortcomings of Angle's classification and its modification. Describe the characteristics of class II division 1 and class II division 2 malocclusion. [MUHS]
11. What are the six keys to normal occlusion? State how Ack-erman-Proffit system is an improvement over Angle's classification. [NTR-OR]
12. Describe Angle's class II division I malocclusion. Discuss how it differs with Angle's class II division 2 malocclusion. [RGUHS-BUHS]
13. Give Angle's classification in detail and mention its drawbacks. [MUHS]
14. Classify various aetiologic factors of malocclusion. Enumerate the different classifications of malocclusion and write the drawbacks of Angle's classification. [TN]
15. Discuss in detail about the aetiology, features, diagnosis and treatment of class III malocclusion. [TN]
16. Enumerate the differences between true and pseudo class III malocclusion. Discuss the list of treatments in mixed dentition. [TN]
17. Give Angle's classification in detail and describe its modification. [MUHS]
18. Enumerate the differences between true class III and pseudo class III malocclusions. Discuss surgical orthodontic procedures in prognathic mandible. [RGUHS-BUHS]
19. Name the different methods of classification of malocclusion. Discuss Simon's classification of malocclusion. [MUHS]

Short Essays

1. Different classifications of malocclusion. [RGUHS]
2. Differences between true and pseudo class III malocclusion. [RGUHS]
3. Characteristics of Angle's class II division II malocclusion. [RGUHS]
4. Enumerate indications and techniques of orthodontic surgeries. [RGUHS]
5. Ackerman-Proffit classification of malocclusion. [NTRUHS]
6. Transient malocclusions. [NTRUHS]
7. Ackerman-Proffit classification. [RGUHS]
8. Angle's class II division I malocclusion.[RGUHS; NTRUHS]
9. Drawbacks of Angle's classification. [RGUHS; MUHS; RGUHS]
10. Angle's classification of malocclusion. [RGUHS]
11. Bilateral posterior crossbite. [TN]
12. Clinical features of class II division 2 malocclusion. [RGUHS]
13. Class II div I versus class II div II malocclusion. [NTR]
14. Bennett classification. [MUHS]
15. Simon's classification of malocclusion. [MUHS; NTRUHS]
16. Features of anterior open bite. [NTRUHS]
17. Dewey's classification of malocclusion. [NTRUHS]
18. Limitations of Angle's classification. [RGUHS]
19. Dewey's modification of Angle's classification. [RGUHS]
20. Pseudo class III malocclusion. [RGUHS]

Short Notes

1. Drawbacks of Angle's classification. [NTR-OR; TN; NTRUHS]
2. Pseudo class III malocclusion. [NTR-OR; TN; RGUHS; NTRUHS]
3. Clinical features of class III malocclusion. [NTR-OR]
4. Bennett's classification. [NTR-OR; RGUHS]
5. Simon's classification of malocclusion. [NTR-OR; MUHS]

6. Validity of Angle's classification. [NTR-OR]
7. Clinical features of class II division 2 malocclusion. [NTR-OR]
8. True class III malocclusion. [RGUHS]
9. Midline diastema. [TN; RGUHS]
10. Angle's class II division 1 malocclusion. [RGUHS]
11. Characteristics of Angle's class II division 2 malocclusion. [RGUHS; TN]
12. Pseudo class III. [RGUHS]
13. Malocclusion. [TN]
14. Rotations. [RGUHS; NTRUHS]
15. Simon's classification. [RGUHS; TN]
16. Distocclusion. [TN]
17. Deep bite. [TN]
18. Handicapping labiolingual deviation index. [TN]
19. Merits and demerits of Angle's classification. [TN]
20. Transient malocclusions. [TN]
21. Features of class II division 1 malocclusion. [TN]
22. Difference between true and pseudo class III. [RGUHS]
23. FH plane. [NTR-NR]
24. Simon's classification. [NTR-NR TN]
25. Frankfurt horizontal plane. [NTR-NR]
26. Lischer's modifications of Angle's classification. [TN]
27. Modifications of Angle's classification. [TN]
28. Ackerman-Proffit classification of malocclusion. [TN; MUHS]
29. Different classifications of malocclusion. [RGUHS]
30. Give differences between true and pseudo class III malocclusion. [MUHS]
31. Enlist various systems of classification of malocclusion. [MUHS]
32. Mention three planes used in Simon's classification and its deviations. [MUHS]
33. Features of Angle's class II division 2 malocclusion. [MUHS]
34. Dewey's modification to Angle's classification of malocclusion. [RGUHS]
35. Ackerman-Proffit classification. [RGUHS; TN]
36. Angle's classification of malocclusion. [RGUHS; BUHS]
37. Pseudo class III malocclusion. [BUHS]
38. Skeletal malocclusion. [NTR-NR]
39. Key ridge. [RGUHS]
40. Borderline case. [NTR-NR]
41. Apertognathia. [NTRUHS]
42. Median diastema. [RGUHS]
43. Dewey's modification of Angle's classification. [RGUHS]
44. Skeletal classification. [TN]
45. Crossbite. [TN; NTR; RGUHS]
46. Angle's classification. [TN; RGUHS]
47. Imbrications. [NTR-NR]
48. Mandibular retrognathism. [NTR-NR]
49. Contributions of EH Angle to orthodontics. [MUHS]
50. Draw a Venn diagram to explain Ackerman-Proffit's classification of malocclusion. [MUHS]
51. Imbrications. [RGUHS; NTRUHS]
52. Causes of midline diastema. [RGUHS]
53. Intrusion. [NTR-OR]

AETIOLOGY OF MALOCCLUSION

Long Essays

1. Enumerate the aetiology of malocclusion. Describe the local factors. [RGUHS]
2. Enumerate and classify the aetiological factors of malocclusion. Describe local factors. [TN]
3. Define malocclusion. Discuss aetiology of malocclusion. [NTR-OR]
4. Describe in detail about the postnatal causes of malocclusion. [TN]
5. Write about the unfavourable sequelae of malocclusion situation. [NTRUHS]
6. Explain in detail about aetiology of malocclusion. [NTR-OR]
7. Classify various factors in the aetiology of malocclusion. Elaborate endocrinal factors. [NTRUHS]
8. Enumerate the prenatal causes of malocclusion. [RGUHS-BUHS]
9. Classify the aetiology of malocclusion. Describe the role of Mouth-breathing in the development of open bite malocclusion. [TN]
10. Classify the aetiology of malocclusion. Discuss general factors in detail. [TN]
11. Discuss the local causes of malocclusion. [NTR-NR]
12. Discuss the general causes for malocclusion. [NTR-NR]
13. Enumerate genetically inherited malocclusion. Discuss crossbite in detail. [MUHS]
14. Classify the aetiologic factors of malocclusions. Discuss the role of habits in causing malocclusion. [TN]
15. Discuss the aetiology, line of treatment and the design of appliances in the correction of anterior crossbite, anterior spacing and open bite. [TN]

16. Discuss in brief about the aetiology, clinical features and treatment of Angle's class II division 1 malocclusion. [MUHS]
17. Discuss the genetic and hereditary factors contributing towards the formation of malocclusion. [MUHS]
18. Classify aetiology of malocclusion. Give aetiology and treatment of midline diastema. [MUHS]
19. What is your opinion about the three most important causes of malocclusion? Describe the orthodontic measures employed to treat them. [MUHS]
20. Classify the various factors in the aetiology of malocclusion and write in detail about the role of habit in causing malocclusion. [RGUHS]

Short Essays

1. Teratogens. [RGUHS]
2. Supplemental teeth. [RGUHS]
3. Buccinator mechanism. [NTRUHS]
4. Unfavourable sequelae of malocclusion. [NTRUHS]
5. Supernumerary tooth. [RGUHS; TN]
6. Importance of genetics in malocclusion. [RGUHS]
7. Mention local factors in the aetiology of malocclusion. [RGUHS]
8. Classify aetiological factors of malocclusion. [RGUHS]
9. Butler's field theory. [TN]
10. Genetic malocclusions. [RGUHS; MUHS]
11. Local factors of malocclusion. [RGUHS]

Short Notes

1. Local factors in the aetiology of malocclusion. [NTR-OR]
2. Ankylosis. [NTRUHS]
3. Local factors causing malocclusion. [NTR-OR]
4. Submerged tooth. [NTR-NR]
5. Supplemental teeth. [NTR-NR]
6. Genetic malocclusions. [RGUHS]
7. How dental caries causes malocclusion? [RGUHS]
8. Supernumerary tooth. [BUHS]
9. Enumerate local factors causing malocclusion (any eight). [MUHS]
10. Enlist the causes of midline diastema. [MUHS]
11. Local causes of malocclusion. [NTRUHS; TN]
12. Causes of midline diastema and its treatment. [RGUHS]
13. Importance of family history in orthodontics. [RGUHS]
14. Mention local factors in the aetiology of malocclusion. [RGUHS]
15. Dilacerated tooth. [NTR-NR]
16. Teratogens. [NTR-OR]
17. Factors causing malocclusion. [NTR-OR]
18. Postnatal causes for malocclusion. [NTR-NR]
19. Prolonged retention of deciduous teeth. [NTRUHS]
20. Postnatal causes for malocclusion. [NTR-NR]
21. Blanch test. [NTR-NR]
22. Acromegaly. [NTR-NR]
23. Aetiology of crowding. [RGUHS]
24. Rotations. [RGUHS]

ORAL HABITS

Long Essays

1. Give aetiology and treatment of mouth-breathing habit. [MUHS]
2. Define abnormal-pressure habits. Write in detail about the classification, clinical findings and treatment of mouth breathers. [TN]
3. Explain the equilibrium theory and write in detail about the clinical features of malocclusion caused by thumb sucking. [TN]
4. Classify habits. How will you manage thumb-sucking habit? [RGUHS]
5. Define a habit. How do you classify habits? Discuss the aetiology, effects and management of thumb sucking. [TN]
6. Discuss the aetiology, clinical picture and management of thumb-sucking habit. [BUHS]
7. Discuss the role of lip and tongue in relation to normal occlusion. [NTR-OR]
8. Enumerate the aetiological factors causing Mouth-breathing and tongue thrust in children and discuss the line of treatment. [NTR-NR; TN]
9. Give aetiology, signs, symptoms and treatment of the following:
   a. Mouth-breathing
   b. Tongue-thrust habit
   c. Lip-biting habit. [MUHS]
10. Describe the effects of the following on developing dentition:
    a. Thumb-sucking habit
    b. Premature loss of deciduous dentition
    c. Mouth-breathing habit. [MUHS]
12. Define a habit. Discuss the aetiology, clinical features and management of thumb-sucking habit. [TN]

12. Define malocclusion. Classify aetiology of malocclusion. Discuss clinical pictures and management of thumb-sucking habit. [NTR-NR]
13. Classify aetiology of malocclusion. Explain in detail about the role of various abnormal habits in causing malocclusions. [RGUHS]
14. Classify habits. Explain the triad of factors affecting habits. Elaborate on lip-biting and nail-biting habits. [NTRUHS]
15. Define habits. Classify and discuss in detail about the features of tongue-thrusting habit and its treatment modalities. [NTRUHS]
16. Discuss the aetiology, clinical picture and management of thumb-sucking habit. [RGUHS]
17. Describe how tongue thrust and thumb-sucking habits cause malocclusion. [RGUHS]
18. Define preventive and interceptive orthodontics. Discuss the management of thumb-sucking habit. [RGUHS]
19. Describe how tongue thrust and thumb-sucking habits cause malocclusion. [BUHS]
20. Define preventive and interceptive orthodontics. Discuss the management of thumb-sucking habit. [RGUHS]
21. Define habit. Discuss any two habits that cause malocclusion. [MUHS]
22. Mention the acquired factors responsible for the development of malocclusion. Describe the effect of loss of deciduous teeth on developing dentition. [MUHS]
23. Describe various oral habits directly responsible for causing malocclusion. Discuss management of one such habit in detail. [MUHS]

Short Essays

1. Bruxism. [RGUHS]
2. Mouth-breathing. [RGUHS; MUHS; TN]
3. Thumb-sucking habit. [RGUHS; TN, MUHS; RGUHS]
4. Mouth-breathing habit. [RGUHS; NTRUHS; NTR]
5. Aetiology and treatment of tongue-thrust habit.[MUHS]
6. Mouth-breathing habit and its effects on the development of occlusion. [RGUHS]
7. Classify tongue-thrust habit. Add a note on its management. [RGUHS]
8. What is adenoid face? [RGUHS]

Short Notes

1. Aetiology of tongue thrust. [RGUHS]
2. Tongue thrust. [TN]
3. Mouth-breathing habit. [TN; NTRUHS; RGUHS]
4. Lip bumper. [TN]
5. Classify tongue-thrust habit. Add a note on management. [RGUHS]
6. Sucking and suckling. [NTR-OR]
7. Tongue-thrusting habit. [NTR-OR; RGUHS]
8. Habit-breaking appliances. [NTR-NR]
9. Management of thumb-sucking habit? [RGUHS]
10. Pernicious oral habits. [TN]
11. Digital sucking springs. [TN]
12. Role of Mouth-breathing in the aetiology of malocclusion. [TN]
13. Mouth-breathing as an aetiological factor of malocclusion. [RGUHS]

ORTHODONTIC DIAGNOSIS

Long Essays

1. What are the diagnostic aids used in orthodontics? Describe anyone of them. [RGUHS]
2. Enumerate various diagnostic aids used in orthodontics. Add a note on study models. [RGUHS]
3. Discuss the importance of intraoral X-rays and study models in orthodontic diagnosis and treatment planning. [RGUHS-BUHS]
4. Discus the various diagnostic aids used in orthodontics. [NTR-OR]
5. Explain the various diagnostic aids used in case analysis. [NTR-OR]
6. Discuss in brief about the various diagnostic aids used in orthodontic case analysis. [NTR]
7. Enumerate various diagnostic aids and elaborate on the various model analysis used for diagnosis and treatment planning in orthodontic practice. [TN; NTRUHS]
8. Discuss supplementary diagnostic aids used in orthodontics. [NTR-NR]
9. Describe the role of X-rays in orthodontic diagnosis. [RGUHS-BUHS]
10. What are the diagnostic aids used in orthodontics? Describe anyone of them? [BUHS]
11. Enumerate essential diagnostic aids. Describe study models in detail. [RGUHS]
12. Enumerate diagnostic aids. Discuss any two in detail. [MUHS]
13. Classify diagnostic AIDS. What are all the essential diagnostic AIDS? [RGUHS]

14. Classify diagnostic AIDS. Discuss in detail about the essential diagnostic aids. [NTRUHS]
15. What are the various diagnostic aids in orthodontics? Write in detail about the clinical examination and case history record. [NTR]
16. What are the study models? Write the uses of the same in orthodontics. [RGUHS]
17. Classify diagnostic aids and write in detail about the case history and examination. [RGUHS]
18. What are the diagnostics aids? Describe in detail about cephalometries and its uses in orthodontics. [RGUHS]
19. Classify diagnostic aids in orthodontics. Describe the uses of roentgenographic cephalometry in orthodantics. [RGUHS]
20. How the orthodontic study model analyses aid in treatment planning? [TN]
21. What is case analysis? Discuss various steps and factors affecting the prognosis of a case. [MUHS]
22. What do you understand by diagnostic aids? Discuss the importance of X-rays in orthodontics. [MUHS]
23. What do you understand by diagnostic aids? Describe the role of cephalometries in orthodontics. [MUHS]
24. Classify the diagnostic aids in orthodontics. Write the importance of study models and enumerate various types of models used in orthodontics. [MUHS]
25. Discuss the utility of radiographical records in orthodontic practices. [MUHS]
26. Describe your procedure for clinical examination of face and intraoral tissue. [MUHS]
27. How will you proceed with the systematic clinical examination of a patient with malocclusion? [MUHS]
28. Discuss in detail about the various diagnostic aids used in orthodontics. [RGUHS]
29. Discuss essential diagnostic criteria used in orthodontics. [NTRUHS]
30. Essential diagnostic aids used in orthodontics. [RGUHS]

Short Essays

1. Intraoral X-rays in orthodontics. [RGUHS]
2. Essential and supplementary diagnostic aids. [RGUHS]
3. Role ofX-rays in orthodontics. [NTRUHS]
4. Study models. [RGUHS; NTR-NR]
5. Trimming of study model. [RGUHS-BUHS]
6. Orthodontics study models. [NTRUHS]
7. Uses of roentgenographic cephalometry in orthodontics. [NTRUHS]
8. Electromyography. [RGUHS]
9. Diagnostic aids in orthodontics. [RGUHS]
10. Uses of radiographs in orthodontics. [RGUHS]
11. What are the study models and uses of the same in orthodontics? [RGUHS]
12. What are orthodontic diagnostic aids? Enumerate them. [MUHS]
13. Hand-wrist radiographs. [NTRUHS]

Short Notes

1. Orthopantomogram. [NTR OR; RGUHS, MUHS]
2. X-rays in orthodontics. [NTR-NR]
3. Facial types. [RGUHS-BUHS]
4. Diagnostic aids. [NTR-NR; RGUHS; NTRUHS]
5. Study models. [NTR-DR; TN; RGUHS]
6. Occlusal X-ray. [NTR-NR]
7. Diagnosis in adult orthodontics. [TN]
8. Study casts. [RGUHS; TN]
9. Path of closure. [RGUHS]
10. Electromyograms. [RGUHS]
11. Intraoral radiograph. [RGUHS-BUHS; TN]
12. Orthodontic study models. [TN]
13. Hand-wrist radiographs. [TN]
14. Carpal radiographs. [TN]
15. Carpal bones. [TN]
16. Diagnostic aids in orthodontics. [RGUHS]
17. What are the study models and uses of the same in orthodontics? [RGUHS]
18. Importance of assessing skeletal age in orthodontic treatment planning. [RGUHS]
19. Incompetent lips. [TN]
20. Facial profile. [RGUHS]
21. Evaluation of smile. [NTR]
22. Facial divergence. [NTRUHS]
23. Lateral cephalogram. [TN]
24. Intraoral periapical radiographs. [RGUHS]
25. Electromyogram as a diagnostic aid. [RGUHS]
26. Hand-wrist X-rays. [TN; RGUHA; NTRUHS]
27. Facial forms. [TN]
28. Bitewing radiographs. [TN; RGUHS]
29. Kesling set-up. [TN; RGUHS]
30. Electromyography. [BUHS; RGUHS; NTRUHS]
31. Radiographs in orthodontics. [MUHS]
32. Lip trap. [MUHS]
33. OPG. [MUHS]
34. Uses of a panoramic radiograph. [RGUHS; NTRUHS]
35. Gnathostatic models. [RGUHS]
36. Uses of study models. [RGUHS]
37. Orthodontic study models. [NTR-NR; NTRUHS]
38. Study models. [RGUHS]
39. Sheldon body type. [NTR-NR]
40. Uses of study models. [TN]
41. Electromyography in orthodontics. [TN]
42. Cephalometric radiology. [TN]
43. Occlusal radiograph. [NTR-OR; TN]
44. Panoramic radiograph. [RGUHS; NTR-NR; MUHS]

CEPHALOMETRIES

Long Essays

1. What is standardization in cephalometries? Discuss Steiner's cephalometric analysis. [MUHS]
2. Discuss cephalometries as a diagnostic aid? [BUHS-RGUHS]
3. Enumerate cephalometric landmarks and elaborate on Steiner's analysis. [NTRUHS]
4. Classify diagnostic aids. Discuss the uses of cephalometries. [RGUHS]
5. Discuss in detail about the clinical implications of growth and development, enumerating the use of cephalometries to study growth. [RGUHS]
6. Short note on:
   a. TMA
   b. EMA
   c. RPE
   d. CSP. [MUHS]
7. Describe the role of cephalometric radiography in orthodontics. Give various planes and angles used in cephalometric analysis. [MUHS]
8. Classify the diagnostic aids. Define cephalometric landmarks and planes. Discuss Steiner's analysis. [TN]
9. Discuss in detail about the clinical implications of growth and development enumerating the use of cephalometries to study the same. [TN]
10. Classify diagnostic aids and write in detail about two cephalometric analysis of your choice used in orthodontics. [TN]
11. What do you understand by diagnostic aids? Describe the role of cephalometries in orthodontics. [MUHS]

Short Essays

1. Y-axis. [RGUHS]
2. Key ridge. [RGUHS; MUHS]
3. Horizontal planes in cephalometry. [RGUHS]
4. Moyers' mixed dentition analysis. [NTRUHS]
5. Bolton's analysis. [NTRUHS]
6. Tweed's triangle. [RGUHS; TN; RGUHS; NTRUHS]
7. Registration point. [RGUHS]
8. Cephalometries. [RGUHS; MUHS]
9. Cephalogram. [RGUHS]
10. Interincisal angle. [RGUHS]
11. Down's analysis. [NTRUHS]
12. Steiner's analysis. [NTR]
13. Uses of cephalometries. [RGUHS]
14. Mandibular plane angle. [RGUHS]
15. What is conventional cephalometries? Give its drawbacks. [MUHS]
16. Write the skeletal measurements of Down's analysis. [MUHS]
17. Define following cephalometric points:
    a. Point S
    b. Point Me. [MUHS]
18. Enumerate five horizontal planes used in cephalometries, and give their uses and significance. [MUHS]
19. How is anteroposterior dimension of maxilla and mandible measured on a lateral cephalogram? [MUHS]

Short Notes

1. ANB angle. [NTR-OR; NTR-NR]
2. FMA angle. [NTR-OR]
3. SNA angle. [NTR-OR; NTR-NR, RGUHS]
4. Cephalometries in orthodontia. [NTR-OR; BUHS]
5. FMA angle. [RGUHS]
6. ANB angle. [RGUHS; TN]
7. Tweed's diagnostic triangle. [TN; MUHS]
8. Uses of cephalometries. [TN; MUHS]
9. Angle SNA. [NTR-NR]
10. Y-axis. [NTR-OR]
11. Y-axis angle. [NTR-NR]
12. Cephalostat. [NTR-OR]
13. Tweed's triangle. [NTR-NR; TN; NTRUHS]
14. S-N plane. [NTR-NR]
15. Uses and limitations of cephalometries. [BUHS; TN]
16. Uses of roentgenographic cephalometry in orthodontics. [RGUHS]
17. EH angle. [NTR-NR]
18. Frankfurt horizontal plane. [NTRUHS]
19. Registration point. [NTR-NR]
20. Bolton plane. [NTR-NR]
21. Mandibular plane. [NTR-NR]
22. Ideal orthodontic plane.
29. 'E'line. [MUHS]
30. SNB angle. [NTR-NR]
31. Angle SNB. [NTR-NR]
32. Interincisal angle. [NTR-NR]
33. Mandibular plane angle. [BUHS]
34. Limitations of cephalometry. [TN]
35. Steiner's analysis. [TN; MUHS]
36. Carey's model analysis. [NTRUHS]
37. 'D' point. [MUHS]
38. Angles—SNA, FMA, ANB. [MUHS]
39. Hand-wrist X-ray. [RGUHS]

40. Occlusal plane. [NTR-NR]
41. Mandibular plane. [NTR-NR]
42. Nasolabial angle. [RGUHS]
43. Computerized cephalometric system. [TN]
44. SNA. [NTRUHS]
45. ANB angle. [NTRUHS]
46. Facial divergence. [NTRUHS]
47. Cephalostat. [NTR]
48. EH Angle and his contributions. [NTR]
49. Ashley Howe's analysis. [NTR]
50. Tweed's analysis. [TN]
51. Registration point. [TN; NTR-NR]
52. VTO (visual treatment objective). [TN]
53. Significance of ANB angle. [TN]
54. Tweed's diagnostic triangle. [RGUHS]
55. Interincisal angle. [NTR-NR]

SKELETAL MATURITY INDICATORS

Long Essays

1. What are the methods of measuring growth. Discuss the importance of the knowledge of growth and development in orthodontics. [TN]
2. Enumerate the various methods of measuring growth. Discuss the clinical importance of the knowledge of growth and development in orthodontics. [TN]

Short Essays

1. Skeletal age. [MUHS]
2. Maturity indicators. [RGUHS]
3. Hand-wrist radiography. [RGUHS; NTR]
4. Microimplants in orthodontics. [NTR]

Short Notes

1. Hand-wrist radiograph. [RGUHS]
2. Skeletal age. [TN]
3. Vital staining. [RGUHS; NTR]
4. Dental age. [RGUHS]
5. Hand-wrist radiography. [NTR-ORA; RGUHS]
6. How are Hand-wrist radiographs useful in orthodontic diagnosis and treatment planning? [RGUHS]
7. Carpel index. [NTR-OR; RGUHS, TN]
8. Hand-wrist X-ray. [NTR-OR]

MODEL ANALYSIS

Short Essays

1. Moyers' mixed dentition analysis. [TN; RGUHS]
2. Nance and Carey's index. [MUHS]
3. Pont's analysis. [RGUHS]
4. Korkhaus analysis. [RGUHS]
5. Bolton tooth size ratio. [RGUHS]
6. LH index or Ashley Howe's index. [MUHS]
7. Pont's index. [TN; MUHS]
8. Bolton's analysis. [RGUHS]
9. Mixed dentition analysis. [RGUHS]
10. Down's analysis. [NTRUHS]
11. Ashley Howe's index. [MUHS; RGUHS]
12. Limitations of Angle's classification. [NTR]
13. Assessment of tooth mass discrepancy. [RGUHS]

Short Notes

1. Nance and Carey's analysis. [NTR-NR; TN]
2. Arch perimeter analysis. [NTR-OR; TN; RGUHS]
3. Model analysis for mixed dentition. [NTR-OR]
4. Bolton tooth size ratio. [RGUHS]
5. Pont's model analysis. [NTR-NR]
6. Pont's analysis. [NTR-NR]
7. Carey's model analysis. [NTR-NR]
8. Kesling tooth positioning. [RGUHS]
9. Nance and Carey's index. [MUHS]
10. Mixed dentition model analysis. [TN; RGUHS]
11. Dental analysis. [TN]
12. Radiographic method of mixed dentition analysis. [TN]
13. Study models. [TN]
14. Pont's index. [TN]
15. Nance and Carey's index. [MUHS]
16. Kesling's diagnostic setup. [TN]
17. Bolton index. [TN]
18. Wit's analysis. [TN]
19. Gnathostatic models. [NTR-NR]
20. Pont's analysis. [NTR-OR; RGUHS]

21. Model analysis. [NTR-OR; RGUHS]
22. Carey's analysis. [NTR-NR, TN; RGUHS]
23. Bolton's analysis. [TN]
24. Bolton tooth size ratio analysis. [TN]
25. Korkhaus analysis. [BUHS]
26. Ashley Howe's index. [MUHS]

BIOLOGY AND MECHANICS OF TOOTH MOVEMENT

Long Essays

1. Discuss the tissue changes and tissue damages incidental to orthodontic treatment. [RGUHS]
2. Define growth and development. Name and describe the various theories of eruption of teeth. [BUHS]
3. Elaborate histology of tooth movement—changes following application of mild and extreme forces. [NTRUHS]
4. Define optimum orthodontic force. Discuss the various theories of tooth movement. [NTRUHS]
5. Discuss the histological changes during orthodontic tooth movement. [NTR]
6. Discuss tissue changes in tipping movement of upper central incisors. [RGUHS-BUHS]
7. What are different theories of tooth movement? Discuss the pressure-tension theory in detail. [MUHS]
8. Enumerate factors necessary for orthodontic treatment and briefly discuss various tissue changes taking place when a tooth is lingually tipped. [MUHS]
9. Describe the various histological tissue changes during active orthodontic treatment. [MUHS; NTRUHS]
10. Describe the tissue changes taking place during palatal movement of upper central incisors. [RGUHS-BUHS]
11. Describe the biochemical principles of orthodontic tooth movement and add a note on undermining resorption. [RGUHS-BUHS]
12. What is an optimum orthodontic force? Describe the tissue reactions to various tooth movements with diagram. [RGUHS]
13. Enumerate factors necessary for tooth movement and briefly discuss tissue changes that take place when a tooth is tipped lingually. [RGUHS-BUHS]
14. Mention various types of tooth movements and write in detail about the pressure-tension theory of tooth movement. [TN]
15. Describe various orthodontic movements that occur when an ideal force is applied. How would you retain a derotated tooth? [MUHS]
16. What is bodily tooth movement? What are the various theories that are involved in the biology of orthodontic tooth movement? Discuss in detail. [MUHS]
17. Enumerate theories of tooth movement and explain one. What are the different types of tooth movement? What are the effects of magnitude of force on tooth movement? [MUHS]
18. Tissue response to orthodontic tooth movement. [RGUHS]
19. Describe the blood flow theory of tooth movement. Describe the tissue reaction in periodontium following application of mild and heavy orthodontic forces. [RGUHS]
20. Define optimum orthodontic force. Explain the biological reactions in response to the application of various types of orthodontic force. [TN]
21. Discuss the biochemical principles involved in orthodontic tooth movement and add a note on undermining resorption. [TN]
22. Discuss the role of force in orthodontics tooth movement. [MUHS]
23. What is optimum orthodontic force? Discuss in detail about various changes that takes place after application of force. [MUHS]
24. Discuss the tissue changes with orthodontic tooth movement. [NTR-OR]
25. Describe the tissue changes consequent to orthodontic forces. [NTR-OR]
26. Discuss the various tissue changes taking place during orthodontic tooth movement. [NTR-NR]
27. Describe the tissue changes subsequent to orthodontic force application. [RGUHS]

Short Essays

1. Undermining resorption. [RGUHS; NTRUHS]
2. Types of tooth movement. [RGUHS]
3. Response of bone and periodontium to orthodontic force. [RGUHS]
4. Discuss various theories of tooth movement. [RGUHS]
5. Compare different types of tooth movements. [RGUHS]
6. Explain frontal resorption. [RGUHS]
7. Enumerate the various types of tooth movement. [RGUHS]
8. Bodily tooth movement. [RGUHS]

Short Notes

1. Undermining bone resorption. [NTR-OR; RGUHS]
2. Wolff's law of transformation of bone. [NTR-OR; RGUHS]
3. Wolffs law. [RGUHS; NTR-NR]
4. Piezoelectric theory. [RGUHS]
5. Undermining resorption. [RGUHS; NTR; TN]
6. Explain frontal resorption. [RGUHS]
7. Types of orthodontic forces. [NTRUHS]
8. Force and couple. [NTRUHS]
9. Piezoelectric theory. [NTRUHS]
10. Root resorption. [TN]
11. Blood flow theory to explain tooth movement. [TN]
12. Optimum orthodontic force. [RGUHS; NTR; RGUHS; NTRUHS]
13. Name the mechanisms of bone formation. [RGUHS]
14. Ideal orthodontic force. [NTR-NR; RGUHS; NTRUHS]
15. Theories of tooth movement. [NTR-OR]
16. Undermining resorption. [NTR-OR; MUHS]
17. Tissue changes following orthodontic tooth movement. [RGUHS; TN]
18. Physiologic tooth movement. [TN]
19. Centre of resistance. [TN]
20. Response of bone and periodontium to orthodontic force. [RGUHS]
21. Frontal resorption. [NTR-NR; TN]
22. Tissue changes on pressure side. [NTR-NR, RGUHS]
23. Trajectories of forces. [RGUHS]
24. Types of tooth movement. [RGUHS]
25. Wolff's law. [RGUHS]
26. Intrusion. [NTR-OR]
27. Bodily movement. [RGUHS-BUHS]
28. Define force and write the characteristics of optimum force. [MUHS]
29. Orthodontic forces. [RGUHS]

ANCHORAGE

Long Essays

1. What is reinforced anchorage? Mention its indications. [RGUHS-BUHS]
2. Define and classify anchorage. Explain in detail about the various types with examples. [TN]
3. Define anchorage. Classify the various types with examples and write briefly about each one of them. [TN]
4. Define anchorage. Write in detail about various types of anchorage. [RGUHS]
5. Define and classify anchorage. Discuss the various anchorage situations in removable and fixed appliances. [TN]
6. Define anchorage. Explain in detail about different types of anchorage with example. [NTR-OR; TN]
7. Define anchorage. Classify orthodontic anchorage and explain with examples. [NTR-NR]
8. Define anchorage. Discuss classification of anchorage. Explain intermaxillary anchorage. [NTR-NR]
9. Define anchorage. Classify different types with examples and write briefly about each one of them. [RGUHS-BUHS]
10. Define, classify and explain anchorage by giving examples. [TN]
11. Define anchorage. Discuss method of reinforcing anchorage. [MUHS]
12. Define anchorage and explain with examples the different types of anchorage in orthodontics. [MUHS]
13. Classify anchorage; explain when, why and how you would like to reinforce it. [MUHS]
14. Define anchorage. Explain the various types of anchorage with examples. [RGUHS]
15. Define orthodontic anchorage. Classify them. Discuss the uses of extraoral anchorage in orthodontics. [RGUHS]
16. Define anchorage. Describe various types of anchorage with suitable examples. [RGUHS]

Short Essays

1. Reinforced anchorage. [RGUHS]
2. Anchorage. [RGUHS; MUHS]
3. Extraoral anchorage. [RGUHS; NTR]
4. Stationary anchorage. [NTRUHS]
5. Intermaxillary anchorage. [RGUHS]
6. Reciprocal anchorage. [RGUHS; NTRUHS]

Short Notes

1. Simple anchorage. [RGUHS; BUHS]
2. Define anchorage. Classify it with respect to number of teeth used. [MUHS]
3. Extraoral sources of anchorage. [TN]
4. Cortical anchorage. [TN, RGUHS]

5. Define anchorage. Enumerate methods of reinforcing anchorage. [MUHS]
6. Anchorage. [NTR-OR; RGUHS, BUHS]
7. Extraoral anchorage. [NTR-OR; TN; RGUHS; NTRUHS]
8. Reciprocal anchorage. [NTR-NR; TN; RGUHS; MUHS]
9. Intermaxillary anchorage. [NTR-OR, RGUHS]
10. Give classification of anchorage. [MUHS]
11. Define anchorage. Give examples of reciprocal anchorage. [MUHS]
12. Define anchorage in orthodontics. Give White and Gardiner's classification. [MUHS]
13. What is reinforced anchorage? Give two examples with diagrams. [MUHS]
14. Stationary anchorage. [TN]
15. Anchorage in orthodontics. [NTR-OR]
16. Baker anchorage. [TN; RGUHS; NTRUHS]
17. Factors affecting anchorage. [TN]
18. Reinforced anchorage. [BUHS, MUHS; NTRUHS]
19. Define orthodontic anchorage. Classify anchorage? [RGUHS]
20. Define anchorage. Give an example of reinforced anchorage. [MUHS]

AGE FACTORS IN ORTHODONTICS

Short Essays

1. Age factor in tooth movement. [RGUHS]
2. Age factors in orthodontics. [RGUHS]

Short Notes

1. Ideal age for orthodontic treatment. [TN]
2. Difference between adult and adolescent patients. [TN]

PREVENTIVE ORTHODONTICS

Long Essays

1. Classify orthodontics. What are the procedures undertaken in preventive orthodontics? Explain in detail. [TN]
2. Define and describe briefly about preventive and intercep-tive orthodontics. [MUHS]
3. Define preventive orthodontics. Discuss the various treatment plans given under the preventive orthodontics. [NTR-OR]
4. Describe space maintainers and space regainers. [RGUHS]
5. Describe in brief about space maintainers and their classification with examples. [BUHS]
6. What are space maintainers? Describe the various types used in orthodontics and their indications. [MUHS]
7. Describe in brief about space maintainers and their classification with examples. [RGUHS]
8. Describe the role of prevention in orthodontic practice. [MUHS]
9. What are the various preventive orthodontic procedures? Explain in detail about the various space maintainers. [TN]

Short Essays

1. Space maintainer. [MUHS; RGUHS; NTRUHS]
2. Features of an ideal space maintainer. [RGUHS]
3. Define serial extraction and write about indications of serial extractions. [NTRUHS]
4. Procedures under preventive orthodontia. [RGUHS]
5. Serial extractions. [NTRUHS]
6. Preventive orthodontics. [NTRUHS]

Short Notes

1. Classification of space maintainers. [RGUHS]
2. Preventive orthodontics procedures. [TN]
3. Oral hygiene measures during orthodontic treatment. [NTR-OR]
4. Space regainer. [RGUHS]
5. Preventive orthodontics. [NTR-OR; TN; RGUHS]
6. Advantages of fixed space maintainer. Give an example. [RGUHS]
7. What are the requirements of space maintainers? [MUHS]
8. Procedure under preventive orthodontia. [BUHS]
9. Define space maintainer and give four types of space maintainers. [MUHS]

10. Distal shoe space maintainer. [NTRUHS; NTR]
11. Nance appliance. [RGUHS]
12. Discuss preventive orthodontic procedures. [NTR-OR]
13. Space maintainer. [NTR-NR; TN; RGUHS]
14. Fixed space maintainer. [NTR-OR]
15. Distal shoe space maintainer. [NTR-OR; RGUHS; TN]

INTERCEPTIVE ORTHODONTICS

Long Essays

1. Define and describe briefly preventive and interceptive orthodontics. [MUHS]
2. Define interceptive orthodontics. Describe in detail about serial extractions. [NTR-OR]
3. Define interceptive orthodontics. Discuss serial extraction procedure. [RGUHS-BUHS]
4. Define interceptive orthodontics. Enumerate the various interceptive orthodontic procedures and describe in detail about serial extraction procedure. [RGUHS-BUHS]
5. Enumerate the various procedures done in interceptive orthodontics. Write in detail about serial extractions. [TN]
6. Define interceptive orthodontics and discuss about the various procedures involved in detail. [TN]
7. Define serial extraction. Discuss in detail about indications, contraindications and procedure of serial extraction. [TN]
8. Enumerate various interceptive orthodontic procedures and describe in detail about serial extraction procedure. [TN]
9. Write all you know about serial extractions. [TN]
10. Define interceptive orthodontics. Discuss the indication, contraindications, advantages and disadvantages of serial extractions. Describe one commonly used sequence of serial extractions. [TN]
11. Describe the indications, contraindications and technique of serial extraction. [RGUHS-BUHS]
12. Define serial extraction. Discuss in detail about the indications and procedure of serial extraction. [RGUHS-BUHS; RGUHS]
13. Classify extractions in orthodontics. Write about therapeutic extraction in detail. [RGUHS]
14. What is serial extraction? Describe various methods of serial extraction. [MUHS]
15. Define serial extraction. Discuss indications and contraindications, and advantages and disadvantages of serial extraction. [MUHS]
16. Serial extraction is an interceptive orthodontic procedure— discuss. [RGUHS]
17. Discuss in detail about extractions in orthodontics. [TN]
18. Define interceptive orthodontics and describe various methods of interceptive orthodontics. [RGUHS]

Short Essays

1. First premolar extractions. [RGUHS]
2. Enforced extraction. [RGUHS]
3. Interceptive orthodontics. [RGUHS]
4. Define serial extraction. Add a note on therapeutic extraction. [RGUHS]
5. Indications and contraindications for serial extraction procedures. [MUHS]
6. Indications for serial extraction. [RGUHS]
7. Serial extractions. [NTR-OR; RGUHS; MUHS]
8. Muscle exercises. [NTR-OR]
9. Classify space maintainers and write briefly on any one fixed space maintainer. [NTRUHS]

Short Notes

1. Advantages of serial extraction. [RGUHS]
2. Disadvantages of serial extraction. [RGUHS]
3. Define serial extraction. Give its contraindications. [MUHS]
4. Serial extraction. [RGUHS; NTRUHS; TN]
5. Muscle exercise. [RGUHS-BUHS]
6. Wilkinson extractions. [RGUHS, NTRUHS, RGUHS]
7. Enumerate various serial extraction procedures. [MUHS]
8. Define serial extraction. Add a note on it. [RGUHS]
9. Define serial extraction and discuss any one method of serial extraction. [MUHS]
10. Indications for second premolar extraction. [NTRUHS; RGUHS]
11. Missing teeth. [RGUHS]
12. Interceptive orthodontics. [BUHS; MUHS]

METHODS OF SPACE GAINING

Long Essays

1. Describe various methods of gaining space. [MUHS]
2. Enumerate various methods of gaining space and discuss extractions in orthodontics. [TN]
3. Discuss various methods of gaining space in treating malocclusion. [TN]
4. What is arch length discrepancy? How will you assess the total discrepancy in a given adult patient? What methods can be used to correct arch length discrepancy? [TN]
5. Enumerate various methods to gain space in orthodontics and write in detail about expansion. [MUHS]
6. Enumerate various methods of gaining space in orthodontics and justify your choice for the best method. [MUHS]
7. Describe various methods to gain space in orthodontics. Give their indications and contraindications. [MUHS]

Short Essays

1. Proximal stripping. [RGUHS]
2. Methods of space gaining in dental arch. [NTR-NR]
3. Methods of gaining space. [RGUHS; NTRUHS]
4. Distal driving of molars. [RGUHS]
5. What are the methods of gaining space in orthodontics. [RGUHS]
6. Methods of gaining space in orthodontics. [NTR]
7. Space regainers. [NTRUHS]

Short Notes

1. Proximal stripping. [RGUHS]
2. Enlist methods of gaining space. [MUHS]
3. Define space regainers and give any two examples. [MUHS]
4. Slenderization. [NTRUHS]
5. Molar distalization. [TN]
6. Proximal stripping. [TN; RGUHS; NTR]
7. Methods of gaining space. [BUHS; TN]
8. Uprighting of molars. [RGUHS]
9. Distalization. [TN]
10. Reproximation of teeth. [RGUHS]
11. Methods of molar distalization. [RGUHS]
12. Enumerate methods of gaining space. [RGUHS]
1. Space regainers. [NTRUHS]
14. What are the methods of gaining space in orthodontics? [RGUHS]
15. Clinical evaluation of facial profile. [RGUHS]

ARCH EXPANSION

Long Essays

1. Explain rapid maxillary expansion in detail. [TN]
2. Classify expansion in orthodontics. Discuss your line of treatment for a case of 12 years with bilateral buccal crossbite. [MUHS]
3. Enumerate various methods to gain space in orthodontics and write in detail about expansion. [MUHS]
4. Enumerate various methods to gain space in orthodontics. Discuss rapid palatine expansion. [MUHS]

Short Essays

1. Rapid maxillary expansion. [RGUHS]
2. Rapid palatine expansion. [MUHS]
3. Expansion screws. [RGUHS; MUHS]
4. Dental versus skeletal expansion. [RGUHS]

Short Notes

1. Dental versus skeletal expansion. [NTR-OR]
2. Coffin spring. [RGUHS; NTR-NR]
3. Arch expansion. [RGUHS; BUHS; TN]
4. Expansion screws. [RGUHS; NTR-NR]
5. Role of expansion as a method of gaining space.[MUHS]
6. RME. [NTR-NR; TN]
7. Indications of rapid palatine expansion. [MUHS]
8. Expansion devices. [TN]
9. Rapid palatal expansion. [NTR-OR; TN; RGUHS]
10. Slow expansion appliance. [NTR-OR]
11. Rapid maxillary expansion. [NTR-NR; TN; MUHS]
12. Expansion appliance. [NTR-NR]
13. What is the pitch of expansion screw? Describe accepted mode of activation for conventional screw. [MUHS]

EXTRACTIONS

Long Essays

1. How will you plan extractions in orthodontic treatment? [RGUHS]
2. Enumerate the reasons for extraction of teeth in orthodontics. [RGUHS; BUHS]
3. Describe in detail about extractions in orthodontics. Give your choice of teeth in extractions with reasons. [NTR-OR]
4. Describe in detail about extractions in orthodontics. [NTR-OR]
5. Describe about extractions in orthodontics with reasons. [NTR-OR]
6. What are the reasons for extractions in orthodontics? Discuss the choice of teeth for extractions. [RGUHS]
7. Classify extractions in orthodontics. Write about therapeutic extractions in detail. [RGUHS]
8. What are the various methods of gaining space? Write in detail about extractions in orthodontics. [TN]

Short Essays

1. Describe the factors that justify extraction of teeth for treating malocclusion. [MUHS]
2. Wilkinson extractions. [MUHS]
3. Serial extractions. [NTRUHS]

Short Notes

1. Impacted canines. [TN]
3. Therapeutic extraction in orthodontics. [NTR-NR]
4. Planning extractions. [TN]
5. Extraction in orthodontics. [NTR-OR; TN]
6. Therapeutic extraction. [NTR-OR; TN]
7. Impacted tooth and its orthodontic correction. [TN]

ORTHODONTIC APPLIANCES: GENERAL PRINCIPLES

Long Essays

1. Compare the merits and demerits of removable and fixed orthodontic appliance. [BUHS; RGUHS]
2. Classify orthodontic appliances. Mention the various types of malocclusion that can be corrected by using appliances using screws. [BUHS-RGUHS]
3. What are the indications and contraindications of removable and fixed orthodontic appliances? Enlist components and functions of each fixed appliance component with diagrams. [TN]
4. Enumerate ideal properties of an orthodontic appliance and describe various methods of canine retraction. [MUHS]
5. What are the advantages and disadvantages of removable and fixed appliances? Classify removable appliances and name the basic parts of an active plate, giving function of each. [MUHS]
6. Define orthodontic appliance. Classify them. State the difference between fixed and removable appliances. [TN]
7. What are the advantages and disadvantages of removable and fixed appliances? Describe the various components of fixed appliances. [MUHS]

Short Essays

1. Compare fixed and removable appliances. [RGUHS]
2. What are the basic requirements of an orthodontic appliance? [MUHS]

Short Notes

1. Optimum orthodontic force. [TN]
2. Force and couple. [NTRUHS]
3. Ideal requisites of orthodontic appliance. [NTR-NR]
4. Frankfurt horizontal force. [RGUHS]

REMOVABLE ORTHODONTIC APPLIANCES

Long Essays

1. Discuss various clasps used in orthodontics. [TN]
2. Discuss the advantages, disadvantages and indications for using removable orthodontic appliance. Describe the construction and use of a removable appliance in the treatment of anterior crossbite of one or two teeth. [TN]
3. Define and classify orthodontic appliances. Discuss the various types of tooth movement and how they, are achieved using removable appliances. [TN]
4. Enumerate ideal properties of an orthodontic appliance and describe various methods of canine retraction. [MUHS]
5. Classify removable appliances and name the basic parts of an active plate, giving function of each. [MUHS]
6. Explain slow and rapid expansion—its indications, contraindications and appliances used. [NTRUHS]
7. Define orthodontic appliance. Classify orthodontic appliances and explain in detail about the components, indications and the various factors to be considered in designing a removable orthodontic forces. [TN]

Short Essays

1. Advantages of removable orthodontic appliances. [MUHS]
2. Catalans appliance. [RGUHS; TN]
3. Anterior biting plane. [NTRUHS]
4. Lip bumper. [NTRUHS]
5. Maxillary anterior bite plane appliance. [NTRUHS]
6. Habit-breaking appliance. [RGUHS]
7. Adams clasp and its advantages. [NTRUHS]
8. Canine retractor. [RGUHS]
9. Springs used for distalizing the canines. [RGUHS; NTRUHS]
10. Requirements of removable orthodontic appliance. [RGUHS]
11. Describe parts of removable appliances and write about salient features of canine retractors. [MUHS]
12. Enumerate various types of clasps used in an orthodontic appliances and describe Adams clasp in brief. [MUHS]
13. Give classification of canine retractors. [MUHS]
14. Adams clasp and its modification. [TN]

Short Notes

1. Roberts retractor. [NTR-OR]
2. Orthodontic springs. [NTR-OR]
3. Removable appliance. [NTR-OR]
4. Z-spring. [NTR-OR; RGUHS]
5. Crozat clasp. [NTR-NR]
6. Adams clasp. [NTR-OR; TN; RGUHS; NTRUHS]
7. Roberts retractor. [RGUHS]
8. Canine retractors. [RGUHS, NTR-NR; MUHS]
9. High labial bows. [RGUHS-BUHS; NTR-NR]
10. Arrowhead clasp. [RGUHS-BUHS]
11. Labial low. [NTR-OR; TN]
12. Canine retractors. [NTR-OR; RGUHS]
13. Springs to bring about mesiodistal movement. [NTR-OR]
14. Self-supporting springs. [NTR-NR; TN]
15. Bite plane appliances. [NTR-NR]
16. Spring. [RGUHS-BUHS, TN]
17. Coffin spring. [RGUHS; NTR-NR; NTRUHS]
18. Labial bows. [RGUHS; NTR-NRA; MUHS]
19. Adams clasp. [RGUHS; MUHS; RGUHS]
20. Canine retraction spring. [RGUHS-BUHS; TN]
21. Double cantilever spring. [RGUHS]
22. Components of removable appliances. [NTR-NR]
23. Orthodontic clasp. [NTR-NR; MUHS]
24. Catalans appliances. [NTRUHS]
25. Hawley appliance. [NTRUHS]
26. Hawley retainer. [NTRUHS]
27. Advantage of removable orthodontic appliance. [RGUHS; NTR-NR; RGUHS]
28. Types of labial bows and their uses. [TN]
29. Active plates. [TN]
30. Lingual appliance. [TN]
31. Requirements of removable orthodontic appliance. [BUHS]
32. Lip bumper. [RGUHS]
33. Inclined plane. [RGUHS]
34. Finger spring. [RGUHS; NTR, RGUHS]
35. Adams clasp and modification. [TN]
36. Cantilever spring. [TN; NTRUHS]
37. Buccal canine retraction. [TN]
38. Springs used for distalizing the canines. [RGUHS]

FIXED ORTHODONTIC APPLIANCES

Long Essays

1. Define optimal orthodontic force. Discuss tissue changes subsequent to light and heavy forces. [TN]
2. Discuss the advantages and disadvantages of fixed appliance over removable appliances. [BUHS-RGUHS]
3. What are the theories of tooth movement? What factors affect the tooth movement? Give an account of tissue changes during orthodontic tooth movement. [TN]

Short Essays

1. Properties of ideal orthodontic wires. [RGUHS]
2. Components of fixed appliance. [RGUHS; MUHS]
3. Angle appliances. [MUHS]
4. Screws. [MUHS]
5. NiTi wires. [MUHS]
6. Rapid palatal expansion. [RGUHS]
7. Quad helix appliance. [RGUHS]
8. Preadjusted edgewise appliances. [RGUHS]
9. Arch wires. [RGUHS]
10. Orthodontic cement. [MUHS]
11. Orthodontic wires. [MUHS]
12. Indirect bonding. [MUHS]
13. Direct bonding. [MUHS]
14. Passive components of fixed appliances. [RGUHS]
15. Classify orthodontic wires and write about 18-8 stainless steel. [RGUHS]
16. Begg appliance. [RGUHS-BUHS]
17. Fixed appliance. [RGUHS]
18. Parts of fixed appliance. [RGUHS]
19. Name a few fixed appliance techniques. Write about anyone technique. [RGUHS]
20. What are the physical properties of orthodontic wires? Write about S-S wires. [RGUHS]
21. Name three fixed appliances. Differentiate between Begg and edgewise technique. [RGUHS]
22. Orthodontic bands. [MUHS]
23. Screw plates. [MUHS]
24. Denholtz appliance. [MUHS]
25. Hyrax screw. [MUHS]

Short Notes

1. Parts of fixed appliance. [NTR-OR]
2. Components of fixed appliance. [NTR-OR; RGUHS, MUHS, RGUHS]
3. Fixed appliances versus removable appliance. [NTR-OR]
4. Piezoelectric theory. [TN]
5. Undermining resorption and hyalinization. [TN]
6. Orthodontic springs. [TN]
7. Root resorption. [TN]
8. Histology of tooth movement. [TN]
9. Derichsweiler appliance. [RGUHS]
10. Enumerate active and passive components of fixed appliances and give role of each. [MUHS]
11. NiTi wires. [RGUHS]
12. Stainless steel. [RGUHS]
13. Elastics. [NTR-OR, RGUHS, RGUHS]
14. Arch wire. [NTR-OR]
15. 18-8 Stainless steel. [NTR-NR]
16. Stainless steel in orthodontics. [NTR-OR]
17. Fixed appliance. [NTR-OR; TN]
18. Fixed functional appliance. [RGUHS; TN]
19. Orthodontic wires. [RGUHS; MUHS]
20. 18-8 Stainless steel. [RGUHS; NTR-NR]
21. Edgewise appliance. [RGUHS]
22. Components of Begg appliance. [RGUHS]
23. Advantages of fixed appliances over removable. [TN]
24. Undermining resorption. [TN]
25. Enumerate the objectives of stage I of Begg technique. [MUHS]
26. Differentiate between Begg and edgewise technique. [MUHS]
27. Molar tubes. [RGUHS; NTRUHS]
28. Fixed retainers. [TN]
29. Hyrax appliance. [NTRUHS]
30. Advantages of fixed appliances. [RGUHS; NTR-NR]
31. Ideal properties of orthodontic wires. [MUHS]
32. Enumerate the ideal requisites of an orthodontic appliance. [MUHS]
33. What are the advantages of bonding over banding? [MUHS]
34. Disadvantages of fixed appliances. [RGUHS]
35. Parts of fixed orthodontic appliances. [RGUHS]
36. Brackets in fixed orthodontic appliance. [RGUHS]
37. Components of fixed appliances. [TN, RGUHS; NTRUHS]
38. Class II elastics. [TN]
39. Preadjusted edgewise appliance. [TN]

FIXED ORTHODONTIC APPLIANCES

Long Essays

1. Mention three myofunctional appliances and their mode of action. [RGUHS]
2. Enumerate the uses of oral screen. How will you fabricate an oral screen? [RGUHS]
3. Classify appliances. Describe functional appliances and about how they work and modify growth. [RGUHS]
4. Define functional appliance. How do you correct class II division 1 malocclusion using functional appliances? [GUHS-BUHS; TN]
5. What are myofunctional appliances? Classify them. Explain about the activator in detail. [TN]
6. Mention three myofunctional appliances and their mode of action. [BUHS]
7. Classify appliances. Describe functional appliances how they work and modify growth. [RGUHS]
8. Classify myofunctional appliances. Describe in detail about its indication, construction and trimming of activator. [RGUHS]
9. Define and classify myofunctional appliances. Discuss the indications, contraindications and steps in fabrication of any one functional appliance. [RGUHS]
10. Explain the steps in the fabrication of oral screen and give its disadvantages. [NTR-NR]
11. Enumerate the uses of oral screen. How will you fabricate an oral screen? [BUHS]
12. Classify myofunctional appliances. Name the components of FR-2 (Frankie 2) appliance and describe its mode of action. [RGUHS; NTR]
13. Describe the fabrication of an activator to correct a case of class II division 1 malocclusion. [RGUHS-BUHS]
14. What are functional appliances? Give examples. Enumerate the mechanism of any one of the functional appliances in detail. [RGUHS; TN]
15. Classify myofunctional appliances. Discuss in detail about the mechanism of action, fabrication and trimming of activator. [RGUHS]
16. What are the functional appliances? Give examples. Discuss any one appliance in detail. [NTR-NR]
17. What are myofunctional appliances? Describe in detail about preparation and uses of oral screen. [NTR-OR]
18. State principles of Andresen appliance. Discuss in detail about its indications, contraindications, uses and construction. [NTR-OR]
19. What are functional appliances? Give examples. Describe the trimming and mechanism of action of Andersen appliance. [NTR-OR; RGUHS]
20. What are myofunctional appliances? Classify them. Explain activator. [NTR-NR]
21. Define the term 'myofunctional appliance'. Classify them and write the mode of action of the activator. [TN]
22. Write about the indications and contraindications of:
    a. Activator
    b. Bionator
    c. Standard edgewise therapy
    d. Begg therapy. [MUHS]
23. Define and classify functional appliances. Write in detail about Frankel appliance. [TN]
24. Define a functional appliance. What are the indications, mode of action and design of 16 FR II appliances? [TN]
25. Classify orthodontic appliances. Discuss in detail about the mode of action of activator. [TN]
26. Write briefly on anterior bite plane. [TN]
27. Define and classify functional appliances. Describe in detail about the activator. [TN]
28. Classify functional appliances. Enumerate the indications for functional appliances and describe about the functional regulator lb. [TN]
29. Define and classify myofunctional appliances. Discuss in detail about any one functional appliance for correction of skeletal class II malocclusion. [TN]
30. What is a myofunctional appliance? Describe any one of the commonly used myofunctional appliance in orthodontic treatment. [MUHS]
31. What is a myofunctional appliance? Describe any one of the commonly used myofunctional appliance in orthodontic treatment—its indications and contraindications. [MUHS]
32. What are functional and myofunctional appliances? Discuss the use of activator in detail. [MUHs]
33. What is the basis of functional orthodontic therapy? Describe in detail about any one functional appliance. [MUHS]
34. What is myofunctional appliance? Discuss about Frankel functional regulator. [MUHS]
35. Classify myofunctional appliances. Discuss activator in detail. [MUHS]
36. Define functional appliances, classify them and state about how the activator acts and enumerate its various modifications. [MUHS]

Short Essays

1. Extraoral force. [MUHS]
2. Twin block appliance. [RGUHS]

3. Catalans appliance. Mention the disadvantages of this appliance. [RGUHS]
4. Functional appliance. [MUHS; NTRUHS]
5. Difference between activator and Frankie appliance. [NTRUHS]
6. Classify myofunctional appliances and enumerate the indications of activator. [NTRUHS]
7. Case selection for functional appliance. [NTRUHS]
8. Face mask therapy. [NTRUHS]
9. Anderson activator. [NTRUHS]
10. Muscle exercise. [MUHS]
11. Catalans appliance. [MUHS]
12. Oral screen and their indications. [RGUHS]
13. Differences in activator and Frenkel's philosophy. [RGUHS]
14. List the important differences between activator and Frankel appliances. [RGUHS]
15. Name the components of functional regulator 2 (Frankel 2) appliances and describe the action of buccal shields. [RGUHS]
16. Frankel II. [RGUHS]
17. Classification and indications of extraoral appliances. [RGUHS]
18. Functional regulator II. [RGUHS]
19. Rapid maxillary expansion. [RGUHS]
20. HYRAX. [RGUHS]
21. Philosophy of Frankel appliance. [RGUHS]
22. Jasper jumper. [RGUHS]
23. Activator. [RGUHS-BUHS]
24. Oral screen. [RGUHS, MUHS; NTRUHS]
25. Frankel appliance. [RGUHS; NTRUHS]

Short Notes

1. Frankel appliance. [NTR-OR]
2. Functional regulators. [NTR-OR]
3. Bionator appliances. [RGUHS, NTR-NR; TN]
4. Frankel appliance. [MUHS]
5. FRII appliances. [NTR-NR]
6. Myofunctional appliance. [RGUHS-BUHS; TN]
7. What are the indications of oral screen? [RGUHS]
8. Headgears in orthodontics. [TN]
9. Differences between activator and Frankel appliance. [TN]
10. Face mask. [TN; NTRUHS]
11. Inclined plane. [TN]
12. Frankel function regulator. [TN]
13. Jasper jumper. [TN]
14. Fixed functional appliance. [TN]
15. Action of functional appliances. [TN]
16. Anterior bite planes. [TN]
17. Face mask therapy. [TN]
18. Activator appliances. [MUHS; TN]
19. Catalans appliances. [RGUHS; TN]
20. Frankel appliance. [RGUHS]
21. Write about activator appliance. [NTRUHS]
22. Contraindications of activator. [RGUHS]
23. Orthopaedic force in orthodontics. [TN]
24. Headgear. [NTR-NR]
25. Give indication and precondition for activator therapy. [MUHS]
26. Mention the parts of FR2 and its uses. [MUHS]
27. Twin block. [NTRUHS]
28. Vestibular screen. [RGUHS]
29. Chin cap. [RGUHS; TN]
30. Extraoral traction. [TN, MUHS]
31. Orthodontic forces in orthodontics. [TN]
32. Chin cap. [NTR-NR]
33. Describe various types of headgears available to control the growth of maxilla. [MUHS]
34. Orthopaedic appliance. [RGUHS]
35. Oral screen. [NTR-OR; TN, RGUHS]
36. Lip bumper. [NTR-NR; RGUHS]
37. Headgears used in orthodontics. [TN]
38. Mode of action of activator. [TN; RGUHS]
39. High-pull headgear. [TN]
40. Classification of functional appliance. [NTR-NR; MUHS; RGUHS]

40. Functional regulator appliances. [RGUHS]

MANAGEMENT OF COMMON MALOCCLUSIONS

Long Essays

1. Classify aetiology of malocclusion. Give aetiology and treatment of midline diastema. [MUHS]
2. Discuss features and management of class I malocclusion. [RGUHS-BUHS]
3. Enumerate the aetiological factors causing spacing and crowding of the teeth. Mention their treatment. [RGUHS-BUHS]
4. A child in the mixed dentition reports to you with crowding in the lower anterior teeth. Discuss your line of treatment. [MUHS]
5. Discuss the causes and treatment of anterior crowding of teeth. [RGUHS-BUHS]
6. What are the causes of midline diastema? How would you correct midline diastema. [RGUHS-BUHS]
7. Describe the causes of midline diastema and explain how would you correct it. [NTR-OR]
8. Describe the causes of median diastema and the measures to correct it. [NTR-OR]

Short Essays

1. Aetiology and treatment of midline diastema. [MUHS]
2. Treatment of midline diastema. [NTRUHS]
3. Self-correcting malocclusion. [RGUHS]
4. Management of midline diastema. [RGUHS]
5. Midline diastema. [MUHS; RGUHS; NTRUHS]
6. Crowding of anterior teeth. [MUHS]

Short Notes

1. Spacing. [RGUHS]
2. Rotation. [RGUHS; NTR-NR]
3. Aetiology and treatment of imbrications. [MUHS]
4. Aetiology of diastema. [RGUHS]
5. Midline diastema. [NTR-OR; TN; RGUHS; MUHS; RGUHS]
6. Derotation of teeth. [RGUHS-BUHS]
7. Imbrication. [TN]
8. Causes and management of midline diastema. [TN]
9. Lower anterior crowding. [NTR-NR]
10. Derotations. [RGUHS]
11. Causes of crowding. [RGUHS]
12. Median diastema. [RGUHS]
13. Abnormal labial frenum. [RGUHS]
14. Maxillary midline diastema. [NTR-NR]
15. Midline diastema—diagnosis and causes. [NTR-OR]

MANAGEMENT OF CLASS II MALOCCLUSION

Long Essays

1. Discuss in brief about the aetiology, clinical picture and treatment of Angle's class II division I malocclusion. [RGUHS]
2. Discuss your treatment choice of appliance for an 8-year-old patient presenting class II division I malocclusion with positive VTO. [RGUHS]
3. Describe the treatment plan for a class II malocclusion cases during mixed dentition period. [TN]
4. Discuss in brief about the aetiology, clinical picture and treatment of Angle's class II division 1 malocclusion. [BUHS]
5. Discuss the treatment plan for Angle's class II malocclusion patients in mixed dentition period. [NTR-OR]
6. Describe the shortcomings of Angle's classification and its modification. Describe the characteristics of class II division 1 and class II division 2 malocclusion. [MUHS]
7. Discuss clinical picture of Angle's class II division 1 malocclusion and its clinical management. [NTR-NR]
8. How would you set out a treatment of a class II division 1 malocclusion case in the mixed dentition with moderated crowding in the anteriors? Justify your modality of treatment. [MUHS]
9. A child in a mixed dentition having a backward placed chin with protrusion and spaces in upper anterior teeth— describe the line of treatment and appliance used. [MUHS]
10. Write the treatment modalities for Angle's class II division 1 malocclusion for a child patient in mixed dentition. [MUHS]
11. Discuss your treatment of appliance for an 8-year-old patient presenting class II division 1 malocclusion with positive VTO. [NTR-OR]
12. Give the features and treatment plan of Angle's class II division 1 malocclusion. [MUHS]

13. Describe the typical clinical features of Angle's class II division 1 malocclusion and discuss your line of treatment for a 12-year-old girl with class II division 1 malocclusion. [NTR-OR]
14. A 12-year-old boy with receding chin, proclined anteriors and deep bite reports to you. Discuss your diagnosis and justify your diagnosis. [MUHS]

Short Essays

1. Characteristics of Angle's class II division 2. [RGUHS]
2. Mandibular retrusion. [RGUHS-BUHS]
3. Extraoral and intraoral features of class II division 2 malocclusion. [RGUHS]

Short Notes

1. Clinical features of class II division I malocclusion. [NTR-NR]
2. Write clinical features of Angle's class II division 1 malocclusion. [MUHS]
3. Features of class II division 1 malocclusion. [RGUHS-BUHS]
4. Define growth modulation and state its methods. [MUHS]
5. Clinical features of class II division 2 malocclusion. [NTR-NR]
6. Growth modification. [MUHS]

MANAGEMENT OF CLASS III MALOCCLUSION

Long Essays

1. Enumerate the differences between true and pseudo class III malocclusion. Discuss your line of treatment in mixed dentition. [RGUHS-BUHS]
2. Enumerate various methods in treating a case of class III malocclusion at an early age. [MUHS]
3. Discuss the clinical picture of skeletal Angle's class III malocclusion and its clinical management. [NTR-NR; RGUHS]
4. Aetiology of class III malocclusion. How would you treat a child with locked incisor teeth? [MUHS]
5. Discuss in brief the aetiology, clinical picture and treatment of Angle's class III malocclusion. [RGUHS-BUHS]
6. A 9-year-old boy reports to the department of orthodontics with a chief complaint of prognathic mandible. Discuss the line of treatment. [MUHS]

Short Essays

1. Treatment of class III malocclusion. [RGUHS; NTRUHS]
2. Aetiology of class III malocclusion. [MUHS]
3. Treatment of midline diastema. [NTRUHS]
4. Angle's class III malocclusion. [MUHS]
5. Aetiology and treatment of pseudo class III malocclusion. [MUHS]
6. Explain treatment procedure in an 8-year-old child with a deficient maxilla, appliance used and mode of action. [RGUHS]

Short Notes

1. Management of mandibular prognathism in adults. [RGUHS]
2. Dental compensation in skeletal class III malocclusion. [RGUHS]

MANAGEMENT OF OPEN BITE, CROSS BITE AND DEEP BITE

Long Essays

1. Aetiology and treatment of open bite. [MUHS]
2. Classify expansion in orthodontics. Discuss your line of treatment for a case of 12 years with bilateral buccal crossbite. [MUHS]
3. Define, classify, give aetiology, clinical features, diagnosis and various methods of treatment of crossbite. Why is it considered an orthodontic emergency? [MUHS]
4. Enumerate genetically inherited malocclusion. Discuss crossbite in detail. [MUHS]
5. Discuss the aetiology, line of treatment and the design of appliance in correction of anterior crossbite and anterior spacing. [BUHS-RGUHS]
6. Define preventive, interceptive and corrective orthodontics. Enumerate about the various modes of bilateral posterior crossbite correction and discuss in detail about any one mode. [RGUHS]

7. An 8-year-old male child is having one of the upper central incisors in anterior crossbite. What can be the probable aetiology? Design an appliance for the correction of the above case. What will be your advice to the patient? [TN]
8. Describe the probable aetiologic factors responsible for anterior crossbite and anterior open bite, and also their treatment. [BUHS]
9. Describe the probable aetiologic factors responsible for anterior crossbite and anterior open bite, and also their treatment. [RGUHS]

Short Essays

1. Lower inclined plane appliances. [RGUHS-BUHS]
2. Catalans appliances. Mention their disadvantages. [RGUHS]
3. Inclined plane appliances. [RGUHS]
4. Open bite. [RGUHS; NTR-NR]
5. Anterior open bite. [RGUHS]
6. Anterior bite plane. [RGUHS]
7. Aetiology and treatment of deep bite. [MUHS]
8. Aetiology of open bite. [MUHS]
9. Aetiology and treatment of open bite. [MUHS]
10. Features of Mouth-breathing. [RGUHS]
11. Catalans appliances. [RGUHS]
12. Anterior crossbite. [RGUHS; MUHS]
13. Aetiology and treatment of crossbite. [MUHS]
14. Inclined plane. [NTR-NR]
15. Posterior crossbite. [NTR-NR]
16. Management of crossbite. [RGUHS; NTRUHS]

Short Notes

1. Causes of anterior open bite. [RGUHS]
2. Anterior crossbite. [NTR-OR]
3. Catalans appliance. [NTR-OR]
4. Treatment of anterior crossbite. [NTR]
5. Crossbite. [NTR-OR; MUHS; TN; RGUHS]
6. Springs to bring about mesiodistal movement. [NTR-OR]
7. Anterior crossbite. [RGUHS]
8. Management of crossbite. [RGUHS]
9. Tongue blade therapy. [RGUHS]
10. Indications of anterior open bite. [MUHS]
11. Catalans appliance. [RGUHS]
12. Anterior bite plane and its mode of action. [RGUHS]
13. Inclined plane. [RGUHS]
14. Deep overbite. [NTR-OR]
15. Anterior deep bite. [NTR-OR]
16. Deep bite. [RGUHS]
17. Sensitization and stabilization of stainless steel.[RGUHS]
18. Apertognathia. [RGUHS]

CLEFT LIP AND PALATE

Long Essays

1. What are the causes of cleft lip and palate? Write about the management. [NTRUHS]
2. Classify cleft lip and palate. Describe the orthodontic management of the same. [NTR]
3. Describe in brief about the malformations of dental arches in cleft lip and palate cases. Write about aetiology and orthodontic management of cleft lip and palate cases. [MUHS]
4. Describe the aetiology, clinical picture and management of cleft lip and palate patients. [RGUHS-BUHS]
5. What are the causes of cleft lip and palate? How will you manage the problems associated with them? [TN]

Short Essays

1. Surgical closure of cleft lip. [RGUHS]
2. Management of cleft palate. [RGUHS]
3. Management of cleft palate. [RGUHS-BUHS]
4. Veau's classification of cleft lip and palate. [RGUHS]
5. Veau's classification of cleft lip and cleft palate. [RGUHS]
6. Briefly discuss the orthodontic treatment protocol from birth to adulthood for a child born with cleft lip and palate. [RGUHS]

Short Notes

1. Cleft lip and palate. [RGUHS; TN]
2. Cleft lip. [NTR-NR; TN; NTRUHS]
3. Cleft lip and palate. [BUHS]
4. Cleft lip and palate. [NTR-NR, MUHS]
5. Orthodontic management of cleft lip and palate. [TN]
6. Cleft lip and palate. [TN]
7. Management of cleft lip and palate. [NTR-NR; TN]
8. Cleft palate. [RGUHS]
9. What is 'team approach' in rehabilitation of cleft lip/palate patients? [MUHS]

SURGICAL ORTHODONTICS

Long Essays

1. What is surgical orthodontics? Enumerate the minor and major surgical orthodontic procedures. Discuss any three minor surgical orthodontic procedures. [TN]
2. Define surgical orthodontics. Give objectives, classification of surgical orthodontics, and discuss in detail about minor surgical orthodontic procedures. [MUHS]
3. Classify surgical orthodontics. Discuss about minor surgical orthodontic procedures. [RGUHS]

Short Essays

1. Pericision. [NTR-NR; BUHS; RGUHS]
2. Genioplasty. [RGUHS]
3. Orthognathic surgery in the maxilla. [RGUHS]
4. Enumerate indications and techniques of orthodontic surgeries. [RGUHS]
5. Sterilization in orthodontics. [NTRUHS]
6. Minor surgical procedures in orthodontics. [NTRUHS]
7. Describe surgical modalities in correction of mandibular prognathism. Describe any one in brief. [MUHS]

Short Notes

1. Frenectomy. [RGUHS]
2. Orthognathic surgery in the maxilla. [TN]
3. Camouflage [RGUHS]
4. Cosmetic surgeries. [RGUHS]
5. Surgical aids in orthodontics. [TN]
6. Piezoelectric theory. [TN]
7. Resection and osteotomies. [TN]
8. Minor surgical procedures. [TN]
9. Minor surgical procedures in orthodontic practice. [TN]
10. Piezoelectric theory in the biologic control of tooth movement. [TN]
11. Blanch test. [RGUHS; NTR]
12. Orthognathic surgery. [TN]
13. Pericision. [NTR-NR; RGUHS; NTRUHS; RGUHS]
14. Surgical orthodontics. [NTR-OR; MUHS]
15. Supracrestal fibrotomy. [NTR-NR]
16. Proximal slenderization/stripping. [NTRUHS]
17. Blanch test. [NTR]
18. Camouflage treatment. [NTR]
19. Impacted upper permanent canine. [RGUHS]

RETENTION AND RELAPSE

Long Essays

1. Enumerate theories of retention. Add a note on causes of relapse. [NTRUHS]
2. Discuss retention and relapse in orthodontics. [RGUHS; NTR-NR]
3. Discuss the causes of relapse in orthodontics. [RGUHS-BUHS]
4. Define relapse. Discuss various methods to prevent relapse. [RGUHS-BUHS]
5. Define retention and relapse. What are the types of retention and enumerate the causes for relapse. [TN]
6. What is retention? Describe in brief about various retention appliances commonly used in orthodontic practice. [MUHS]
7. Discuss in detail about the various theories of retention. [RGUHS]
8. Write about the theories and types of retention. [RGUHS]
9. Define retention and relapse. Write briefly about causes of relapse. [RGUHS]
10. What is relapse? Give its causes, classify retention appliances and describe in detail about the Hawley retainer. [MUHS]
11. Define retention and relapse in orthodontics. What are the causes of relapse and how would you prevent them? [RGUHS; TN]
12. Discuss the role of periodontium and growth in causing relapse. Write in brief about four other causes of relapse. [RGUHS]
13. Define stability. Mention the various causes of relapse and enumerate the retention appliances. [TN]
14. What are the causes for relapse? Write in detail about the theories and types of retention. [TN]
15. Explain in detail about retention after treatment of malocclusion. [RGUHS]
16. Define retention and relapse. Explain in detail about the causes and methods of preventing relapse in orthodontics. [TN]
17. Define retention and relapse. Write the various causes of relapse and how to prevent them. [RGUHS]

18. Define retention and relapse. Explain the various causes of relapse and methods of preventing relapse in orthodontics. [TN]
19. Discuss the causes of relapse following orthodontic treatment. What are the theories of retention? [RGUHS]
20. Discuss the role of periodontium and growth in causing relapse. Write in brief about four other causes of relapse? [RGUHS]
21. Define retention and discuss theories of retention. [MUHS]
22. Describe various orthodontic movements that occur when an ideal force is applied. How would you retain a derotated tooth? [MUHS]

Short Essays

1. Relapse and retention. [MUHS]
2. Relapse in orthodontics. [RGUHS; NTRUHS]
3. Define retention. Explain the schools of retention. [RGUHS]
4. Relapse. [MUHS]
5. Retention. [RGUHS]
6. Permanent retention. [RGUHS]
7. What is relapse? How can we prevent it? [RGUHS]
8. Define retention. Add a note on the role of third molars in causing relapse. [RGUHS]
9. Fixed retainer. [NTR-NR; TN]
10. Theories of retention. [MUHS; RGUHS]
11. Retention in orthodontics. [MUHS; NTRUHS]
12. What is retention period? [MUHS]

Short Notes

1. Retention appliance. [NTR-OR; RGUHS]
2. Retention and relapse. [NTR-OR; TN]
3. Retention and retainers. [NTR-OR]
4. Upper Hawley appliance. [NTR-OR]
5. Name different schools of thought for retention.[MUHS]
6. Riedel's theorems of retention and relapse. [TN]
7. Theories of retention. [RGUHS]
8. Causes of relapse in orthodontics. [TN]
9. Causes of relapse. [TN]
10. Relapse in orthodontics. [RGUHS]
11. Retainers. [RGUHS-BUHS]
12. Relapse. [NTR-OR; RGUHS]
13. Hawley retainer. [NTR-OR]
14. Permanent retention. [NTR-OR; NTRUHS; RGUHS]
15. Hawley appliance. [RGUHS; NTRUHS]
16. Hawley retention. [RGUHS-BUHS]
17. What is the role of the third molar in causing the relapse. [RGUHS]
18. Adjunctive periodontal surgeries to minimize relapse. [TN]
19. Types of retention. [TN; RGUHS]
20. Define retention. [TN]
21. Natural aids to retention. [RGUHS]
22. What is relapse? How to prevent relapse? [RGUHS]
23. Define retention. Add a note on the role of third molars in causing. [RGUHS]
24. Define and classify retention, giving examples. [MUHS]
25. Retention and retainers. [MUHS]

GENETICS IN ORTHODONTICS

Short Essays

1. Twin studies. [MUHS]
2. Importance of genetics in orthodontics. [RGUHS]

Short Notes

1. Dentofacial disturbances of genetic origin. [TN; RGUHS]
2. Mutation. [TN]
3. Chromosomes. [RGUHS]
4. Teratogens. [NTR-OR]
5. Pedigree studies. [RGUHS]
6. Importance of genetics in malocclusion. [TN; RGUHS]
7. Genetic disorders. [TN]
8. Genetics in orthodontics. [NTR-OR]
9. Role of heredity in malocclusion. [NTR-OR]
10. Role of genetics in aetiology of malocclusion. [TN]

LAB PROCEDURES

Long Essay

1. What are the study models? Write the uses of the same in orthodontics. [RGUHS]

Short Essays

1. Soldering and welding. [RGUHS]
2. 18-8 Stainless steel. [RGUHS]
3. Solder and flux. [NTR-NR; TN]
4. Soldering and spot welding. [MUHS]
5. Study models. [RGUHS; NTR-NR]
6. Properties of an ideal wire. [RGUHS]
7. Ideal orthodontic plane. [RGUHS]
8. Slenderization. [RGUHS]
9. Dental spot welder. [NTR-NR]
10. Uses of study models. [RGUHS]

Short Notes

1. Orthodontic study models. [NTR-NR; NTRUHS]
2. Soldering. [RGUHS]
3. Soldering. [NTR-OR; MUHS]
4. Soldering and welding. [NTR-OR; NTR-NR; RGUHS; TN]
5. Welding in orthodontics. [NTR-OR]
6. Cold cure acrylic resins. [RGUHS-BUHS]
7. Study models. [RGUHS]
8. Uses of study models. [RGUHS]
9. Soldering and welding. [RGUHS, TN]
10. Welding and soldering. [TN; RGUHS]
11. Flux and antiflux. [RGUHS; TN; NTRUHS]
12. Trimming of study model. [RGUHS-BUHS]
1. Shape memory alloy. [TN]
14. Soldering, welding and braking. [TN]
15. Spot welding. [RGUHS; TN; NTRUHS]
16. Antiflux. [RGUHS; NTRUHS]
17. Direct bonding. [TN; NTR-OR]
18. Heat treatment of orthodontic wire. [TN]
19. Soldering in orthodontic wires. [TN]
20. Piezoelectric theory. [NTRUHS]
21. Gases used for soldering. [NTRUHS]
22. Solder and flux. [TN]
23. CSF procedure. [TN]
24. Sensitization and stabilization. [RGUHS]
25. Braided and twisted wires. [TN]
26. Properties of ideal orthodontic wires. [TN]
27. Irreversible hydrocolloids. [TN]
28. Solders of stainless steel. [TN]
29. Wrought cobalt-chromium-nickel alloys. [TN]
30. Nickel-titanium wires. [TN]
31. Spot welder. [NTR-OR; TN]
32. Study models. [NTR-OR]
33. Sterilization in orthodontics. [TN]
34. Soldering in orthodontic practice. [TN]

MATERIALS USED IN ORTHODONTICS

Short Notes

1. Shape memory alloy. [RGUHS]
2. Elgiloy wires. [TN; NTRUHS]
3. Shape memory alloy. [RGUHS; TN; NTRUHS]
4. Glass ionomer cements. [RGUHS]
5. Nitinol wires. [TN]
6. 18-8 Stainless steel. [TN; NTRUHS]
7. Nickel-titanium alloy. [TN]
8. Stainless steel. [NTRUHS]
9. Orthodontic impressions. [NTRUHS]
10. Uses of alloy in orthodontics. [TN]
11. Irreversible hydrocolloids. [NTRUHS]
12. Molar tubes. [NTRUHS]
13. Irreversible hydrocolloids. [NTR-NR]
14. Tensile strength. [RGUHS]
15. Stainless steel in orthodontic practice. [TN]
16. Wires used in orthodontics. [TN]
17. NiTi wires. [RGUHS]
18. Superelasticity. [RGUHS]